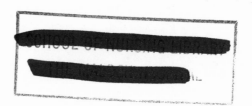
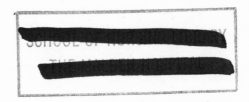

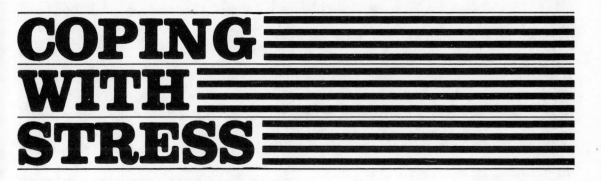

COPING WITH STRESS

A Nursing Perspective

Doris C. Sutterley, R.N., M.S.N.
and
Gloria F. Donnelly, R.N., M.S.N.
Editors

A Collection from:
Advances in Nursing Science
Critical Care Quarterly
Family & Community Health
Topics in Clinical Nursing

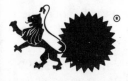

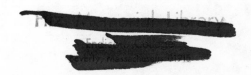

AN ASPEN PUBLICATION®
Aspen Systems Corporation
Rockville, Maryland
London
1981

Library of Congress Cataloging in Publication Data
Main entry under title:

Coping with stress.

Bibliography: p. 321
Includes index.
1. Stress (Psychology)   2. Stress (Physiology)
I. Sutterley, Doris Cook.   II. Donnelly, Gloria Ferraro.
BF575.S75C658   155.9′16′024613   81-17599
ISBN 0-89443-650-3   AACR2

Library of Congress Catalog Card Number: 81-17599
ISBN: 0-89443-650-3

Printed in the United States of America

1 2 3 4 5

Table of Contents

Preface

Stress and ways of coping are currently of intense interest to nurses perhaps because of the stressful nature of practice in today's health care system. Articles and studies on stress and coping have proliferated the health care literature during the past five years. Research findings in the area of stress are requiring that we expand our perspective on the mind–body relationship and on how the human organism has more potential for self-regulation than was once believed. For example, the promising new research in psychophysiology (particularly, the immune system) is sensitizing health professionals to the notion that the organism responds on a physiological level to life events and that caring, including self-care, ameliorates the negative effects of stress.

The purpose of this anthology on stress and coping is to bring together current selections from the nursing literature that will (1) increase the practitioner's knowledge of the stress response; (2) sensitize the practitioner to the relationship between stress and illness; and (3) introduce caring, particularly self-care interventions for use with clients and caregivers.

To accomplish our purpose we begin with selections that describe models of stress, coping and adaptation. A model is a way of organizing what we see or experience so that we might speculate on the relationship between the phenomena and predict what will happen under varying conditions. Guzzetta and Forsyth in "Nursing Diagnostic Pilot Study: Psychophysiologic Stress," discuss the development of nursing diagnostic categories with which to describe manifestations of stress in acutely ill clients. They suggest that the diagnostic labeling process will direct the plan of therapy and be instrumental in evaluating the effectiveness of nursing actions. Other articles in Part I detail ways of conceptualizing stress, coping and adaptational processes in the human organism that might have implications for nursing intervention.

Part II, Stress and Life Events, includes articles that emphasize the relationship between life events and the stress response. Hefferin in "Life-Cycle Stressors: An Overview of Research" summarizes major studies dealing with life-cycle stressors, such as separation and loss, developmental stages and transitions, and various life crises.

The relationship of stress to illness is highlighted in Part III. The manifestations of stress in clients experiencing health problems such as kidney failure, respiratory failure, cardiac problems and burn trauma are examined. The authors, who have worked closely with acutely ill clients, recommend coping strategies that have proven effective during periods of high level stress.

Part IV represents an interesting cross section on self-regulation modalities currently used to deal with stress and stress-related problems. Sutterley in "Stress and Health: A Survey of Self-Regulation Modalities" proposes an original definition of stress that encompasses the major theoretical perspectives on stress. Nutrition, exercise and a variety of noninvasive self-care modalities such as relaxation techniques and acupressure are discussed with specific directions given for application. Other articles deal with the specifics of biofeedback and hypnosis and how health education promotes self-care.

The final section of the anthology (Part V) is specifically for the caregiver. The overriding theme in "Stress and the Caregiver" is that caregivers are most effective when they have learned to care for themselves. Specific strategies such as assertiveness, time management, self-confrontation and peer support are presented for dealing with the stressors of work.

It is our hope that this compilation of articles on stress and coping will stimulate the reader to examine whether or not current practice in the health care system is conducive to the amelioration of the negative effects of stress to health and to healing. This volume is also a challenge to the practitioner to search for new ways to potentiate the human capacity for self-regulation and healing.

Doris C. Sutterley
Gloria F. Donnelly
November 1981

Part I
Models of Stress

A Stress-Coping Model

Diane W. Scott, R.N., Ph.D.
Nurse Scientist

Marilyn T. Oberst, R.N., Ed.D.
Director

Mary Jo Dropkin, R.N., M.S.N.
Research Associate
Department of Nursing Research
Memorial Sloan-Kettering Cancer Center
New York, New York

A MODEL or scientific paradigm, according to Thomas Kuhn,[1] is a set of interrelated assumptions about classes of phenomena. Models have a heuristic value, in that they have a closely linked protocol or set of procedures for observing and analyzing the phenomena. For an applied discipline such as nursing, models can be useful because they combine theoretical assumptions, research-based knowledge, diagnostic problem-solving, and clinical intervention. A model is a link between concept and action, and can function as a tool to coordinate the structure and process of a research program designed to improve the effectiveness and therapeutic value of nursing practice.

Development of a stress-coping framework or model for nursing research has been attempted by Goosen and Bush,[2] and Roy.[3] Numerous other frameworks with possible utility for nursing exist.[4, 5-22] However, as Wild and Hanes[21] indicate, framework development is incomplete given the lack of continuity of basic theo-

4

retical and operational constructs. Few attempts have been made to develop a dynamic model—one which maps the entire adjustive process and recognizes the complete interaction between individual and environment.

One stress-coping model, described later, has been developed as a conceptual framework for a department of nursing research in an acute care cancer center and will be used as a theoretical foundation for studies the department undertakes.

BACKGROUND

Stress

Stress arises from a transaction between individual and environment when the individual construes stimuli as damaging, threatening, or challenging. In general, stress situations involve awareness of demands that tax or exceed available resources as appraised by the individual. Demands can be of several types: social, cultural, psychological, and physiological, but basically each represents a change in balance between the demand and the resources to deal with it. Stressors, or stimuli that produce stress, differ in quality and intensity for each individual, and they may act together to augment, intensify, or reduce the total effect. Stress threshold and tolerance levels differ with each person, and depend on genetic and constitutional make-up, past experience, self-concept and other factors. Stress is particularly important in health because it has the potential to impair human functioning.[23]

Beginning with the work of Hans Selye,[24] researchers have sought, over the past three decades, to describe and analyze the effects of stress. Selye and others found that the demands imposed on a person by internal and external environments can cause difficulty, fatigue, exhaustion, and even death, if not counterbalanced by forces that contribute to maintaining his or her integrity. How the human organism maintains integrity was the subject of further research in the 1970s. From that work a science of stress, coping, and adaptation has evolved.

A substantial branch of stress research has addressed itself to the physical and physiological manifestations of stress. In the initial phase of stress exploration, Selye[24] proposed and demonstrated a general syndrome arising from the application of specific physical stresses to animals. His *general adaptation syndrome* and its characteristic physiology dominated the experimental domain until recently. Mason et al[25] proposed more specific responses based on the type of stressor and the associated functioning of specific hormonal axes and their many related substrates.

The trend in stress analysis research is heavily in favor of a cognitively based

---

The trend in stress-analysis research is heavily in favor of a cognitively based theory.

---

theory.[26-30] Stress is a generic entity involving many variables working in concert rather than any one specific negative emotion, stimulus, or response. This idea has moved stress research from an emotion or arousal context to one in which the individual's interpretation and evaluation of a stimulus-filled environment becomes the basis for a response to the stress experience, and in which emotions and physiological responses are viewed as by-products of cognition.

The cognitive branch of stress research is based on Piaget's developmental psychology, according to which innate schemata are the underlying basis for growth and life. Piaget described the interaction between person and environment as an assimilation-accommodation process whereby people assimilate the environment and accommodate their own structure to learn and survive.[31] Using this framework, other cognitive psychologists suggest that a mental operation underlies and affects the physiological level of response.

Some researchers using a cognitive approach identify levels of awareness or consciousness and their variations over time and experience in humans in the normal course of living. Levels of consciousness, information, representation (imagery, conceptualization and language), and the chemical and structural bases of memory are basic components of the cognitive process.[32] Proponents of the cognitive interpretation of stress such as Averill and Opton,[33] Lazarus,[4,23] Monat and Lazarus[34] and others have outlined an appraisal process whereby the individual continuously scans the environment for stimuli and then operates upon it through a careful and continual evaluation of threat to system survival.

The essential point of the cognitive approach is that in the critical progression of events occurring after stressor-person impact, cognitive functioning occurs which encompasses all neurological levels of system control, autonomic regulation, elicitation of feeling states, sensory selection processes, and individual and species preservation; and the cortical structure contributions of memory and mental operation. The latter two functions, taken together, form a basis for thought and evaluation.

Coping

Study of the dynamics of adaptation has focused on the natural counterpart to stress, known as coping. The multiplicity of coping strategies utilized to bring about change and growth is seen as the linkage between stressor impact and adaptation. Lazarus,[23] in his systematic model of the stress-coping process, identifies two elements of coping: (1) problem-solving and (2) regulation of emotion. He emphasizes that cognitive appraisal of the stress situation occurs as a primary condition, and that emotional and other response categories follow the appraisal.

A constellation of coping strategies, rather than any single one, ultimately brings about adaptation and growth—the maintenance of integrity. Initial direction of the process is controlled by cognition, but the total coping response is comprised of cognitive activity, emotions, and physiological response *in interaction*. Therefore, in the development of a model, literature will be reviewed in terms of cognitive, emotional, and physiological responses to stressor impact and the known options within each.

6   LITERATURE REVIEW

Cognitive Response to Stress

Although information about the environment is largely processed at the level of the cerebral cortex, subcortical areas of the brain contain important structures through which information processing and arousal are mediated. The cerebral cortex handles memory, symbolic representation, and thinking and reasoning. Several subcortical structures direct sensation to the cortex and are source structures for generalized arousal, certain specific emotions, and visceral regulation for somatic survival. These structures receive feedback through chemical signals from the pituitary gland and autonomic nervous system via the hypothalamus, and some information from the internal and external environment directly.[18] The role of the subcortical nervous system structures as sources of arousal, certain emotions, and somatic integrity has been demonstrated.[35-41] The concept of cognition, then, is expanded to incorporate the broader context of neural control, rather than solely cortical control of emotion and physiological responses. However, coping responses are governed principally by cortical level integration.

Posner[42] has identified two major components of thinking and reasoning ability: (1) mental structure and (2) mental operations. The structure of thinking and reasoning ability includes long- and short-term memory systems and their codes, and the capacity for abstraction and concept formation. Memory has three qualitative codes: (1) imagery, the internal representation of sensory experience; (2) enactive, the learning, reproduction, and preservation of motor skills and movement; and (3) symbolic, the representation of language and other characters that represent reality in another form. Memory is organized so that input can be selected, organized, changed, and retrieved with varying amounts of effort. Abstraction and concept formation allow people to move from the immediate sensation of form, color, and size to identification of patterns and their differences.

Mental operations are considered the dynamic components of thinking and reasoning and include:

1. Tools of symbolic logic: deduction, inference, evaluation, interpretation, and understanding the unstated assumptions with which people operate on perceived stimuli.

2. Levels of consciousness: facilitating both sensory and motor systems and implied by the degree of alertness or changes in performance and brain activity. Generally the more reflexive mental operations are preserved as consciousness decreases. Thatcher and John[32] have identified six levels of information input and processing that correlate with the extent of cortical activity and progressively higher levels of consciousness or awareness: (1) sensation, or reflex response; (2) perception, or interaction between sensation and memory; (3) reorganization of basic processes; (4) processing of multisensory perception as experience; (5) sequential or long-term memory; and (6) symbolic representation and critical thinking. Diurnal patterns, pharmacologic depressants and stimulants, and internal and external environmental conditions,

such as amount and rate of stimulus input, age, and physical condition may affect level of cognitive functioning. To comprehend an individual's cognitive coping pattern, understanding of his or her position on the awareness scale described above is essential.

3. Problem solving: the global process by which a person moves from problem identification to solution and evaluation. The objective of problem solving is to achieve new representations through the performance of mental operations.[42] The process includes identifying the problem or initial representation, collecting information or using search strategies, operating on the information or incubation, and determining a solution or termination. Neisser[43] summarizes the process well when he defines cognition as the way in which sensory inputs are "transformed, reduced, elaborated, stored, reconciled and used."

Lazarus[23] has outlined the cognitive process during primary appraisal of the stress situation. The individual's initial evaluation of the stress situation in terms of his or her well-being produces one of three possible appraisals of the stressor: (1) irrelevant; (2) benign, resulting in positively toned emotions; or (3) stressful, resulting in negatively toned emotions. If the stimuli are appraised as stressful, further differentiation occurs and includes: (1) harm or loss, injury or damage already done; (2) threat, anticipated trauma has not yet occurred, assuming a hostile and dangerous environment with the self as lacking in resources to master it; or (3) challenge,

opportunity for growth, mastery, or gain, assuming the demands are difficult but not impossible, using existing or acquirable skills. The cognitive phase of the primary appraisal determines the intensity and quality of emotional response to any transaction.

Emotional Response to Stress

The literature reflects considerable disagreement among researchers regarding concepts of emotion. While there is agreement that different emotions exist and are initiated by cognitive processes, many different interpretations of the fundamental dynamics of emotions exist. Researchers also disagree about the exact relationship between outward expressions and their underlying emotions. No consensus exists on whether emotion is a symptom secondary to cognition or an independent entity,[44] but there is growing recognition that affect and cognition are closely linked.

Plutchik et al[45] have developed a systematic model of emotion, identifying four pairs of basic bipolar emotions: (1) fear-anger, (2) joy-sadness, (3) acceptance-distrust, and (4) expectancy-surprise. A constellation of defense mechanisms, diagnostic categories, and behaviors is associated with each bipolar pair. Although Plutchik et al are psychoanalytically oriented, their model does imply that thinking and judgment go into the choice of emotion, and that the specific emotion felt is a product of some objective on the part of the individual.

For the purposes of the present stress-coping model, the defense mechanisms that Plutchik et al associate with specific

8 **Table 1.** Emotion, Defense, and Behavior

Emotion	Defense	Behavior
Joy	Reaction formation	Hyperactivity
Sadness	Compensation	Attempts to regain loss
		Takes on characteristics of loss
Acceptance	Denial	Overlooks or ignores
Distrust	Projection	Uses blame
Surprise	Regression	Crying
	Fantasy	Daydreaming
	Acting out	Impulse-activity
Anticipation	Intellectualization	Redefines, recategorizes
	Rationalization	Makes excuses
	Undoing	Cancels out
	Sublimation	Transforms direction of energy
Fear	Repression	Forgetting, loss of memory
	Introjection	Nonadmission
	Isolation	Lack of feelings
Anger	Displacement	Attack-like
		Aggressive

Source: Adapted from Plutchik R, Kellerman H, Conte HR: A structural theory of ego defenses and emotions, in Izard CE (ed): *Emotions in Personality and Psychopathology.* New York, Plenum Press, 1979, pp 227–260.

emotions will be considered general labels for the behavioral response as shown in Table 1.

The model of Plutchik et al differentiates the eight specific emotions qualitatively from anxiety. Anxiety is regarded as general energy arousal that, over time and experience, is refined into specific dominant emotions.

Emotions can vary in both duration and intensity. When an emotion is prolonged over time, according to Weisman,[46] it becomes a *mood;* when prolonged over an even longer period of time, to the extent that the emotional state becomes almost a trait fixed in the personality, it becomes an *attitude.* Arieti[47] has devised a similar classification, but calls the groupings *first-, second-,* and *third-order emotions.* Intensity might be defined as complexity or a tightly woven set of emotions that present themselves as a syndrome. Conflict and guilt are examples of the complex interaction of several emotions and represent another dimension of the nature of emotion.

Current understanding of emotion, then, suggests that (1) emotion occurs as a consequence of the person's evaluation of the environment; (2) emotion is a feeling state with physiologic parameters; (3) emotion is experienced initially in global form and later refined into specific basic emotions; (4) emotions may be classified according to type, duration; and intensity—characteristics that change over time and events.

Following the cognitive evaluation of a stressor, a person determines the degree of threat and the resources available to meet the demand. Almost simultaneously, a fluctuation in general anxiety takes place, followed by a refinement of the energy into one or more specific emotions. The resultant response is a translation of the emotion into a behavior. Over time and many reappraisals an emotional response may become increasingly fixed and trait-like within the personality, and may play an important role in determining the ultimate adaptation. For the purpose of this model, emotion will be considered an intervening variable having a powerful and direct effect on behavioral response.

Physiological Response to Stress

The literature identifies three major physiologic transmitters of stress reaction: (1) hormonal stimulation, (2) sympathetic activation, and (3) end-organ response. All three are interrelated and interdependent.

The early work of Cannon,[48] later extended by Euler,[49] laid the groundwork for understanding the sympathetic-adrenal-medullary system and its responsiveness to emotion.[26,50] Recent work by Frankenhauser,[51] Levi,[52] and Mason[53] has explored the role of physiology in adaptation to stress in more detail. The sympathetic nervous system provides for neural activation and neurotransmission of chemical substrates through multiple pathways and many levels of integration that assure, by convergence and redundancy, appropriate functional responses when the organism is thrown off balance.[54]

Mason[53,55] has identified a number of neuroendocrine axes, each responding to different emotions and different stressors. The multiple endocrine secretory changes involve growth hormone, prolactin, ACTH and cortisol, luteinizing and follicle-stimulating hormones (androgens, estrogens), thyroid-stimulating hormone and thyroxine, vasopressin, oxytocin, epinephrine and norepinephrine, and insulin. To determine the effect of each axis, Mason used tests of 17-OHCS, epinephrine, norepinephrine, butanol-extractable iodine (thyroid index), growth hormone, insulin, testosterone, ERIO (androgen metabolite), estrone, and urinary volume. Variances in levels of each of these substances in relation to one another have begun to produce certain predictive patterns in response to certain stressors and emotions. In carefully controlled studies, Mason stressed primates with four discrete stressors (heat, cold, hunger, and exercise) and found different patterns or profiles of hormonal excretion in response to each. This finding is important evidence to support a theory of *specific* adaptational response in opposition to Selye's notion of a general arousal response common to all emotion and stress situations. Although Mason and associates have also documented unique hormonal profiles in studies with parents of leukemic children and in army recruits undergoing basic training,[56,57] much more research is needed in this area.

Neural activation by hormonal secretion and sympathetic passage terminates in end-organ response. The classic end-organ reactions are cardiac changes, dilation of coronary vessels, vasodilation in voluntary muscles, vasoconstriction in the intestinal tract, decreased peristalsis, and metabolic actions that mobilize glucose and fat metabolism.[54] In the stress-coping model, neurotransmission occurs simultaneously with emotional response. End-organ changes are considered to be behavioral outcomes of the process.

STRESS-COPING MODEL

A stress-coping model has been developed by the authors to provide theoretical direction for a department of nursing research and as a foundation for generat-

---

A stress-coping model has been developed by the authors to provide theoretical direction for a department of nursing research and as a foundation for generating research proposals.

---

ing research proposals. This model represents what Kuhn calls a "class of phenomena" with its set of interrelated assumptions, including those of structure and process.[1]

Structure of the Model

The structure of the stress-coping model is represented by a set of definitions of model components.

Stress: A situation in which environmental demands, internal demands, or both tax or exceed the adaptive resources of an individual, social, or tissue system.[34]

Coping: A process characterized by continuous use of goal-directed strategies that are initiated and maintained over time and across encounters by means of cognitive appraisal and regulation of emotion and physiologic response.[23] Modes of coping include motor and expressive behaviors aimed at neutralizing the stressor(s), and regulation of emotional and

physiologic response aimed at preservation of integrity.

Appraisal: The total comprehension of stress including related coping strategies, neurocognitive activity, affective and physiologic responses, and behavioral outcomes. Primary appraisal focuses on evaluation of the stressor array; secondary appraisal and later reappraisals concentrate on effectiveness of coping responses and changes in stress configuration.

Neurocognitive activation: Evaluation of a stimulus array at any given moment in time utilizing the neurocognitive apparatus for stress interpretation.

Affective response: Arousal of a feeling state as a consequence of neurocognitive activation. Characteristics include type, intensity, and duration with close linkage to simultaneously occurring biochemical and physiologic changes. Primary appraisal involves a generalized global anxiety reaction. Secondary appraisal refines the general response into more specific emotions associated with the stress situation. Later reappraisals and ultimate adaptation may reflect mood states and attitudinal development.

Physiological response: Changes in secretion of substances and activation of sympathetic nervous system pathways in response to the cognitive "fight," "flight," or "freeze" command. The pattern of activation generally coordinates with affective response and occurs as a function of neurocognitive evaluation. Primary appraisal reflects a generalized response where pituitary-adrenal axis activity predominates. Secondary appraisal and subsequent reappraisals reflect interaction patterns of multineuroendocrine axes secretion. Ultimate adaptation may reflect cellular, tissue, organ, and system effects of physiologic response over time. Immediate results are measured directly or indirectly through end-organ response.

Behavioral response: All neurocognitive, affective, and physiologic responses to the stress situation may be measured by direct observation of expressive and motor actions, self-report indices, or end-organ response levels. Primary appraisal includes behaviors in response to the stressor impact. Secondary appraisal and subsequent appraisals focus behavior on initial coping strategies and their effectiveness in neutralizing the stress situation.

Adaptation: The result of coping efforts to maintain integrity by establishing balance between demands and the power to deal with them.[23] Desirable outcomes include minimum impairment of human functioning; economical balance among demands, power or resources, and cost; strengthening of assimilation and accommodation modes within the system; growth and learning; achievement of acceptable goals.

The Stress-Coping Process

The process of stress-coping is depicted in the model as a flow of events occurring over time and across encounters. Coping with stress represents a gradual movement toward specified goals and is a necessary characteristic of growth. Coping strategies consist of the neurocognitive, affective, and physiologic responses to a stress situation and may be observed in the behavioral response dimension.

Figs 1 to 3 depict the stress-coping process in increasingly specific terms. Fig 1 shows the process in its broadest, most general form.

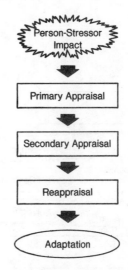

Fig 1. Stress-coping process (over time and events).

The first phase of coping includes a primary appraisal consisting of a neurocognitive evaluation of the stress configuration, the initial affective response, the corresponding physiologic response, and

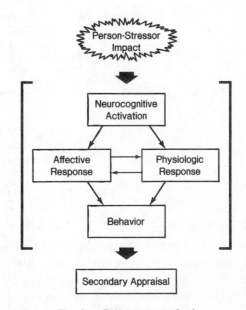

Fig 2. Primary appraisal.

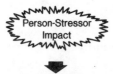

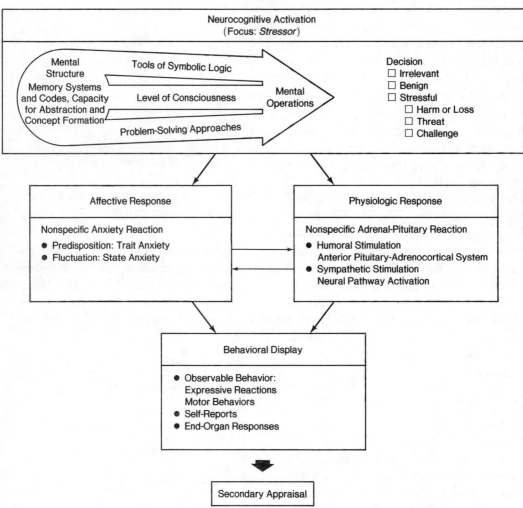

Fig 3. Coping phase 1: primary appraisal.

the resultant composite coping behaviors that occur as precursors to the secondary appraisal or second neurocognitive evaluation.

Fig 2 demonstrates the connections among cognitive appraisal as defined by Lazarus,[23] the affective response based on the work of Izard,[44] Plutchik et al,[45] Weisman,[46] and others, and the physiologic response from the findings of Frankenhauser,[51] Mason,[53] and Sigg.[54]

Fig 3 amplifies the major components of primary appraisal.

Fig 4 depicts the next phase of coping

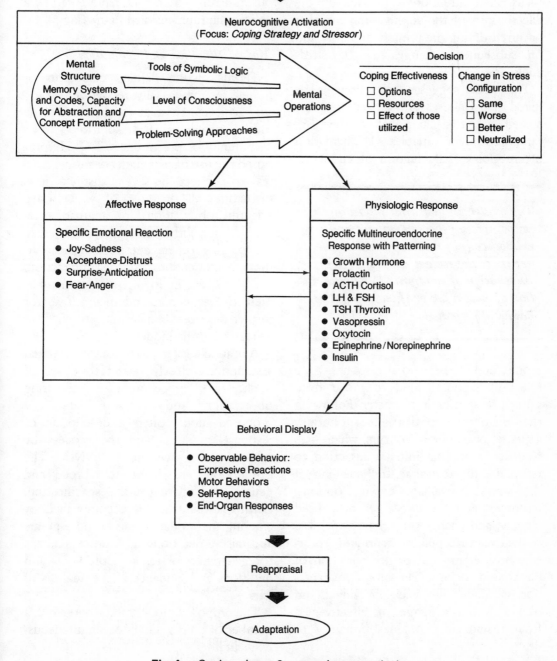

Fig 4. Coping phase 2: secondary appraisal.

14

where a secondary appraisal occurs using the same operational sequence as the primary appraisal, but with a different focus. Here attention is focused on the effectiveness of the coping strategies that occurred during the primary appraisal and on subsequent changes in the stress configuration.

The model suggests that following the initial person-stressor impact and its related cognitive interpretation, there are three dependent variables: (1) fluctuation of emotion, (2) fluctuation of endocrine

---

The model suggests that following the initial stressor-person impact and its related cognitive interpretation, there are three dependent variables: (1) fluctuation of emotion, (2) fluctuation of endocrine profile, and (3) behavioral response.

---

profile, and (3) behavioral response. As a rule, all responses tend to move from general to specific in character. Following the primary appraisal, a secondary appraisal or reappraisal occurs, which uses feedback from the initial transaction to reappraise the relevance and meaning of the stressor; evaluate coping options, resources, and the effect of those used initially; and change the primary appraisal of the event. Reappraisal continues repeatedly until adaptation or neutralization of the stressor occurs. The ultimate adaptation is unique for each individual and occurs within a range of effectiveness from maintenance of ideal integrity to death.

It should be noted that the time required for the entire process varies with each person and each event. The process, from primary appraisal to adaptation, is continuous in nature, and can be represented by a helical, multidimensional figure (Fig 5).

Model Utilization and Evaluation

Thomas Kuhn defined paradigms or models as "universally recognized scientific achievements that for a time provide model problems and solutions to a community of practitioners."[1(pviii)] He proposed the use of paradigms or models as a way to connect the several distinct views of nature—all or most of which have scientific, observational, or pragmatic merit—held by youthful sciences.

Modeling orders questions relating to fundamental entities and their interaction, seeks answers in logical and sometimes predictive sequence, and then allows for further discovery, expansion, growth, and validation of the model.

A model is a class of interrelated assumptions closely linked to a set of methods or procedures for measuring observations and analyzing data. The proposed model offers a description of response to stress and the process by which one grows and survives. The assumptions are deliberately broad and general, thus inviting further specification. Further specification is accomplished by entering the model at one or more points and raising questions. This process allows for generation of research problems and questions and guidance in the analysis of data.

The proposed model can be entered at a number of points, singly or simultaneously, including:

• Nature of the stressor,

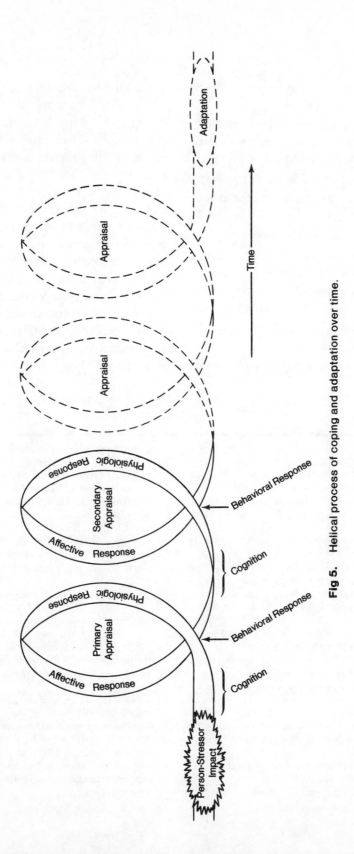

Fig 5. Helical process of coping and adaptation over time.

16

- Exploration of the entire coping response or parts thereof,
- Exploration of a mediating variable or its relationship to another (regulation of emotion, physiological response),
- Identification of adaptive outcomes,
- Multiple determinants of the stress-coping process,
- Tool or instrument development,
- Exploration of one or more variables in the behavioral response dimension and the patterning of those responses,
- Outcome of primary appraisal,
- Further definition of secondary appraisal, and
- Exploration of modes of coping: information-seeking, direct action, inhibition of action, intrapsychic.

Regular, periodic evaluation of the model, with further specification through research, will generate new knowledge and provide new direction for nursing diagnoses and intervention. The knowledge and insights generated and reinvested in the model will allow for further specification of component parts and continuous expansion of the entire form. The original idea of the model is dynamic in that it becomes increasingly complex, generating an extension of knowledge that allows for further problem identification, and, more importantly, solutions that may be applied in practice.

REFERENCES

1. Kuhn T: *The Structure of Scientific Revolutions.* Chicago, University of Chicago Press, 1970.
2. Goosen GM, Bush HA: Adaptation: A feedback process. *Adv Nurs Sci* 1:51–65, 1979.
3. Roy C: The Roy adaptation model: Testing the adaptational model in practice. *Nurs Outlook* 24:682–691, November 1976.
4. Lazarus RS: *Psychological Stress and the Coping Process.* New York, McGraw-Hill, 1966.
5. Appley MH, Trumbell R: *Psychological Stress.* New York, Appleton-Century-Crofts, 1967.
6. Bandura A: Self-efficacy: Toward a unifying theory of behavioral change. *Psychol Rev* 84:191–215, March 1977.
7. Beck H: Minimal requirements for a biobehavioral paradigm. *Behav Sci* 16:442–455, September 1971.
8. Becker BJ: A holistic approach to anxiety and stress. *Am J Psychoanal* 36:139–146, Summer 1976.
9. Bern DO: Psychological adaptation and development under acculturative stress: Toward a general model. *Soc Sci Med* 3:529–547, April 1970.
10. Cox T: *Stress.* Baltimore, University Park Press, 1978.
11. Ashby WR: *Design for a Brain.* London, Science Paperbacks, 1960.
12. Hermann MG: Testing a model of psychological stress. *J Pers* 34:381–396, 1966.
13. Hesketh JL: Development of a normative model of performance and satisfaction in individual decision making: An empirical test of initiative, need for power, self-esteem, intelligence, decisiveness, need for achievement and grade point average as predictive factors. *Diss Abstr Int* 35:4242, February 1975.
14. Kagan A: Epidemiology, disease and emotion, in Levi L (ed): *Emotions: Their Parameters and Measurement.* New York, Raven Press, 1975.
15. Lazare A: Hidden conceptual models in clinical psychiatry. *N Engl J Med* 288:345–351, February 1973.
16. Levine S, Scotch NA: *Social Stress.* Chicago, Aldine, 1970.
17. McGrath JE: *Social and Psychological Factors in Stress.* New York, Holt Rinehart & Winston, 1970.
18. Mechanic D: Illness behavior, social adaptation and the management of illness: A comparison of educational and medical models. *J Nerv Ment Dis* 165:79–87, August 1977.
19. Schor AG: Acute grief in adulthood: Toward a cognitive model of normal and pathological mourning. *Diss Abstr Int* 35:2447, November 1974.
20. Vogel W, et al: A model for the integration of hormonal behavior, EEG and pharmacological data in psychopathology, in Landahn G, Herrman WH (eds): *Psychotropic Action of Hormones.* New York, Spectrum 1976, pp 121–134.

21. Wild BS, Hanes C: A dynamic conceptual framework of generalized adaptation to stressful stimuli. *Psychol Rep* 38:319-334, February 1976.

22. Yusin AS: Analysis of crises using a stress-motivation-response model. *Am J Psychother* 28:409-417, July 1974.

23. Lazarus RS: The stress and coping paradigm. Paper presented at the conference on the critical evaluation of behavioral paradigms for psychiatric science, University of Washington, Seattle, November 1978.

24. Selye H: *The Story of the Adaptation Syndrome.* Montreal, Acta, 1952.

25. Mason JW: A re-evaluation of the concept of nonspecificity in stress theory. *J Psychol Res* 8:323-333, August 1971.

26. Von Euler US, et al: Cortical and medullary adrenal activity in emotional stress. *Acta Endocrinol* 30:567-573, April 1959.

27. Beck AT: Cognition, affect and psychopathology. *Arch Gen Psychiatry* 24:495-500, June 1971.

28. Dember WN: Motivation and the cognitive revolution. *Am Psychol* 29:161-168, March 1974.

29. Mandler G: *Mind and Emotion.* New York, John Wiley & Sons, 1975.

30. Weiner B (ed): *Cognitive Views of Human Emotion.* New York, Academic Press, 1974.

31. Piaget J, Inhelder B: *The Psychology of the Child.* New York, Basic Books, 1969.

32. Thatcher RW, John ER: *Foundations of Cognitive Processes.* New York, John Wiley & Sons, 1977.

33. Averill JR, Opton EM, Jr. Psychophysiological assessment: Rationale and problems, in McReynolds P (ed): *Advances in Psychological Assessment.* Palo Alto, Calif, Science & Behavior Books, 1968, pp 265-288.

34. Monat A, Lazarus RS (eds): *Stress and Coping: An Anthology.* New York, Columbia University, 1977.

35. Gellhorn E, Loofbourrow GN: *Emotion and Emotional Disorders: A Neuro-Physiological Study.* New York, Harper & Row, 1963.

36. Gray J: *The Psychology of Fear and Stress.* London, Werdenfild & Nicolson, 1971.

37. Hebb DO: Drives and the conceptual nervous system. *Psychol Rev* 62:243, 1955.

38. Hess WR: *The Functional Organization of the Diencephalon.* New York, Grune & Stratton, 1957.

39. Lindsley DB: Psychological phenomena and the electroencephalogram. *Electroencephalogr Clin Neurophysiol* 4:443, November 1952.

40. MacLean PD: The limbic system in relation to psychoses, in Black P (ed): *Physiological Correlates of Emotion.* New York, Academic Press, 1970.

41. Moruzzi G, Magoun HW: Brainstem reticular formation and activation of the EEG. *Electroencephalogr Clin Neurophysiol* 1:455, 1949.

42. Posner MI: *Cognition: An Introduction.* Glenview, Ill, Scott, Foresman, 1973.

43. Neisser U: *Cognitive Psychology.* New York, Appleton-Century-Crofts, 1967.

44. Izard CE: Emotions in personality and psychopathology: An introduction, in Izard CE (ed): *Emotions in Personality and Psychopathology.* New York, Plenum Press, 1979.

45. Plutchik R, Kellerman H, Conte HR: A structural theory of ego defenses and emotions, in Izard CE (ed): *Emotions in Personality and Psychopathology.* New York, Plenum Press, 1979.

46. Weisman AD: *Coping with Cancer.* New York, McGraw-Hill, 1979.

47. Arieti S: Cognition and feeling, in Arnold MB (ed): *Feelings and Emotions.* New York, Academic Press, 1970, pp 135-143.

48. Cannon WB: New evidence for sympathetic control of some internal secretions. *Am J Psychiatry* 2:15-30, July 1922.

49. Von Euler US: *Noradrenalin: Chemistry, Physiology, Pharmacology, and Clinical Aspects.* Springfield, Ill, Charles C Thomas, 1956.

50. Von Euler US, Lundberg U: Effects of flying on the epinephrine excretion in air force personnel. *J Appl Physiol* 6:551-555, March 1954.

51. Frankenhauser M: Experimental approaches to the study of catecholamines and emotion, in Levi L (ed): *Emotions—Their Parameters and Measurement.* New York, Raven Press, 1975, pp 209-234.

52. Levi L (ed): *Emotions—Their Parameters and Measurement.* New York, Raven Press, 1975.

53. Mason JW: Endocrine parameters and emotion, in Levi L (ed): *Emotions—Their Parameters and Measurement.* New York, Raven Press, 1975, pp 143-181.

54. Sigg EB: The organization and functions of the central sympathetic nervous system, in Levi L (ed): *Emotions—Their Parameters and Measurements.* New York, Raven Press, 1975, pp 93-122.

55. Mason JW: The scope of psychoendocrine research. *Psychosom Med* 30(pt 3):565-808, 1968.

56. Friedman SB, Chodoff P, Mason JW, et al: Behavioral observations on parents anticipating the death of a child. *Pediatrics* 32(pt 1):610-625, October 1963.

57. Mason JW, et al: Pre-illness hormonal changes in army recruits with acute respiratory infections. *Psychosom Med* 29:545, 1967.

Adaptation: A Feedback Process

Geraldine M. Goosen, M.S.
Doctoral Student
University of Tucson
Arizona

Helen A. Bush, Ph.D.
Associate Professor
Coordinator of Curricula
Texas Woman's University
Dallas Center
Dallas, Texas

NURSING PRACTITIONERS, researchers, scientists and educators are continually trying to establish a body of knowledge for the nursing profession. One area receiving increasing attention in this search for a body of knowledge is adaptation. As the link between health and adaptability becomes more evident, nursing intervention directed toward assisting the client to adapt to an ever-changing environment may become a unique theoretical framework for nursing. A new awareness, a clarified consciousness regarding the relationships between and among the individual person, the person's environment, nursing's involvement with the person and the individual's adaptation or health are imperative.

THEORIES AND THE CONCEPT OF ADAPTATION

Since the 1930s there has been a wealth of publications regarding theories and concepts of change, stress, coping and

20 adaptation. This information has been used by professional nurses who have recognized the potential for each concept in the daily lives of individuals.

The words *stress, adaptation* and *coping* have various, unclear meanings. For most persons, the word *stress* implies pressure or load which is being experienced at a given time. *Adaptation* and *coping* are frequently used to describe adjustment or acceptance behaviors. Similar usages are found in the literature, with some authors giving a separate interpretation to each of the two words while others use coping and adaptation synonymously.

Change

Society exists in an environment of rapid change. Toffler describes this environment as "a stream of change so accelerated that it influences our sense of time, revolutionizes the tempo of daily life, and affects the very way we 'feel' about the world around us."[1(p17)] Meyer has compiled a chart of important events in a person's life which evoked or are associated with some adaptive or coping behavior on the part of the individual. These events may be socially desirable or undesirable and include such occurrences as change in residence, entry into school, graduation or dropping out, changes in employment and dates of important phenomena such as births or deaths in the family.[2(p52-56)] These changes require an alteration from the existing steady state and disrupt the life patterns of the individual.[3(p825)] It is important to note that change per se, not the desirable or undesirable aspects, should be assessed for accurate evaluation of stressfulness on the individual.

The state of health or disease for individuals in our society is based upon the ability to adapt to changes in life events. The health or disease state is synonymous with success or failure experienced by the individual in the effort to respond adaptively to environmental challenge.[4(p344-368)]

The relationship between the inability to respond favorably to change and the onset of illness is discussed throughout scientific nursing and medical literature. Good health habits, the possession of social assets, identified value system, personal

---

Good health habits, the possession of social assets, identified value system, personal goals and psychological well-being are a few of the balancing factors that assist individuals to withstand high levels of change in their lives.

---

goals and psychological well-being are but a few of the balancing factors that assist individuals to withstand high levels of change in their lives, thus diminishing the possibility of illness, disease or injury.[5(p71), 6(p345)] The quality and quantity of human life are influenced by the universal characteristics of human nature; the transitory conditions which humans encounter; and the human ability to determine need priorities, identify options, decide upon a course of action and accept the decision regardless of the outcome.[4(p259)]

Stress

The most classic definition of stress is Selye's "nonspecific response of the body to any demand made upon it." Selye's theories regarding the need for stress to maintain life are widely accepted.[7(p13)] If the nonspecific response increases the need for readjustment, the demands placed on the body may be excessive and damaging.

Selye's concepts are centered around the General Adaptation Syndrome and describe the body's physiological response to stressors. Stressors may arise from sorrowful or joyful situations which present in varying degrees of intensity, thus requiring varying degrees of response for readjustment. When faced with these stressful situations the individual can respond through the neurological, immunological or phagocytic, and hormonal mechanism.[8(p39)]

Since the origin of stressors varies individually, as do the responses, it has been difficult for health professionals to determine the relationships between the phenomenon known as "stress" and the concept of illness. Levi proposed that stress could be measured by identifying and evaluating the cause of the stress; by studying the behavioral reactions of a homogeneous group to different stressors; and by identifying commonalities in descriptions of feelings indexed by stressors in an interview or questionnaire (this is done through projective tests and stress reaction or response measurements). The length of time during which the stress responses persist after the initial impact is also uncertain and varies among and within individuals. This individual response factor presents another hurdle in evaluating the impact of stressors.[9]

Adaptation

The attention that has been given to the adaptation process equals the importance of adaptation to human existence in a changing world. Murray and Zentner equated adaptation to health. They define health as a "purposeful, adaptive response physically, mentally, emotionally and socially to internal and external stimuli in order to maintain stability and comfort."[10(p7)]

The dynamic but finite quality of adaptation is related to the aspect of change which is inherent in adaptation. Murphy viewed change as "constant and universal." She states that humans are continuously "faced with the unchanging law that change will occur"—change within the human environment, between humans and the environment, among humans and within humans themselves.[11(p46)]

Toffler warns about the limits to adaptability:

> When we alter our life style, when we make and break relationships with things, places or people ... we adapt; we live. Yet there are finite boundaries; we are not infinitely resilient. Each adaptive reaction exacts a price, wearing down the body's machinery bit by minute bit.... Thus man remains a biosystem with a limited capacity for change.[1(p324)]

Mechanic referred to the importance of viewing adaptation as a transactive process between people and their life situation. The process of adaptation depends on the degree of fitness between the skills and capacities of individuals and the type of challenges with which they are confronted. To the extent that capacities are fitted well to the challenges, the flow of events is routine and ordinary.[12]

Lazarus states that as environmental change is perceived, the individual cognitively appraises the situation to determine the significance of the change. This

22

appraisal will determine the quality and quantity of the emotional stress state which will occur as a result of the environmental change. Coping methods, or self-regulatory processes as Lazarus calls them, as well as cognitive appraisal, are key mediators of the individual's stress reaction. Psychological and concomitant physiological response to threat by humans is neither uniform nor simple. The stimulus must first be perceived, then interpreted in the context of prior experience, and finally if read as a threat it is still to be confronted by psychological barriers known as coping methods. Lazarus suggests that the key mediator of Selye's General Adaptation Syndrome may be psychological. The pituitary cortical response to a stressor may require that the individual first recognize the threat and cognitively appraise the potential impact.[13(p146)]

Coping

Coping refers to efforts to master conditions of harm, threat or challenge. Lazarus defines coping mechanisms as "those direct active tendencies aimed at eliminating or minimizing a stressful event which are task and reality oriented."[13(p8)]

Freud refers to defense mechanisms as a unifying process rather than discrete entities, and identifies five of their most important properties: defenses are a major means of managing instinct and effort; they are unconscious; they are discrete from one another; although after the hallmark of major psychiatric syndromes, defenses are dynamic and reversible, and they could be adaptive as well as pathological.[14(p77)]

Vaillant defines the "ego mechanisms of defense" as "unconscious and sometimes pathological, mental processes that the ego uses to resolve conflict among the four lodestones of our inner life: instincts, the real world, important people and the internalized prohibitions presented by our consciences and our culture."[14(p75-90)]

Nursing Management and Adaptation

In Rogers's view, adaptation means the promotion of harmony between humans and the environment with the ultimate goal for the individual and nursing being the achievement of the highest state of health for the individual. Nursing strategy must consider the wholeness of humans and "derives its safety and effectiveness from a unified concept of human functioning."[15(p224)]

The importance of this statement for nursing cannot be overemphasized or overamplified; here Rogers is advising what system science has taught—that all known factors which concern an event or a process must be located and specified, and only in that way can the investigation be secure in the correctness of conclusions. For nursing, the caution denotes the need for a complete perception of unitary humans utilizing three principles of homeodynamics. These principles are named complementarity, helicy and resonancy, and clearly support the concept adaptation in that each of the three terms postulates humans' inevitable interrelationships with the environment. *Complementarity* is "the continuous, mutual, simultaneous interaction process between human and environmental fields."[16(p8)] *Helicy* refers to the unitary nature of the human-environment relationship by involving rhythmicity and negentropic evaluation as components of the innovative changes that take place in a spiral fashion. *Resonancy* refers to the fact that changes in the pattern and organization of the human field and the environmental field are propagated by waves.

The Roy Adaptation Model designates humans and their interaction with the environment as the units of analysis of nursing assessment. Nursing intervention takes the form of manipulating parts of the system of humans or the environment. The four subsystems of humans are delineated as physiological needs, self-concepts, role function and interdependence.[17]

Rogers and Roy affirm the wholeness of humans; that humans are open systems with a pattern and regularity; that they are tied to the environment and that the total human—physiological, psychological, sociocultural and developmental—must be considered. The two nurse scientists acknowledge that the nurse can provide support at various levels and at all places on the continuum or spiral in the adaptive and readaptive process of living. There is agreement here about the meaning of the concept and nature of humans and human adaptation, and the concept and nature of nursing. It is this feature of the scientific endeavor—achieving agreement on the meaning of terms that is "more important than the actual form of the definition."[18(p48)]

This applies not only to nurse scientists but to the other scientists who have been discussed above. Though the terminology and approach to adaptation vary with these scientists, there is unification in the thought that humans are in constant interaction with a changing environment. This

Though the terminology and approach to adaptation vary among scientists, there is unification in the thought that humans are in constant interaction with a changing environment.

environment precipitates stimuli or stressors, which necessitates activity or response on the part of the individual.

ASSUMPTIONS AND VALUE ORIENTATION OF THE CONCEPT ADAPTATION

The following are assumptions basic to the process of adaptation (see Appendix for definitions of terms).

1. Adaptation is necessary for all persons, at all times, in varying degrees.
2. The mind controls the body.
3. The perception of the extent to which a particular stimulus or life event is stressful is idiosyncratic, differing from individual to individual.
4. Similar stimuli, both quantitative and qualitative, will elicit different responses in the same individual.
5. Qualitatively different stimuli of equal toxicity do not necessarily elicit the same syndrome in different people.
6. The value system of the individual has an influence on adaptation to stimuli.
7. Clients' personal endeavors are requisite for their own adaptation.
8. The value system of the nurse will

24

affect the adaptation process of the client.

9. Nurses and other health personnel are uncertain of their role and responsibility in the client's adaptation to stimuli.

ADAPTATION—A CONCEPT FOR NURSING

The process of adaptation is viewed as a feedback system with five possible phases. (See Figure 1.) Following perception of a stimulus, in the first phase the stimulus, which may be an internal or external variable, is **appraised** or evaluated within the cerebral cortex for its magnitude and potential impact on the individual's internal and external environment. If the stimulus can be analyzed and resolved **cognitively,** adaptation occurs at this initial phase. If the stimulus is perceived as threatening it is then acknowledged as a stressor requiring further activity to achieve a satisfactory degree of resolution.

The second phase incorporates the **coping mechanisms** of the individual. The manner in which the individual reacts intuitively and spontaneously to stimuli evolves over a period of time. The pattern viewed as successful to the individual may not consistently lead to adaptation; nevertheless, the tried and tested behavior will usually be implemented precipitously after a stressor is perceived. The limbic

FIGURE 1. A FEEDBACK PROCESS OF ADAPTATION

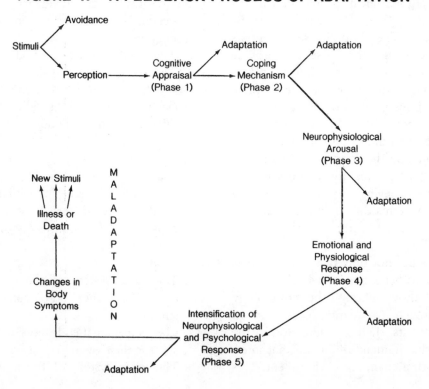

system, which is more complex than the diencephalon, is believed to be the portion of the brain which may trigger the responses and behaviors classified as defense mechanisms. The limbic system is frequently referred to as the visceral brain. It is considered an "old part of the brain in terms of evolution and involves the regulation of basic biological or visceral function."[19(p48)]

The coping mechanisms designated within this phase of the model include the stages or levels identified by Vaillant in his report of a 32-year study on adaptation. Vaillant selected 18 mechanisms which he organized into four levels. The behaviors which denote these mechanisms are open to interpretation.

1. Level I, Psychotic Mechanisms, includes denial, distortion and delusional projection. These mechanisms may be observed in children prior to age five and are also identifiable in the dreams and fantasy lives of adults. Outside this realm, the consistent use of these three mechanisms would denote nonacceptable behaviors and require further demands upon the body for resolution.

2. Level II, Immature Mechanisms, includes fantasy, projection, hypochondriasis, passive-aggressive behavior and acting-out. These mechanisms are commonly seen in children and adolescents as well as in adults with physical and depressive illness and addiction. Behaviors resulting from these mechanisms are not socially acceptable.

3. Level III, Neurotic Mechanisms, includes intellectualization, repression, reaction-formation, displacement and dissociation. These mechanisms are commonly used in children and adults as neurotic hang-ups or defenses. Those patterns that are established as frequently used methods for responding to stimuli can readily be converted to more effective mechanisms through professional guidance and counseling or through individual introspection and analysis of behavior.

4. Level IV, Mature Mechanisms, includes altruism, humor, suppression, anticipation and sublimation. These mechanisms commonly facilitate adaptation for individuals from adolescence to old age.[14(p383-386)]

Stimuli which elicit a mature response are resolved within this phase, thus facilitating adaptation. Stimuli or stressors which are not resolved precipitate a neurophysiological arousal. This arousal may be the result of a major stressor which does not trigger or initiate a coping mechanism or the mechanisms from Level I, II or III having been utilized unsuccessfully.

The third phase is **neurophysiological arousal** which occurs when the hypothalamus alerts the autonomic nervous system and the endocrine system to an invading stressor. Impulses received by the autonomic system are transmitted by reflex back to the organs, thus initiating a complex series of neurophysiological and biochemical changes in the body. The sympathetic nervous system is responsible for the changes occurring in the body—changes which are indicative of neurophysiological arousal. The body is prepared either to defend itself against the stressor or to resolve and incorporate the stressor into the body system. If adapta-

26 tion does not occur during this arousal phase, the body responds in many varying ways.

The fourth phase incorporates the **emotional and physiological responses** of the body to the neurophysiological arousal. These responses include sympathetic responses, endocrine responses, immune responses and emotional responses. Within the fourth phase the results of sympathetic nervous activity are clearly observable. The occurrence of adaptation during this phase initiates the parasympathetic response, inducing a state of relaxation. If the body has not adapted to a stimulus-stressor at this time, it is obvious that the body will be called upon to provide more intense efforts to solve the problem.

The fifth phase includes **intensification of neurophysiological and psychological response.** Body responses to stimuli from the sympathetic and parasympathetic systems are indicative of the efforts exerted. It is highly desirable for adaptation to occur during this phase since the failure of adaptive response will initiate changes in body symptoms heralding maladaptation or illness. Such changes precipitate new stressors for the body provided death does not occur.

The reticular system, a "column of cells" occupying the central portions of the mid-brain, is the communicator between all cognitive and neurophysiological activities. This system is viewed as the integration between cortical and subcortical functions. Adaptation to stimuli occurring at any of the five phases is announced to the major regulating components of the body. The reticular system is viewed as a constant stimulus to the brain, sending messages that are perceived as relevant and rejecting those that are irrelevant. This system also controls, tempers and refines muscular activity and contributes to high mental processes through focusing of attention, introspection and reasoning.[19(p51)]

ANTECEDENTS AND CONSEQUENCES

Each phase of the adaptive process is governed by physiological, psychological and sociocultural variables which provide the basis for stimuli perception, interpretation and subsequent holistic unique response. Some of these antecedents and consequences within the process of adaptation are shown in Figure 2. The variables are identified for each possible phase of adaptation.

These variables should provide some insight into the type of data that must be obtained from the client to evaluate the adaptive process, and are the basis for observable empirical and clinical referents. Many of the variables are applicable to each of the phases; nevertheless, these are perceived as the major variables which are incorporated in the adaptive potential for each phase. Each phase of the feedback model for adaptation is proposed as a

---

The reticular system, a "column of cells" occupying the central portions of the mid-brain, is the communicator between all cognitive and neurophysiological activities.

FIGURE 2. ANTECEDENTS AND CONSEQUENCES WITHIN THE PROCESS OF ADAPTATION

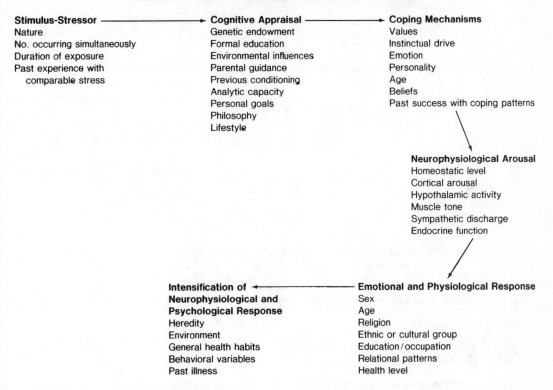

Stimulus-Stressor ——————→ **Cognitive Appraisal** ——————→ **Coping Mechanisms**
Nature   Genetic endowment   Values
No. occurring simultaneously   Formal education   Instinctual drive
Duration of exposure   Environmental influences   Emotion
Past experience with   Parental guidance   Personality
   comparable stress Previous conditioning   Age
                               Analytic capacity   Beliefs
                               Personal goals   Past success with coping patterns
                               Philosophy
                               Lifestyle

Neurophysiological Arousal
Homeostatic level
Cortical arousal
Hypothalamic activity
Muscle tone
Sympathetic discharge
Endocrine function

Intensification of ←—————— **Emotional and Physiological Response**
Neurophysiological and   Sex
Psychological Response   Age
Heredity   Religion
Environment   Ethnic or cultural group
General health habits   Education/occupation
Behavioral variables   Relational patterns
Past illness   Health level

potential operation through which stimuli are resolved and incorporated to increase the individual's utility, performance and pleasure within the chosen environment.

EMPIRICAL AND CLINICAL REFERENTS

Empirical and clinical referents, which are measurable and verifiable in reality for each phase, are identified in Figure 3. Through testing of the model it is anticipated that additions and/or deletions will be made to this beginning list of referents. Clinical referents which are indicative of sympathetic, endocrine, immune and emotional responses are listed in Table 1.

Failure of adaptation to occur at any of the five phases results in illness or maladaptation. Prior to a diagnosed illness, nonspecific signs and symptoms are detectable, which may indicate to the nurse that the client is in a state of maladaptation. These include complaints of pain, increased corticoids, increased hydrochloric acid in the stomach, increased eosinophils, allergic type responses such as sneezing and rhinorrhea, and decreased kidney function.

Diagnosed illnesses which are frequently classified as psychosomatic in origin include peptic ulcers, ulcerative colitis, asthma, dermatosis, angioneurotic edema, hay fever, arthritis, Raynaud's disease,

FIGURE 3.   CLINICAL AND EMPIRICAL REFERENTS
FOR THE PROCESS OF ADAPTATION

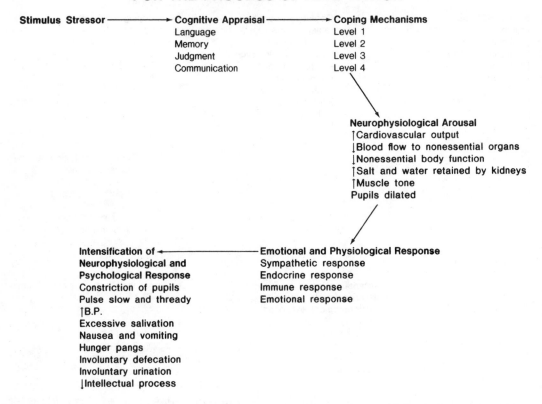

hypertension, hyperthyroidism, amenor-rhea, enuresis, paroxysmal tachycardia, migraine, impotence, insomnia, alcoholism and cancer.[19(p7),20]

TYPES OF RELATIONSHIPS BETWEEN THE CONCEPTS OF THE FEEDBACK PROCESS

In order to develop systematic explanations of phenomena, relationships between theoretical concepts and empirical referents should be investigated. Hardy declared that, "although the identification of causal relationships in the health sciences is the reason for considerable success in disease prevention, relationships that are stochastic and relationships that are conditional are valuable in the prediction and control of disease-related events and hence should be identified rather than ignored."[21(p102)] Adaptation and its referents, which have been shown in Figures 1 to 3, may be examined for their relationships using the types given by Hardy. These types are: symmetrical, asymmetrical, causal, probabilistic, time order, concurrent, sufficient, conditional and necessary.

Using the first two concepts in the feedback process of adaptation—perception of stimuli and cognitive appraisal—an

Table 1
Clinical Referents for Emotional and Physiological Responses

Sympathetic Response	↑ Respiration
Dilated pupils	↑ Glucose
↓ Gastrointestinal function	↑ Electrolytes
Tight throat	↑ Temperature
Cool-perspiring hands	
Locked diaphragm	**Immune Response**
Rigid pelvis	Corticosteroids
Numb genitals	Imbalance of immune
Tight anus	factors
↑ Pulse	
Tense neck	**Emotional Response**
Shallow respirations	Fear
Tense upper back	Rage
Flexor muscles in	Hate
legs contracted	Euphoria
Extensor muscles in	Joy
legs inhibited	Relief
	Love
Endocrine Response	Passion
↑ Blood pressure	Hunger
↑ Heart rate	Sleep pattern alterations
↑ B.M.R.	Eating pattern alterations

explanation of relationships is shown. A symmetrical relationship is found in the following statement: if perception of stimuli exists then cognitive appraisal of degree of threat exists; if cognitive appraisal of degree of threat then perception of stimuli. Another meaning identifies a causal relationship: if perception of stimuli then *always* cognitive appraisal of degree of threat. Stating this in another manner denotes a sufficient relationship: if perception of stimuli then cognitive appraisal of degree of threat *regardless of anything else.* A concurrent relationship exists between these two concepts: if perception of stimuli then *also* cognitive appraisal of degree of threat. Lastly, when the statement is altered to read in this manner the relationship is a necessary one: if perception of stimuli *and only if* perception of stimuli then cognitive appraisal of degree of threat.

The following cases may help clarify the analysis of adaptation. The first case offers a model for adaptation. The second case is the same subject with a multitude of unresolved stressors depicting maladaptation.

Adaptive Case

The subject is a 25-year-old insurance adjuster who has been divorced for one year after a first marriage of four years. She has no children, has a bachelor of science degree in home economics, owns a car, and has hospitalization and medical coverage through her employer's plan. She is Caucasian and a Catholic. She has a boyfriend who is married but is planning to divorce within a short period of time.

Lifestyle Determinants: A wanted child, lived overseas when father in army. Has one living brother four years younger than she. Mother described as strong person. Father died of heart attack when she was ten. Mother remarried four years later. Physical growth and development normal. Family went to church regularly and seemed to be a happy group generally. Family lives across the country from subject.

Lifestyle: Within the next three months boyfriend will be divorced and he and subject will marry. Subject would like to have two children and keep her position with the insurance company. Believes she is smart, can be assertive and aggressive, and will be able to combine a career with marriage and motherhood. At the present time she is self-sufficient. Thinks the world is an O.K. place and says people generally

30 can be trusted. Feels stealing is wrong unless food is needed and money is lacking; totally against child abuse; thinks adultery is probably wrong but has done it herself; feels people should work and support themselves.

Tasks: Believes work is very important and desires financial security. Likes sex and has sexual relationship with married boyfriend. Has close relationship with girlfriend, boyfriend and mother—they are her best friends. She is able to verbalize her ideas and beliefs with them. Discusses problems with the appropriate person, and these three persons assist her in decision making; she believes her relationship with each of them is a reciprocal one. She takes at least one class or course each year for personal and professional fulfillment and upgrading. Goes to church every Sunday because she believes it is the right thing to do. Votes in every election. Belongs to a Women's Club and is a member of a health club. She plays tennis fairly regularly.

Coping Mechanisms: Uses rationalization and denial to an acceptable degree. Plans for the future using short- and long-term goals. Is able to postpone immediate gratifications if necessary or desirable. Uses tennis and activities at health club to achieve a desired level of health and as recreation. Is able to discuss fears, worries, problems with those she respects.

Physical Assessment and Review of Systems: Is allergic to penicillin; weight is normal for height. Sleeping and eating patterns are regular and sufficient to her needs. Does not take medications other than birth control pills. Drinks alcoholic beverages very infrequently; does not smoke and drinks very little coffee or tea, but does take one to two soft drinks each day. Wears glasses for reading. The review of systems is negative.

Mental Status Examination: Is carefully and appropriately dressed. Has good posture and appropriately expressive face and voice. Is logical, oriented, alert and above-average intelligence. Possesses insight and good judgment.

Maladaptive Case

The subject is a 25-year-old secretary-typist who has been divorced for one year after a first marriage of four years. She has no children, has a bachelor of science degree in home economics and owns a car. She is Caucasian and a Catholic. The subject has hospitalization and some medical coverage through her employer's plan, but does not have coverage for psychotherapy on outpatient basis.

Complaints: Feels tense, nervous, hassled. Has episodes of shakiness, tension, sweating, heart palpitations two to three times each week and feels overwhelmed. Has problems with work supervisors and boyfriend who is married and does not appear to be getting a divorce. She does not know what to do and has not tried anything to help herself, just cries. Is able to go to work and function.

Lifestyle: Does not know what to expect in next five to 15 years. Has no further educational goals but would like to get a better job. Does not like home economics field. Would like to get married and have a "couple of kids." Believes the best situation for her would be to be wealthy, happily married with two children and have a good job. Believes she is smart, can be aggressive and is a selfish person. Says she is too heavy. Wants to become self-sufficient. Thinks the world is a neutral-hostile place and says people can never be trusted. Feels stealing is wrong unless food is needed and money is lacking; totally against child abuse; thinks adultery is probably wrong but has done it herself; feels people should work and support themselves.

Tasks: Believes work is very important; desires financial security. Likes sex and has sexual relationship with married boyfriend. Married because she was pregnant, then miscarried at two and one-half months. Has close relations with girlfriend, boy-friend and mother—they are her only friends. Her girlfriend told her to go to a clinic for help and she did go. Subject believes her boyfriend is the cause of all her problems; she cannot tell him how she feels and does not know where she stands with him. Does not do anything with her spare time except wait for boyfriend to call or may do something with girlfriend who is also divorced. Has not gone to church in past three months, but went regularly before that because it was the right thing to do. Did not vote in last election.

Coping Mechanisms: If she gets "upset" she sits and cries or gets depressed. Recently dreamt her boyfriend left her. Feels way to improve current situation is to "have more control over my life."

Physical Assessment and Review of Systems: Had gallbladder attack one year ago; put on bland diet but no medications. Had abortion (illegal) at age 18 and miscarriage at age 20. Had spinal meningitis at three years. Is allergic to penicillin. Is currently sleeping poorly. Has difficulty getting to sleep; wakes early and cannot get back to sleep. This occurs one to three times each week. Has seen M.D. and is on Etrafon-Forte (4-25) i h.s. Takes aspirin for tension headaches and takes birth control pills. Has smoked marijuana on occasion. Drinks on weekends when she goes to bars with boyfriend. Drinks very little coffee or tea; normally takes one or two soft drinks each day. "Heart pounds" when anxious. Has cough (smokes two packs of cigarettes each day); has frequent URI. Has anorexia alternating with excessive appetite; has irregular eating habits and has had "nervous stomach for years." Wears glasses for reading.

Mental Status Examination: Is carefully dressed, wears heavy eye make-up and has very long polished finger nails. Has slightly slouched posture. Is tearful at intervals, cooperative. Facial expression is apprehensive, voice expressive. Has labile affective state. Verbal content reveals sadness, fear. Mood fluctuates between depression and anxiety each day. Has logical sentences and organized ideas. Is oriented and has good memory. Is alert and has average or above-average intelligence. Insight—has some knowledge of what problems are, usually faulty judgment and pattern of poor decisions in past. Perception—is uncertain about what she is really like; knows she wants to have more control of her life. Is uncertain as to how others really see her.

TESTING

The value and efficacy of the feedback process of adaptation can be clarified through clinical nursing practice and nurs-

32

Historical studies to determine the process of adaptation through selected eras of our society would provide some insight into the evolution of current conditions in the environment and the adaptive patterns which individuals used to meet the existing challenge.

ing research. The three major methods of research—historical, descriptive and experimental—can each be employed to test the model. Historical studies to determine the process of adaptation through selected eras of our society would provide some insight into the evolution of current conditions in the environment and the adaptive patterns which individuals used to meet the existing challenge. Within the descriptive method, an exploratory, phenomeno-logical approach could be used in answering the following types of questions. What are the common elements in the daily experiences of adaptation? When neurophysiological arousal occurs within the feedback process of adaptation, how frequently does adaptation occur? The experimental method may be directed at identifying response patterns to stimuli controlled for type, amount and frequency. The stimuli could be directed toward samples varied by age, sex and race.

The ability to adapt to the ever-changing environment is requisite to life, but the degree to which individuals are able to incorporate change into the maturation process and day-to-day living varies. Knowledge of adaptability will provide nurses with data to evaluate clients' status of adaptability, or their health status.

REFERENCES

1. Toffler, A. *Future Shock* (New York: Random House 1970).
2. Meyer, A. "The Life Chart and the Obligation of Specifying Positive Data in Psychopathological Diagnosis" in Winters, E., ed. *The Collected Papers of Adolph Meyer* vol. III (Baltimore: The Johns Hopkins Press 1951).
3. Petrich, J. and Holmes, T. "Life Change and Onset of Illness." *Med Clin N Am* 61:4 (July 1977) p. 825-838.
4. Dubos, R. *Man Adapting* (New Haven: Yale University Press 1965).
5. Holmes, R. and Masuda, M. "Psychosomatic Syndrome: When Mothers-in-Law or Other Disasters Visit, a Person Can Develop a Bad, Bad Cold or Worse." *Psychol Today* 5:11 (April 1972) p. 71-72+.
6. McNeil, J. "Keeping People Well Despite Life Change Crisis." *Public Health Reports* 92:4 (July-August 1977) p. 343-348.
7. Selye, H. *The Stress of Life* (New York: McGraw-Hill Book Co. 1976).
8. Selye, H. "A Code for Coping with Stress." *AORN J* 25:1 (January 1977) p. 35-47.
9. Levi, L. *Stress, Sources, Management and Prevention* (New York: Leveright Publishing Co. 1967).
10. Murray, R. and Zentner, J. *Nursing Concepts for Health Promotion* (Englewood Cliffs, N.J.: Prentice-Hall 1975).
11. Murphy, J. *Theoretical Issues in Professional Nursing* (New York: Appleton-Century-Crofts 1971).
12. Mechanic, D. "Stress, Illness and Illness Behavior." *J Human Stress* 2:2 (June 1976) p. 2-7.
13. Lazarus, R. "Cognitive and Coping Process in Emotion" in Monat, A. and Lazarus, R., eds. *Stress and Coping: An Anthology* (New York: Columbia University Press 1977).
14. Vaillant, G. *Adaptation to Life* (Boston: Little, Brown and Co. 1977).
15. Rogers, M. *An Introduction to the Theoretical Basis of Nursing* (Philadelphia: F. A. Davis Co. 1970).
16. Rogers, M. "Nursing Science: A Science of Unitary Man." Supplementary Material for Nursing Theorists

General Session—The Second Annual Nurse Educator Conference 1978, New York, N.Y. p. 8.
17. Riehl, J. and Roy, C. *Conceptual Models for Nursing Practice* (New York: Appleton-Century-Crofts 1974).
18. Reynolds, P. *A Primer in Theory Construction* (Indianapolis: Bobbs-Merrill Co. 1971).
19. Pelletier, K. *Mind as Healer, Mind as Slayer* (New York: Dell Publishing Co. 1978).
20. LeShan, L. "Psychological States as Factors in the Development of Malignant Disease: A Critical Review." *J Nat Cancer Inst* 22:1 (January 1959) p. 1-16.
21. Hardy, M. "Theories: Components, Development, Evaluation," *Nurs Res* 23:2 (March-April 1974) p. 100-107.

Appendix
Definitions of Terms

Following are definitions for key words used in the concept analysis of adaptation. Other words or terms which are not defined will maintain the common usage as interpreted by the reader.

Adaptation—those constant, positive alterations which individuals make in their patterns of interaction to stimuli within the environment. These alterations perpetuate the survival of the individual and increase the individual's utility, performance and pleasure within the chosen environment.

Maladaptation—alterations that the individual makes to internal and external stimuli; these alterations result in illness or a state of disharmony for the individual and the environment.

Stimuli—factors, events or variables arising inside and/or outside the body which constitute a change from the usual, thus necessitating some degree of response from the individual.

Stressor—a stress-producing factor determined as such by the cerebral cortex during the analysis of stimuli.

Stress—the nonspecific responses of the body to any demands made upon it; these responses can be associated with pleasant or unpleasant experiences.[8(p39)]

Holistic—the inextricable interaction between the person and the psychosocial environment. Mind and body function as an integrated unit including physical, psychological and spiritual components.[19(p11)]

Health—a purposeful, adaptive response (physically, mentally, emotionally and socially) to internal and external stimuli in order to maintain stability and comfort.[10(p7)]

Illness—a disturbed adaptive response to internal and external stimuli resulting in disequilibrium and inability to use the usual health-promoting resourses.[10(p7)]

External Variables—changes or alterations that occur outside the body and may be physical, biological, social or cultural in nature.

Internal Variables—include personal structural characteristics, psychological processes, physical growth and development, body repair mechanisms and resulting behavior.

Cognitive Appraisal—knowledge from personal views or experiences which provides a basis for estimating value.

Coping Mechanisms—conscious or unconscious methods used by the individual to eliminate, minimize or incorporate a stimulus or event.

A Challenge to the
Concept of Adaptation as "Healthy"

Paula M. Sigman, R.N., M.S.
Nurse Consultant
Methodist Hospitals of Dallas
Doctoral Candidate, Texas Woman's University
Dallas Center
Dallas, Texas

NURSING LITERATURE abounds with writings on adaptation and its relationship to health and illness. Models have been and continue to be devised, and theories continue to be postulated concerning adaptation and nursing practice. While interest in conceptual analysis, model and theory development originated with but a few of nursing's leaders, this interest has erupted into a growing commitment by the profession to the pursuit of scientific thought and investigation. A key feature of this commitment seems to be nursing's growing alignment with and stress upon the concept of health or wellness as essential to defining nursing's role within the health care field. While medicine is said to emphasize illness and the "not-well-man," nursing has capitalized upon this by directly aligning itself with the concept of wellness or health. Understandably, then, concepts basic to nursing model development are defined as essentially healthy, positive.

While the concept of adaptation easily

36 lends itself to nursing as nursing attempts to define itself and move toward theory formation, the concept of adaptation as "healthy" *can* be challenged. Nurses need to critically analyze the concept before incorporating it into nursing practice.

DEFINITION OF ADAPTATION

Adaptation, as presently defined, is a process by which people, in groups or individually, *constructively cope* with conditions imposed internally or externally in order to meet their needs.[1(p158)] Such conditions may be entirely beyond their control or may result from the freedom to choose between alternatives.[1(p158)] Adaptation is the constant adjustment of the homeostatic, biological and other internal mechanisms to the outside environment in order to survive better or to change the environment.[2(p11)] This change can be viewed as *forward-moving change* which allows adaptation to be accomplished *without a loss of long-range goals* or *values* and without psychological disintegration or disruption of a person's overall functioning.[3(p157)]

Adaptation, then, both influences and defines the individual's level of health, with "health" being a strongly positive concept since it is not only polar to illness on a health/illness continuum but is a state which we in nursing help the patient obtain or maintain. Intervention by nurses is utilized to prevent, modify or reduce harm or dysfunction that induces new or additional illness and leads the individual away from the health end of the continuum. In essence, nursing intervention can be understood in terms of health, and, consequently, adaptation.

REGRESSION—AN ELEMENT OF ADAPTATION

The concept of adaptation as a process of forward-moving change that results in constructive behavior implies that regression, or behavior viewed or labeled as either deviant or destructive, cannot be an element of adaptation, of positive health change, of survival. However, regression or "unhealthy" behavior *can* be denoted as part of adaptation. The classical example of individual and mass adaptation in Europe's concentration camps of the 1930s and 1940s, where psychological disintegration and changes in values were indeed evident, illustrates this phenomenon.

The Concentration Camp Experience

The German concentration camp experience became a total adaptation experience, a way of life. Whatever helped individuals survive was considered good, and whatever threatened survival was to be avoided: "Everything is permissible as long as it contributes to helping me survive in camp."[4(p130)] Essential to the prisoners' survival was adaptation.

There are three factors which are said to reveal the thoroughness of change and adaptation experienced by individuals: (1) overall resistance becomes minimal to nonexistent; (2) suicide, the utmost escape from the need to adapt in order to survive, is infrequently adopted; and (3) hatred toward the powerful is absent.[5(p110-115)] Studies of concentration camp prisoners have recorded the thoroughness of their adaptation in terms of these three factors. "With few exceptions, when led to execution, either singularly, in groups or in masses, (they) never fought back ... death was accepted without a fight."[6(p284)] For the majority of prisoners the basic simplicity of the survival urge made suicide incomprehensible, "yet they could, when commanded ... go to their death without resistance."[5(p114)] Finally, hatred toward the S.S. guards was for the most part absent.

The behaviors exhibited by the prisoners were regressive, deviant from society's expectations (including European society in the 1930s and 1940s); personalities were dramatically changed, with old values and goals being discarded and "new" values being assimilated. And these changes were long lasting. Behaviorally, liberated prisoners frequently admitted that they could no longer visualize themselves "living outside the camp, making free decisions and taking care of themselves and their families."[7(p439)] In adapting to life (survival) in a camp, a prisoner "had to change his personality so as to accept as his own the values of the Gestapo."[7(p447)] Under such acute stress, an entire new set of standards was necessary for the old values to disappear.[8(p136)] The prisoners developed types of behavior which were characteristic of infancy or early youth, and it was this infantile regression to childlike dependency, due in part to shock or acute depersonalization, that also led to "identification with the aggressor"[9(p121)] and internalization of Gestapo values.[7(p141)]

The concentration camp prisoners existed in a closed system, which eliminated any possibility for environmental change. By choosing the most constructive behavior available in order to survive, goals were lost, old values were abandoned and new values were assimilated. Although psychological disintegration did not take place,

In the hospital setting, adaptation is seen as focal to the nursing process. However, blanket acceptance of adaptation as the "way to go" can create conflict.

regressive behavior and psychological adaptation did occur.

The experience of the concentration camp involved then a detachment both from prior standards of behavior and from prior values. This was essentially a process of adaptation to a standard of accepted (social) normalcy, through drastic change and with a relatively short onset. As a result of internalizing the attitudes of the significant others (the S.S. guards) the concentration camp prisoners unquestioningly obeyed and did not revolt against the controlling S.S. guards. Many liberated prisoners practiced the role pattern of the significant others as an adaptive behavior for survival even after leaving the concentration camps. Was this "healthy" according to the present definition of adaptation? Or would this behavior be labeled unhealthy, maladaptive or something else?

Adaptation in the Hospital Setting

In the hospital setting, adaptation is seen as focal to the nursing process. However, blanket acceptance of adaptation as the "way to go" can create conflict. For example, the physiological needs of a patient may conflict with the psychological needs; and nursing intervention, aimed at psychological adaptation, can create additional strain and conflict.

38   In the case of a post-mastectomy patient, conflict occurred when several nurses urged the patient to achieve an optimum level of physical wellness. The patient refused to help herself become independent and self-sufficient. Contractures occurred and she lost the ability to use either arm to any significant degree. Numerous nurses from the hospital setting, from private duty to public health nursing, tried various approaches to help this client adapt and arrive at some individually optimum level of wellness. However, while the patient continued to suffer physiologically, emotionally she "was never happier"; her troubled marriage stabilized since her husband now felt needed and wanted to help his wife as much as possible. For years, the husband, a disabled veteran, had felt insignificant and insecure because of his wife's success and independence; the wife spent years struggling between a desire to be cared for and a need to financially provide for the family. Now, retired and due to her "illness," she could "sit back and be taken care of."

Once again, according to the composite definition of adaptation, while the encouragement of adaptation to social customs, expectations and the like and the discouragement of deviance from the accepted norm may decrease discord and adverse effects, they are not necessarily "healthy." Coping constructively with imposed conditions and forces beyond an individual's control may be necessary for survival, but is the adaptation healthy? At the least it may not be ethical. And humans may adapt best when change is neither sudden nor requires much expenditure of energy; but is this realistic?

With the survival instinct basic to human nature, do nurses expect too much of patients to have them adapt in a "healthy" way? There is physical health, psychological health, spiritual health and moral health. When the process of adaptation begins, change results. But, as shown above, whether this change and the concept of adaptation are predominantly health concepts is debatable.

REEVALUATING ADAPTATION

According to the definition of adaptation given, adjustment is similar to adaptation. Adjustment, however, refers to minor and often temporary changes in customary behavior to meet crises and present life problems. For example: the Donner Party survivors adjusted in a temporary way to survival via cannibalism; adolescents adjust to normal changes internal and external to them; disaster survivors adjust to temporary leadership without surrendering values. Contrary to the accepted definition of adaptation, value changing can occur with adaptation; this may be a reaction to manipulation or a response to power or the expectations of culture. Considered a relatively lengthy process, while adjustment is short,[10(p137)] no adaptation is considered permanent.[3(p158)] Is not some permanent change both "healthy" and fostered by nursing? Then perhaps it is neither adaptation nor adjustment which is the health concept basic to both defining nursing and theory formation for nursing. Could it be accommodation? Crate has stated, "It is not the role of the nurse to attempt to change the basic life pattern of a person but to support and guide him as he moves toward a way of life that accommodates his illness and needs."[11(p72)] Focusing on the accommodation aspect of adaptation might eliminate problems inherent to the concept of adaptation as "healthy."

The concept of adaptation is not an "exclusive means of understanding all processes which the individual undergoes."[12(p53)] Neither is it the same as adjustment nor the opposite of maladjustment. While often a useful means by which to understand some relationships between individuals and their environment, adaptation as it relates to health and illness is not necessarily "healthy." Confusingly, adaptation is also not synonymous with illness (or "unhealthy"). It is a phenomenon that exists and (as defined to date) should not, without more critical analysis, be accepted as a health concept upon which nursing science can be based for its model development and theory formulations.

REFERENCES

1. Boland, M. M., et al. "Application of Adaptation Theory to Nursing" in Murray and Zentner, eds. *Nursing Concepts for Health Promotion* (Englewood Cliffs, N.J.: Prentice-Hall, Inc. 1973) p. 157-205.
2. Lough, M. et al. "Basic Considerations in Health and Illness" in Murray and Zentner, eds. *Nursing Concepts for Health Promotion* (Englewood Cliffs, N.J.: Prentice-Hall, Inc. 1973).
3. Murray, R. and Zentner, J. *Nursing Concepts for Health Promotion* (Englewood Cliffs, N.J.: Prentice-Hall, Inc. 1973).
4. Lingens-Reiner, E. *Prisoners of Fear* (London: Gollancz Publications 1948).
5. Elkins, S. M. *Slavery* (Chicago: University of Chicago Press 1969).
6. Kogon, D. *The Theory and Practice of Hell* (New York: Farrar-Straus 1946).
7. Bettelheim, B. "Individual and Mass Behavior in Extreme Situations." *J Abnorm Psychol* 38 (October 1943) p. 424-466.
8. Cohel, E. *Human Behavior in Concentration Camps* (New York: The Norton Press 1953).
9. Freud, A. *The Ego and Mechanisms of Defense* (London: Hogarth Press 1948).
10. Bronowski, T. *The Ascent of Man* (Boston: Little, Brown and Company 1973).
11. Crate, M. A. "Nursing Functions in Adaptation to Chronic Illness." *Am J Nurs* 65 (October 1965) p. 72-76.
12. Martin, H. W. and Prange, A. J. "Human Adaptation" in Auld and Birum, eds. *The Challenge of Nursing: A Book of Readings* (St. Louis: The C. V. Mosby Co. 1973) p. 47-57.

SUGGESTED READINGS

Aquilera, D. C. et al. *Crisis Intervention Theory and Methodology* (St. Louis: The C. V. Mosby Co. 1970).

Alexander, L. "War Crimes: Their Social-Psychological Aspects." *Am J Psychiatry* 55 (September 1948) p. 173-178.

Barnes, H. E. *An Existential Ethics* (New York: A. A. Knopf, Inc. 1967).

Beland, I. L. Clinical Nursing. *Pathophysiology and Psychosocial Approaches* (London: MacMillan Co. 1971).

Bok, S. Lying. *Moral Choice in Public and Private Life* (New York: Pantheon Press 1978).

Cohen, Y. A. *Man in Adaptation: The Bisocial Background* (Chicago: Aldine Publishing Co. 1968).

Cohen, M. and Nagel, E. *An Introduction to Logic and Scientific Method* (New York: Harcourt, Brace Jovanovich, Inc. 1962).

Davis, J. H. *Group Performance* (Boston: Addison-Wesley Pub. Co. 1969).

Dollard, J. *Castle and Class in a Southern Town* 2nd ed. (New York: Harper & Row 1949).

Dubos, R. *Man Adapting* (New Haven, Conn.: Yale University Press 1965).

Engel, G. L. "Homeostasis, Behavioral Adjustment and the Concept of Health and Disease" in Grinker, R. L., ed. *Mid-Century Psychiatry* (Springfield, Ill.: Charles C Thomas Publisher 1953) p. 33-59.

Ewing, A. C. *Ethics* (New York: The Free Press 1953).

Kant, I. *Fundamental Principles of the Metaphysics of Morals* (New York: Liberal Arts Press 1953).

40   Lindberg, G. et al. *Sociology* 4th ed. (New York: Harper & Row 1973).

Mead, G. H. *Mind, Self and Society* (Chicago: University of Chicago Press).

Riehl, J. P. and Roy, S. C. *Conceptual Models for Nursing Practice* (New York: Appleton-Century Crofts 1974).

Sagan, C. *The Dragons of Eden* (New York: Random House 1977).

Yousef, M. et al. *Physiological Adaptation* (New York: Academic Press 1972).

Nursing Diagnostic Pilot Study: Psychophysiologic Stress

Cathie E. Guzzetta, R.N., Ph.D., CCRN
Assistant Professor
School of Nursing
Catholic University
Washington, D.C.

Garyfallia L. Forsyth, R.N., Ph.D.
Associate Professor
College of Nursing
Rush University
Chicago, Illinois

NURSING THEORISTS, researchers and practitioners embrace the goal of defining a scientific body of knowledge in and for nursing.[1-6] Until recently the reciprocal interdependence of the three aspects of scientific inquiry was not fully appreciated. The circular process of theory, research and practice and the way in which each contributes to the establishment of knowledge may be internalized through involvement in each of the component parts.

This current project is a report of a pilot study concerned primarily with nurses' systematic and logical organization of observable events. This may be called nursing diagnosis, since the ability to make a diagnosis and to prescribe actions is closely related to the organizing and labeling of the phenomena about which diag-

The authors thank Sharon Butler, R.N., M.S.N., Aeries M. Eberhart, R.N., M.S.N., Margaret Ann Isaacs-Skelton, R.N., M.S.N. and Patty P. Lillis, R.N., M.S.N. from the Medical College of Georgia School of Nursing for their assistance in the preparation of this article.

42 nostic and therapeutic judgments are made. Developing a classification of diagnoses is one approach to describing the domain of nursing by building first-level or factor-isolating theory.[7]

The definition of nursing is expected to result from the compilation of the efforts of many. Thus, it will represent "what is" rather than "what ought to be." Once a representative description is made, tested and disseminated to all practitioners, the problems of nursing education, communication, research and theory building may begin to be resolved.

The process of nursing diagnosis involves placing a patient in a diagnostic category for the purpose of identifying and directing nursing management. A diagnostic category has three parts, including: (1) the state of the patient, the problem or the category label, (2) the probable cause of the problem and (3) the signs and symptoms. Gordon has identified this system as the Problem-Etiology-Sign/Symptom (P-E-S) format.[8(p1299)]

The pilot study was directed toward assuming the responsibility for developing a typology of stress as observed in patients with acute illness. The diagnostic process was divided into three phases: (1) the conceptual phase, in which the theoretical framework was described, the concept of stress was analyzed, the etiologies of stress were identified and the signs and symptoms consistent with the stress response were determined; (2) the empirical or clinical phase, in which the process was tested; and (3) the interpretative phase, in which the process was analyzed, evaluated and validated.

THE CONCEPTUAL PHASE

A Description of the Theoretical Framework

The concept of stress is often defined, investigated and analyzed in terms of its physiologic or psychologic characteristics. This framework reflects Cartesian philosophy. It views the human being as divisible into body and mind. The framework has been beneficial to the growth of science, allowing the researcher to objectively investigate the human organism without confounding the data with variables related to the soul.[9] When Descartes defined the human being as divisible into two parts "as if" he were both a mind and a body, a prolonged confusion arose over the centuries until the "as ifness" of the body–mind duality was lost.

Getting rid of the old duality which separated the patient into disconnected compartments is a difficult task after the philosophy has dominated thinking for so long. Viewing the mind and body as operating on a continuum, however, reflects a holistic framework and allows the patient to be seen as a biopsychosocial unit. The interconnection of mind and body is reflected in changes of emotions and physiology. The psychophysiological association reflects that a change in the physiological state will be related to an appropriate change in the psychological state and likewise, a change in the psychological state will be related to an appropriate change in the physiological state. These interconnections are considered invariable.[10(p3)]

From this level of understanding, body-mind relatedness is a concrete idea. One can attempt to define it, teach it, practice it and measure it. When we begin to deal with the "spirit" of the body-mind-spirit, however, we encounter difficulty.

"Spirit" may be thought of in a number of diverse ways. To some nurses, the idea of spirit may suggest human virtues such as caring, love, empathy and understanding. Others may conceive of spirit as a quality of transcendence, of a guiding force or as something outside of the self and beyond the individual nurse or patient. To others, spirit may suggest purely mystical feeling. From this viewpoint, it defies words. It is ineffable. If one could describe the spirit, then it would not be the spirit. It is indefinable yet it is a vital life force profoundly felt by the individual. It is capable of affecting one's life and behavior.

As nursing begins the work of describing and explaining those things which nurses diagnose in patients, they must operate from a body-mind-spirit approach. The framework of holism directed the development of this study. It provided the basis for investigating the psychophysiologic aspects of stress which emphasize the oneness of an organism and convey the belief that the psychological being and the biologic being are not separate but function as a unit.

Analysis of the Concept of Stress

A review of the literature was necessary during this phase to provide the investigators with the knowledge necessary to conceptually analyze stress. Concept analysis allows one to clearly examine the phenomena under study and focuses attention on what must be described and analyzed.[2(p5)]

Because of the increasing interest and research in the area of stress, a variety of definitions and explanations have developed, resulting in confusion about the concept. Stress is defined by the physicist in terms of a "cohesive force or molecular resistance in a body opposing the action of applied external force."[11(p4)] This definition does not incorporate meaning for living systems. Sciences dealing with living beings, however, do not have a precise and universal definition of stress. The confusion is compounded further in the area of life sciences when the concept is divided between physiological and psychological stress as discussed earlier.

Selye had defined the concept of stress in physiologic terms as "the state manifested by a specific syndrome which consists of all the nonspecifically induced changes within a biologic system."[12(p54)] This definition implies that stress is found within living beings, that it has no particular cause and it is a state manifested by a syndrome.

A stressor is defined as that which produces stress. A stressor is an alarming

A stressor is an alarming stimulus which, in turn, causes the condition of systemic stress in which extensive areas of the body manifest changes from their normal resting state.

44 stimulus which, in turn, causes the condition of systemic stress in which extensive areas of the body manifest changes from their normal resting state.[12(p64)] In an attempt to deal with the stress, the body uses adaptive responses. These responses or defense mechanisms are reflected in alterations in the individual's thoughts, feelings, endocrine and autonomic processes.

Physiologically, the kidneys, adrenals, liver, blood vessels, heart, brain, nerves, thyroid, pituitary, connective tissue and white blood cells all play a part in the adaptive role when responding to stressors.[11,12]

From a psychological viewpoint, stress is a much more abstract concept. Thus it is difficult to measure, quantify and predict. Researchers use the affective response of anxiety as an index of psychological stress. Anxiety can be conceptualized as a response which is produced by a stressor. It can be defined as an unpleasant emotional state related to the subjectively associated quality of fear which is directed toward the future.[13(p48)] Anxiety is, in effect, a signal that some catastrophic conflict is threatening to break into consciousness. It is a diffuse apprehension, unspecific and vague. It is this very vagueness that makes anxiety such a terrifying experience. Acutely anxious patients feel themselves, their values and their entire backgrounds being threatened.[14]

Anxiety is a response to what *may* happen. The individual is anxious before the event, regardless of what it may be. Anxiety shows no cyclic pattern. It is a continuous, diffuse phenomenon which begins, stops and is finished.[15]

From the literature review, we conceptualized psychophysiological stress as a response which is caused by or related to the presence of a stimulus or stressor. The response is an adaptive mechanism which is reflected in both physiological manifestations and psychological alterations which are interrelated and connected. The diagnostic label of psychophysiological stress represents the first part of the diagnostic category using the P-E-S format.

Identification of the Etiologies of Stress

The second part of the diagnostic category used in the P-E-S format deals with the factors which cause or contribute to the patient's unhealthful response. A specific patient problem may have multiple causes or may exist under different conditions or situations.[8(p1298),16(p81)] The etiology of the problem will determine the treatment. Different causes will have different treatments.

The etiology or contributing factors identified in the assessment indicate what areas the nurse will plan to change. They direct nurses' attention to those things which are maintaining an undesirable patient response and can be independently managed and treated by nurses.

The next step in our nursing diagnostic experience was to determine the specific nature of the stressors producing the stress response. Before proceeding, however, it was necessary to identify a specific patient population, not only to observe the stress response but also to determine which stressors were in operation.

To fully evaluate the concept, researchers must find naturally occurring stressful situations. The advantage of this method is that naturally occurring stressors may be quite intense and may be more powerful than those that could be ethically produced in a laboratory. The disadvantage of this procedure is related to the many variables confounding the situation which cannot be controlled.

Our study sample consisted of acutely ill patients admitted suddenly to the coronary care unit (CCU) with an admission diagnosis of acute myocardial infarction. This specific illness appears to have profound impact on the body–mind–spirit relationship.[17,18]

From our past and present clinical experience and information obtained from the literature, we began to identify and name stressors capable of producing the psychophysiological stress response in acutely ill patients hospitalized with the diagnosis of acute myocardial infarction. As we began our naming, it soon became apparent that the stressors were falling into discrete, although sometimes overlapping, categories. Shortly thereafter, the classifications of physiological, psychological, environmental and sociocultural stressors were defined.

Determination of Signs and Symptoms

For each clinical situation requiring classification, large numbers of patients are surveyed. All the pertinent clinical properties are noted as present or absent for each patient.[19(p178)] These properties are signs and symptoms. They are also termed assessment parameters or empirical referents. Parameters serve as guidelines in selecting what to observe to determine

whether or not the pertinent characteristics are present. They direct the diagnostician's attention toward the signs, symptoms, behavior or condition of the patient that should be assessed to determine the validity of the diagnosis being considered.[20(p59)]

Characteristics, on the other hand, represent the limits of the parameter. They provide the criteria or the operational definition for each parameter which affirms the existence of the diagnosis.[20(p59)] Heart rate, for example, identifies a specific parameter associated with the nursing diagnosis of psychophysiological stress. The characteristics, which would define the limits of heart rate, might include a rate greater than 100 beats/minute. Dysrhythmias may represent the assessment parameter. The criterion of greater than 10 premature ventricular contractions per minute indicates the characteristics of the parameter.

Once a nursing diagnosis has been selected, significant parameters must be identified to complete the third part of the diagnostic category. To rule in or rule out the parameter, characteristics must be established as measurement devices. This process of inclusion or exclusion of parameters involves decision making and will lead toward the definition of clusters of parameters which form subsets of the diagnosis under study.

As we began to review the literature, we quickly realized that there were no comprehensive and systematic empirical referents which thoroughly described the parameters and characteristics of the psychophysiologic stress response. We proceeded by synthesizing the parameters

46

which were identified in various review and research articles related to stress.

When a physiological, psychological, environmental or sociocultural stressor is present, the sympathetic nervous system (SNS) releases norepinephrine. An increase in heart rate results as does an increase in atrial and ventricular contractility.[21,22] There is also an increase in myocardial oxygen consumption and a drop in coronary venous oxygen saturation resulting from coronary vasoconstriction. Peripheral vascular resistance is increased, raising the blood pressure. Vasoconstriction of most blood vessels—especially those of the abdominal viscera and extremities— occurs. Other SNS mechanisms include dilatation of the pupil, increased glucose release from the liver, excitation of mental activity and stimulation of adrenomedullary function.[11,13,14,21-23]

Sympathetic nervous system stimulation of the adrenal medulla in turn causes the release of large amounts of epinephrine and norepinephrine.[24] These hormones are carried to all areas of the body by way of the circulating blood system and have almost the same effect as the direct SNS stimulation except that they last ten times as long. The only significant difference results from the specific effects of epinephrine which include: (1) constriction of the arterioles, (2) augmentation of the rate and force of myocardial contraction, (3) dilatation of bronchioles, (4) increased serum glucose and (5) stimulation of adrenocorticotropic hormone (ACTH) which in turn stimulates the adrenal cortex.

Under stress conditions, the hypothalamic–pituitary system is activated.[17,25,26] The hypothalamus releases corticotropin-releasing hormone (CRH) to the anterior pituitary, causing the release of ACTH. Adrenocorticotropic hormone in turn stimulates the receptor sites in the adrenal cortex to produce glucocorticoids (primarily cortisol) and mineralocorticoids (aldosterone). Cortisol stimulates gluconeogenesis and increases serum glucose levels. Amino acids and free fatty acids are mobilized and increased in the plasma concentration. Aldosterone, on the other hand, enhances the tubular reabsorption of sodium and chloride, which are exchanged for potassium and hydrogen ions excreted in the urine.

The rise in the serum electrolyte concentration of sodium and chloride further stimulates the osmoreceptors in the hypothalamus to increase their rate of neuronal discharge. These impulses are transmitted to the posterior pituitary gland to release antidiuretic hormone (ADH). Stimulation of ADH causes a marked reabsorption of water from the collecting and distal tubules, diluting the ionic concentration of

---

Neuroendocrine changes and sympathetic overactivity produce observable signs, symptoms and behaviors consistent with the psychophysiologic stress response.

---

the blood and increasing the extracellular fluid. An augmentation in cardiac output and arterial pressure is produced.[21] (See Figure 1.)

Neuroendocrine changes—regulated by the central nervous system—and sympathetic overactivity—regulated by the au-

FIGURE 1. THE DIAGNOSTIC PROCESS IN PSYCHOPHYSIOLOGIC STRESS

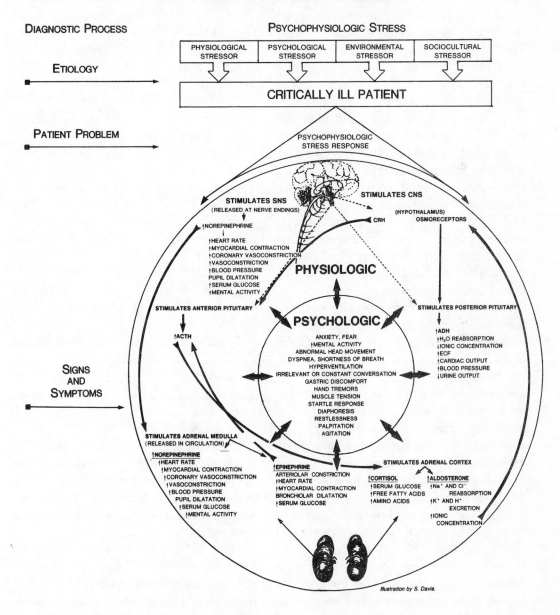

Note: The conceptualization of stress is paralleled with the nursing diagnostic process using the P-E-S format.

48 tonomic nervous system—produce observable signs, symptoms and behaviors consistent with the psychophysiologic stress response. Patients may squirm, pace the floor or show signs of hand tremors. They may be observed to have tic-like head movements or show signs of restlessness, agitation or nonpurposeful activity.[13-15] Respirations may be rapid and deep and may be associated with an inability to get enough air. Additional parameters include diaphoresis, clenched fists, startle responses, expression of fears or anxiety, irrelevant conversation, rapid speech or constant conversation, loud or high-pitched speech, complaints, disinterest or strained faces.[11-14,23] Patients may further complain of palpitations, gastric discomfort, belching or an increase in defecation or micturition.[11,13]

After we had identified specific parameters obtained from the literature, we compared the parameters with scientific research investigations dealing with the psychophysiologic stress response. We attempted to discover which parameters were sensitive and clinically useful in measuring stress and to determine the characteristics or operational definitions of each.

Physiological parameters were systematically classified according to major body systems including cardiovascular, respiratory, gastrointestinal, renal and neuroendocrine systems. This type of classification provided an open method of organization which permitted the selection, inclusion or exclusion of parameters based on clinical utility and/or new investigative findings. (See Table 1.)

From the selected psychological responses identified in the literature, the investigators found that the majority of these parameters were contained within the Holland-Sgroi-Solkoff Anxiety-Depression Scale (A-D Scale).[27] The A-D Scale can be used to assess anxiety and depression and can be utilized in the psychological study of medically ill patients in general as well as of patients in intensive and coronary care.

Most scales available for measuring anxiety are lengthy. Thus, their use is not appropriate for acutely medically ill patients. The A-D Scale depends more upon the observation of the patient and less on the answering of lengthy questions. Validation and reliability studies have been successfully carried out on this scale.[28,29] Only the anxiety part of this instrument was used in the pilot study. (See Table 2.)

There are four possible answers to each question. The minimum obtainable score for anxiety is 15 while the maximum is 60. The range and mean of anxiety scores assessed in various patients using the A-D Scale are found in Table 3.

In an attempt to objectively define the psychophysiological stress response, operational definitions (characteristics) were derived for each parameter. The physiological characteristics for each parameter were identified and defined from the research related to stress and from the investigators' clinical experience. Because the operational definitions had already been defined for the A-D Scale, the investigators believed the criteria to be adequate.

TABLE 1
Selected Physiological Parameters and Characteristics of Stress

Physiological Parameters (P_x)		Characteristics (Ch_x)
A. Cardiovascular		
P_1 Heart rate	Ch_1	a rise of greater than 10 beats/minute over 3 observation periods
P_2 Heart sounds	Ch_2	abnormal S_1 or S_2; presence of S_3, S_4 or murmurs due to acute infarction
P_3 Dysrhythmias	Ch_3	PVCs, PJCs, PACs >5/min or in salvos, multifocal PVCs; exit block; arrest, asystole, heart blocks, bradydysrhythmias, tachydysrhythmias
P_4 ECG changes from initial insult	Ch_4	12-lead ECG changes of additional ischemia, injury or infarct
P_5 Blood pressure	Ch_5	a rise of systolic blood pressure greater than 10 mm Hg over 3 observation periods
B. Respiratory		
P_6 Respiratory rate	Ch_6	a rise of greater than 10/minute over 3 observation periods
P_7 Breath sounds	Ch_7	abnormal sounds suggestive of cardiac decompensation, defined as rales, wheezes, rhonchi
C. Gastrointestinal		
P_8 Nausea/vomiting	Ch_8	subjectively expressed symptom of nausea or documented observation of vomiting
P_9 Defecation	Ch_9	increase in number of BMs/day. Determine baseline number/day/week from history
P_{10} Bowel sounds	Ch_{10}	increase in peristaltic activity, listen to abdomen with stethoscope for 1 full minute and grade bowel sounds according to: 3+-hyperactive; 2+-normal; 1+-hypoactive; 0-none. If greater than 2+-abnormal
D. Genitourinary tract		
P_{11} Urinary output	Ch_{11}	rise in urinary output. Determine intake from output and allow 600cc for insensible loss. Check for sudden weight loss or hypernatremia due to excessive urinary output
P_{12} Urinary cortisol	Ch_{12}	24° urine specimen analyzed by competitive protein binding—radio-assay for unconjugated cortisol. Normal range—23-89 μg with an average of 48 μg/24 hours
E. Neuroendocrine		
P_{13} Herpes zoster/simplex	Ch_{13}	presence of fever blisters or shingles
P_{14} Temperature	Ch_{14}	temperature 1 degree above baseline
P_{15} Pupil size	Ch_{15}	observe pupils in normal, indirect lighting and grade

$$\circ \quad \circ \quad \circ \quad O \quad O \quad O \quad O \quad O$$
$$2 \quad 3 \quad 4 \quad 5 \quad 6 \quad 7 \quad 8 \quad 9$$

If >5 = abnormal

TABLE 2
Selected Psychological Parameters and Characteristics of Stress

Psychological Parameters (P_x)		Characteristics (Ch_x)
A. Parameters from A-D Scale		
P_{16} Voluntary motor activity	Ch_{16}	1. normal and unaccompanied by tremors
		2. normal but accompanied by fine tremulousness of hands
		3. characterized by frank shaking of hands with abrupt jerky movements impairing attempted purposeful activity
		4. grossly tremulous with inability to perform voluntary movements
		NOTE: no CNS disease apparent
P_{17} Voice pitch	Ch_{17}	1. within normal conversational limits
		2. elevated at times during interview
		3. frequently higher than normal throughout interview
		4. persistently shrill
P_{18} General behavior	Ch_{18}	1. calm and composed
		2. composed but mildly apprehensive and uneasy
		3. distressed with moderate apprehension and fear
		4. extremely frightened with loss of emotional control
P_{19} Muscle tone	Ch_{19}	1. relaxed appearance
		2. characterized by a moderate amount of tension in muscles though lying still
		3. characterized by generalized tension in muscles with tightening of muscles, fists and jaws
		4. extreme tension; extremities held absolutely taut with no intervals of relaxation; head may be held off pillow
P_{20} Shortness of breath	Ch_{20}	1. none
		2. occasional episodes of shortness of breath during interview
		3. conversation interrupted by frequent shortness of breath
		4. constant shortness of breath during interview
		NOTE: no medical basis
P_{21} Speech	Ch_{21}	1. spontaneous and appropriately conversational with examiner
		2. verbose, giving lengthy answers
		3. overtalkative without allowing examiner to conduct interview
		4. constantly talking with disregard for examiner
P_{22} Volume level of speech (loudness)	Ch_{22}	1. compatible with conversational level
		2. somewhat louder than usual conversational level
		3. very much louder than usual conversational level
		4. shouting throughout interview
P_{23} Expression of anxiety	Ch_{23}	1. no concern expressed
		2. mild anxiety about condition with concern as to outcome
		3. genuine fear as to outcome but emotional control retained

TABLE 2 (continued)

Psychological Parameters (P_x)		Characteristics (Ch_x)
P_{23} Expression of anxiety	Ch_{23}	4. panicked that might not survive
P_{24} Rate of speech	Ch_{24}	1. within normal limits
		2. faster than normal speech but clear
		3. accelerated sufficiently to make meaning unclear at times
		4. so rapid that speech was largely unintelligible
P_{25} Motor activity (rate and amount)	Ch_{25}	1. within normal limits for physical condition
		2. characterized by restless and fidgety movements
		3. hyperactive with frequent changing of position and gross movements of arms and legs
		4. characterized by ceaseless nonpurposeful activity of all extremities
P_{26} Reaction to surroundings	Ch_{26}	1. normal for physical condition
		2. characterized by startle responses to ordinary noises (e.g., telephone, loud speaker, etc.)
		3. characterized by startle responses accompanied by episodes of fear (excessive for stimulus)
		4. frank panic reactions to a normal event in surroundings, e.g., pupils widely dilated, exaggerated sudden "jump" of whole body with temporary inability to continue conversation
P_{27} Increased respiration	Ch_{27}	1. no hyperventilation during interview
		2. occasional episodes of hyperventilation during interview
		3. frequent episodes of hyperventilation during interview
		4. continuous hyperventilation throughout interview NOTE: without known medical basis
P_{28} Facial appearance	Ch_{28}	1. responsive with full range of appropriate expression
		2. strained and tense
		3. fearful and distressed
		4. panicky with dilated pupils, widened palpebral fissures and tremulousness of mouth and jaws
P_{29} Diaphoresis	Ch_{29}	1. normal dry palms
		2. moist cool palms
		3. moist palms and beads of perspiration on face
		4. beads of perspiration on face, neck and extremities and patches of perspiration on gown
P_{30} Sensation of tachycardia	Ch_{30}	1. no sensations of tachycardia or palpitations
		2. occasional sensations of tachycardia or palpitations
		3. frequent sensations of tachycardia or palpitations
		4. constant sensations of tachycardia or palpitations NOTE: check #1 if there appears to be medical basis for these sensations

Source: Sgroi, S.M., Holland, J. C. B. and Solkoff, N. "Development of an Anxiety-Depression Scale for Use with Medically Ill Patients." Mimeograph. Department of Psychiatry, School of Medicine, State University of New York at Buffalo 1970.

TABLE 3
Range and Means of Anxiety Scores
Using A-D Scale for
Various Patients

| | Anxiety Scores | |
	Range	Mean
Normal	15–22	16.77
Intensive care	15–32	18.19
Medically ill	15–32	19.25
Psychiatric	22–41	27.27

EMPIRICAL PHASE

Objectives

Once we had gathered the essential information related to the patient's state or the psychophysiologic stress response, the etiology and the associated parameters and characteristics, we felt we were ready to pilot test the diagnostic process in the clinical setting. The purpose of the clinical phase was to develop a method of identifying the etiology, parameters and characteristics of stress. Hopefully, a useful clinical diagnostic classification system of the psychophysiologic stress response would be generated with the ultimate goal of determining and directing nursing intervention and management. Specifically, the objectives were to:

1. identify the nature of the stressors which may be present during hospitalization of the patient with an acute myocardial infarct;
2. assess the clinical utility and sensitivity of each of the psychophysiologic parameters reflective of the stress response;
3. determine the reliability and validity of the operational definitions (characteristics) for each parameter;
4. isolate clusters of parameters reflective of the stress response; and
5. derive a method of determining the level of the patient's psychophysiologic stress response based on the patient's total clinical picture.

Stressor/Parameter Assessment Sheet

As a means of systematically assessing the psychophysiologic stress response in the clinical setting, a stressor/parameter (St_x/P_x) assessment sheet was created. (See Figure 2.) The sheet was designed to assess stress for each patient during several separate observational periods. It was used to identify operant stressors and to assess the absence or presence and degree of the parameters reflective of stress.

Both physiologic and psychologic parameters were used. If the patient's physiologic signs and symptoms did not meet the criteria operationalized for each parameter, the data were placed in the 0 column for the time segment. If the patient did exhibit physiologic signs and symptoms which fell within the limits of the criteria, the data were recorded on the left side of the box under column 1 and a corresponding score of 1 was assigned and placed at the right side of the box. All psychological parameters were similarly scored under column 1 and assigned a number from 1 to 4 as specified by the operational definitions of each parameter.

Methodology

Five patients admitted to the CCU with the presumptive diagnosis of acute myo-

NAME: Mr. R. P.   AGE: 60   Dx: _____ ROM

DATE
(CCU) 7/7
(transfer) 7/14
(CCU) 7/28

(St₁) STRESSORS

Physiologic
St₁ – Acute Myocardial Insult
St₂ – Severity of Illness
St₃ – Related Heart Complications
St₄ – Severity of Symptoms
St₅ – Previous Hx Heart Disease
St₆ – Other Coexisting Illness
St₇ – Other Complications
St₈ – REM Sleep
St₉ – Other

Psychologic
St₁₀ – Fear of Death
St₁₁ – Fear of Hospital Procedure
St₁₂ – Weakness
St₁₃ – Alterations in Body Image
St₁₄ – Loneliness
St₁₅ – Powerlessness
St₁₆ – Hopelessness
St₁₇ – Helplessness
St₁₈ – Loss of Virility
St₁₉ – Transfer from CCU
St₂₀ – Other

Environmental
St₂₁ – Observation of Cardiac Arrest
St₂₂ – Observation of Other Patients
St₂₃ – Lack of Structure/Boredom
St₂₄ – Lack of Privacy
St₂₅ – Sensory Deprivation/Overload
St₂₆ – Inability to Sleep
St₂₇ – Untidy Surroundings
St₂₈ – Unpleasant Odors
St₂₉ – Frightening Noises
St₃₀ – Multiple Sounds
St₃₁ – Lack of Windows/Clocks
St₃₂ – Frightening Machines
St₃₃ – Restricted Visiting
St₃₄ – Altered Daily Routine
St₃₅ – Other

Sociocultural
St₃₆ – Age
St₃₇ – Social Class
St₃₈ – Financial Status
St₃₉ – Ethnic Origin
St₄₀ – Religious Beliefs
St₄₁ – Education
St₄₂ – Fear of Family Reaction
St₄₃ – Family Conflicts
St₄₄ – Concern for Self
St₄₅ – Concern for Family
St₄₆ – Interpretation of Symptoms
St₄₇ – Loss of Peer Respect
St₄₈ – Inability to Work
St₄₉ – Other Beliefs/Attitudes
St₅₀ – Other

(Px) PARAMETERS

Physiologic
Cardiovascular
P₁ – Heart Rate
P₂ – Heart Sounds
P₃ – Dysrhythmias
P₄ – ECG Changes
P₅ – Blood Pressure

Respiratory
P₆ – Respiratory Rate
P₇ – Breath Sounds

Gastrointestinal
P₈ – Nausea/Vomiting
P₉ – Defecation
P₁₀ – Bowel Sounds
P₁₁ – Urinary Output
P₁₂ – Urinary Cortisol

Neuroendocrine
P₁₃ – Herpes Zoster/Simplex
P₁₄ – Temperature
P₁₅ – Pupil Size

Psychologic
P₁₆ – Voluntary Motor Activity
P₁₇ – Voice Pitch
P₁₈ – General Behavior
P₁₉ – Muscle Tone
P₂₀ – Shortness of breath
P₂₁ – Speech
P₂₂ – Volume Level of Speech
P₂₃ – Expression of Anxiety
P₂₄ – Rate of Speech
P₂₅ – Motor Activity
P₂₆ – Reaction to Surroundings
P₂₇ – Hyperventilation
P₂₈ – Facial Appearance
P₂₉ – Diaphoresis
P₃₀ – Sensation of Tachycardia

Physiologic Parameter data

Parameter	July 7 (CCU)	July 14 (transfer)	July 28 (CCU)
P₁ – Heart Rate	110	84	120
P₂ – Heart Sounds	S₁ + S₂ + S₃	S₁ + S₂	S₁ + S₂
P₃ – Dysrhythmias	15 PBC/min Ischemia on admission	None	12 PBC/min Ischemia
P₅ – Blood Pressure	140/90	116/76	152/88
P₆ – Respiratory Rate	24	12	26
P₇ – Breath Sounds	Rales	Normal	Normal
P₈ – Nausea/Vomiting	Documented	None	None
P₉ – Defecation	Normal	Normal	Normal
P₁₀ – Bowel Sounds	2+	2+	2+
P₁₁ – Urinary Output	Normal	Normal	Normal
P₁₂ – Urinary Cortisol	47 µg	52 µg	30 µg
P₁₃ – Herpes Zoster/Simplex	None	None	None
P₁₄ – Temperature	98°F	98°F	98°F
P₁₅ – Pupil Size	3+	3+	4+
Physiologic Score	7	0	6
Psychologic Score	26	23	35
PPSS	33	23	40

54 cardial infarction were assessed and evaluated by the investigators in a large teaching hospital in the South. A data base was obtained for each patient using a biopsychosocial history and physical assessment. During each assessment period, the investigators attempted to identify the etiology of the manifest stress. They collected information from the patient, family, the patient's history, physical examination, chart and care plan as well as from the health team members to determine specific physiological, psychological, environmental or sociocultural stressors. During the same time period, the psychophysiologic parameters and characteristics of stress were assessed. Following the assessment period, all information was tabulated on the St_x/P_x assessment sheet and a physiologic and a psychologic score were determined.

This procedure was used for each patient admitted initially to the CCU, repeated for each patient shortly after transfer from the CCU to the floor, and repeated again shortly before discharge from the hospital.

Description of a Sample Subject

The assessment sheet of Mr. R. P. (Figure 2) illustrates the diagnostic methodology. Mr. R. P. was a 60-year-old married male admitted to the CCU with a two-hour history of substernal chest pain which radiated to the left arm and was associated with shortness of breath. He had complained of additional chest pain lasting for ten minutes and associated with nausea and vomiting 20 hours after admission. The patient had been in the CCU 24 hours prior to this assessment.

The patient was a high school graduate who worked five days a week as a custodian for the local school district. He had one daughter living at home and had been married for 20 years. He was 15 pounds overweight and had smoked one pack of cigarettes per day for 25 years. The patient had no previous history of heart disease. He had not previously taken any medications. His family history was noncontributory. This was the patient's first hospitalization.

Upon initial examination, the patient appeared alert, diaphoretic, anxious and in no acute distress. His apical heart rate was 110, respirations 24, blood pressure 140/90, temperature 99 F. He was found to have a third and fourth heart sound summation gallop, a II/VI systolic ejection murmur at the left sternal border, midclavicular line and bibasilar rales. His electrocardiogram revealed anterior ischemia and frequent premature ventricular contractions. His cardiac enzymes were slightly elevated.

During the assessment period, Mr. R.P. talked frequently of dying. He had requested and received the last rites the evening before. He stated he had been unable to sleep since admission and admitted that the cardiac monitor, intravenous (I.V.) line and CCU were frightening. All data were recorded on the St_x/P_x assessment sheet. (See Figure 2.) Mr. R. P. was found to have a physiologic score of 7 and a psychologic score of 26. The diagnosis of psychophysiologic stress was confirmed by the existence of the observed clinical manifestations and was related to the following stressors (St_x):

St_1 = acute myocardial insult;
St_3 = related heart complications;
St_{10} = fear of death;

St_{11} = fear of hospital routine;
St_{24} = lack of privacy;
St_{26} = inability to sleep;
St_{29} = frightening noises;
St_{32} = frightening machines; and
St_{44} = concern for self.

INTERPRETATIVE PHASE

Classification of Stress Levels

After the data had been tabulated for all patients, the classifications of low, moderate and high stress levels were defined. The investigators used the following classification system:

1. Low psychophysiological stress was identified when a score of 2 or less was derived from physiologic parameters and a score of 15 to 22 was obtained for the psychologic parameters;
2. Moderate psychophysiologic stress was identified when a score of 3 to 6 was obtained from the physiologic parameters and a score of 23 to 28 was obtained from the psychologic parameters; and
3. High psychophysiologic stress was identified when a score of greater than 6 was obtained from the physiologic parameters and a score of greater than 28 was obtained from the psychologic parameters.

When the investigators tried to apply this diagnostic classification system to the patients included in the study it did not work. As an example of our inability to apply this system, Mr. R. P., during his first assessment period, was found to have a physiological score of 7, placing him in the high category, while he had a psycho-logic score of 26, placing him in the moderate category as well.

In an attempt to solve this problem, it was decided to derive a total psychophysiologic stress score (PPSS) based on the summation of the physiologic and psychologic scores as follows:

1. low stress level identified by a PPSS of 15 to 24;
2. moderate stress level identified by a PPSS of 25 to 31; and
3. high stress level identified by a PPSS of greater than 31.

When applying this classification system to the data collected, it was discovered that three levels were not adequate to define the levels of observed stress. Mr. R. P., for example, had a total anxiety score of 33 during the first observation period, placing him in the high category. Three days prior to discharge (third assessment period) Mr. R. P. developed substernal chest pain lasting 30 minutes. His electrocardiogram revealed new ST segment elevation and T wave inversion in leads V_{2-5}. He was transferred back to the CCU. During this observational period, the CCU nurses stated the patient refused to follow the physician's orders related to restricted activities and bedrest. Matches were found under his pillow and the nurses had smelled smoke in the room. The patient told the investigators that he did not know why he was back in the CCU. He stated he felt great, denied the previous episode of chest pain and said, "I'm going to get my wife to get the doctor to let me go home. I'll climb out of the window if I have to." Mr. R. P. was assessed and was found to have a PPSS of 40. He was placed in the high category. Clinically, however, Mr. R. P. exhibited a higher level of stress at this time than during his first observational period when he had a score of 33. However he was placed in the high category both times.

As a result, the investigators decided to add a fourth category of extreme anxiety to the other three levels. A new diagnostic classification evolved:

1. low stress level = 15 to 24 PPSS;
2. moderate stress level = 25 to 31 PPSS;
3. high stress level = 32 to 38 PPSS; and
4. extreme stress level = greater than 38 PPSS.

Results and Discussion

The results of the clinical project validated the existence of 31 out of 50 (60%) operant stressors in the patients assessed during three different observational periods. The primary stressors identified during the time segment in CCU were related most frequently to physiologic and environmental causes. The majority of stressors identified after transfer from the CCU and before discharge to home were associated with psychologic and sociocultural factors. There appeared to be an inverse relationship between the numbers of operant stressors and the length of hospitalization (except in the case of Mr. R. P.). Patients were found to have lower PPSS scores after transfer and before discharge than during their stay in the CCU.

The operational definitions for each physiologic parameter were validated and found to clinically measure the stress response. The choice of physiologic parameters, however, indicated that some were more substantive and sensitive than others to clinical measurement of the stress response. These included heart rate, dysrhythmias, blood pressure, respiratory rate, nausea/vomiting and pupil size. Defining the number of parameters to include only those which are useful would lead to a more efficient and effective assessment tool, saving both the patient and the diagnostician time and effort.

The A-D Scale appeared to be clinically useful in assessing and measuring psychological stress. When the physiologic score was added to the psychologic score to derive the PPSS, a workable and holistic diagnostic classification system evolved, allowing the categorization of low, moderate, high and extreme levels of psychophysiologic stress to be identified.

The levels of low, moderate, high and extreme psychophysiologic stress provide a diagnostic label which is clear and concise and sufficiently specific to be clinically useful. Additionally, the labels represent an operational level of abstrac-

---

The levels of low, moderate, high and extreme psychophysiologic stress provide a diagnostic label which is clear and concise and sufficiently specific to be clinically useful.

---

tion reflecting an identifiable clinical entity which has value for directing appropriate nursing actions.

The investigators did not observe clusters of signs and symptoms as previously anticipated when subjects were compared. Although the St_x/P_x assessment sheet was not impressive based on the small number of patients studied, it was found to be a valuable tool for identifying and measuring psychophysiologic parameters as related to specific etiologic stressors based on a given observation time period. Moreover, the assessment sheet incorporated the potential for comparison and contrast of the stress responses over time and appeared to be adaptable to statistical analysis.

Once a diagnostic category is established, it will direct the plan of therapy. The next phase in this process, although not included in this project, would be to validate the effectiveness of nursing actions based on the outcomes of the patient's response.

Take for example, Mr. A. B., who was placed in the diagnostic category of high psychophysiologic stress based on the findings from the St_x/P_x assessment sheet. His PPSS score was found to be 36 and was related to three physiologic and two environmental stressors. His plan of care and nursing management would then be identified and implemented based on the etiology of his stress and the level of the response exhibited. If nursing interventions were effective in reducing the level of psychophysiologic stress, one would expect to see a reduction in the PPSS score, as well as the number of operant stressors. This process would be repeated for a large number of patients exhibiting various levels of stress related to various etiologies. Ultimately, the results will validate prescriptions for effective nursing actions which will control the outcomes of patient care.

RECOMMENDATIONS FOR FURTHER STUDY

It is recommended that the empirical phase of this project be replicated with a large sample of subjects. Operant stressors should continue to be identified, labeled and validated for patients with acute myocardial infarction, as well as those with other types of illness. Nursing actions capable of controlling, reducing, eliminating or preventing the stress response should be identified, implemented and evaluated. The direction of this work should be communicated, synthesized and collaborated with the efforts of the National Group for Classification of Nursing Diagnoses.

REFERENCES

1. Bush, H. A. "Models for Nursing." *Advances Nurs Science* 1:2 (January 1979) p. 13-21.
2. Chinn, P. L. and Jacobs, M. K. "A Model for Theory Development in Nursing." *Advances Nurs Science* 1:1 (October 1978) p. 1-11.
3. Ellis, R. "The Practitioner as a Theorist." *Am J Nurs* 66:7 (1969) p. 1434-1438.
4. King, I. *Toward a Theory for Nursing: General Concepts of Human Behavior* (New York: John Wiley & Sons 1971).
5. Moore, M. "Nursing, a Scientific Discipline." *Nurs For* 7:4 (1968) p. 340-348.
6. Woolridge, P. J., Skipper, J. K. and Leonard, R. D. *Behavioral Science, Social Practice, and the Nursing Profession* (Cleveland: Case Western Reserve University 1968).
7. Kritek, P. B. "The Generation and Classification of Nursing Diagnoses: Toward a Theory of Nursing." *Image* 10:2 (June 1978) p. 33-40.
8. Gordon, M. "Nursing Diagnosis and the Diagnostic

58

Process." *Am J Nurs* 76:8 (1976) p. 1298-3000.

9. Kenner, C., Guzzetta, C. E. and Dossey, B. *Critical-Care Nursing: Body-Mind-Spirit* (Boston: Little, Brown, and Co. forthcoming).

10. Green, E., Green, A. and Walters, E. "Voluntary Control of Internal States: Psychological and Physiological." *J Transpersonal Psychol* 2:3 (1970) p. 3-10.

11. Wolf, S. and Goodell, H. *Stress and Disease* (Springfield: Charles C Thomas 1968).

12. Selye, H. *The Stress of Life* (New York: McGraw-Hill Book Co. 1956).

13. Hill, O. W. *Modern Trends in Psychosomatic Medicine* (New York: Appleton-Century-Crofts 1970).

14. Lader, M. and Marks, I. *Clinical Anxiety* (New York: Grune and Stratton 1971).

15. Janis, I. L. *Psychological Anxiety* (New York: Academic Press 1974).

16. Henderson, B. "Nursing Diagnosis: Theory and Practice." *Advances Nurs Science* 1:1 (October 1978) p. 75-83.

17. Vetter, N. J. et al. "Initial Metabolic and Hormonal Response to Acute Myocardial Infarction." *Lancet* 10 (1974) p. 284-289.

18. Guzzetta, C. E. "Relationship Between Stress and Learning." *Advances Nurs Science* 1:4 (July 1979) forthcoming.

19. Feinstein, A. R. *Clinical Judgment* (New York: Robert E. Krieger Publishing Co. 1967).

20. Gebbie, K. M. and Lavin, M. A. *Classification of Nursing Diagnoses* (St. Louis: The C. V. Mosby Co. 1975).

21. Guyton, A. C. *Textbook of Medical Physiology* (Philadelphia: W. B. Saunders Co. 1976).

22. Hurst, J. W. and Logue, R. B. *The Heart* (New York: McGraw-Hill Book Co. 1978).

23. Levi, L. *Society, Stress and Disease* (New York: Oxford Press 1971).

24. Mason, J. "A Review of Psychoendocrine Research on the Sympathetic Adrenal-Medullary System." *Psychosom Med* 30 (1968) p. 631-653.

25. Cope, C. L. *Adrenal Steroids and Disease* (Philadelphia: J. B. Lippincott Co. 1972).

26. Davidson, I. and Bernard, J. *Todd-Sanford Clinical Diagnosis by Laboratory Methods* (Philadelphia: W. B. Saunders Co. 1974).

27. Sgroi, S. M., Holland, J. C. B. and Solkoff, N. "Development of an Anxiety-Depression Scale for Use with Medically Ill Patients." Mimeograph. Department of Psychiatry, School of Medicine, State University of New York at Buffalo 1970.

28. Holland, J. C. B. et al. "The ICU Syndrome: Fact or Fancy." *Psychiat Med* 4:3 (1973) p. 241-249.

29. Froese, A. et al. "Validation of Anxiety, Depression, and Denial Scales in a Coronary Care Unit." *J Psychosom Res* 18:3 (1974) p. 137-141.

The Multiple Dimensions of Stress

Marita Frain, R.N., Ed.M.
Coordinator, Lower Division of Nursing
  and Assistant Professor of Nursing
Villanova University, College of Nursing
Villanova, Pennsylvania

Theresa M. Valiga, R.N., Ed.M.
Assistant Professor of Nursing
Georgetown University
Washington, D.C.

ONE SEES SPECIAL news reports about it. One sees an outpouring of nonprofessionally oriented books and articles about it. One sees an explosion of programs and conferences about it. The topic of so much attention is, of course, stress.

As discussed in Sutterley's chapter, the potential for human "wear and tear" caused by out technological, competitive, fast-paced society has become an area of great concern for each of us. Stress is a state manifested by the specific syndrome which includes all the nonspecifically induced changes within a human system. To one degree or another, it is usual in all of us at all times, and it can be positive or negative in nature, serving as an enriching experience from which one grows ("eu-stress") or as a damaging experience which inhibits growth ("distress").

60   STRESS AND MULTIDIMENSIONAL
MAN

Stress is a phenomenon which involves all aspects of "multidimensional man"[1] to some extent; it involves the entire organism. This coordinated response of the individual occurs as a result of a stressor, the agent or stimulus which initiates this "unified defense mechanism," and the response prepares the individual to deal with unexpected or unavoidable events. Thus stress cannot and should not be avoided entirely. Selye has termed the entire stress syndrome, namely, the threat and the individual's reaction to it, as the General Adaptation Syndrome (GAS).[2]

As stated, stress is a usual part of our lives. It is the human system's response to demands which are placed upon it, demands to which that holistic system reacts. Coping with stress successfully requires adaptation, the process by which the human system responds to its environment. Adaptation must be flexible. The human organism must either change itself to achieve harmony with its surroundings or alter the environment so it is synchronous with the organism. For example, in situations of lengthy exposure to high altitudes, human organisms change their hemoglobin levels to achieve environmental harmony. But in situations of an environment polluted by industrial manufacturers, the human organism can respond by helping enact environmental controls, thereby changing the environment.

The purpose of such mutual adaptive responses between the organism and its environment is to achieve and maintain a state of health, which then serves as an energy resource for the organism to do what it wants or needs to do; in the case of human beings, this energy is used to set and meet life goals.

Stress is greater at certain times than at others. Individuals deal with stress in many different ways, some of which may be effective, resulting in coping and growth, and some of which may be ineffective, resulting in a lack of growth.

Those persons engaged in helping relationships—nurses, physicians, teachers, counselors, parents—must consider that they as well as their clients are constantly assaulted by a number of stressors. The helper and client each adapt to stress in different ways, and this requires a dual awareness on the part of the helper.

THE MECHANISM OF THE GENERAL ADAPTATION SYNDROME

According to Selye, the GAS evolves in three stages: alarm reaction, resistance and exhaustion.[3] During the alarm phase, the individual's defensive forces are mobilized and the person is prepared for "fight or flight." The resistance phase reflects the adaptation of the individual to the stressor as the individual fights back, and usual functioning returns. If the stress is overwhelming or is not removed, or if the individual is continually ineffective in dealing with it, a state of exhaustion ensues where there is "no more give in the system"; in such a state, disease can occur and death is the final outcome. This three-stage GAS is depicted in Figure 1.[4]

FIGURE 1. SELYE'S GENERAL ADAPTATION SYNDROME

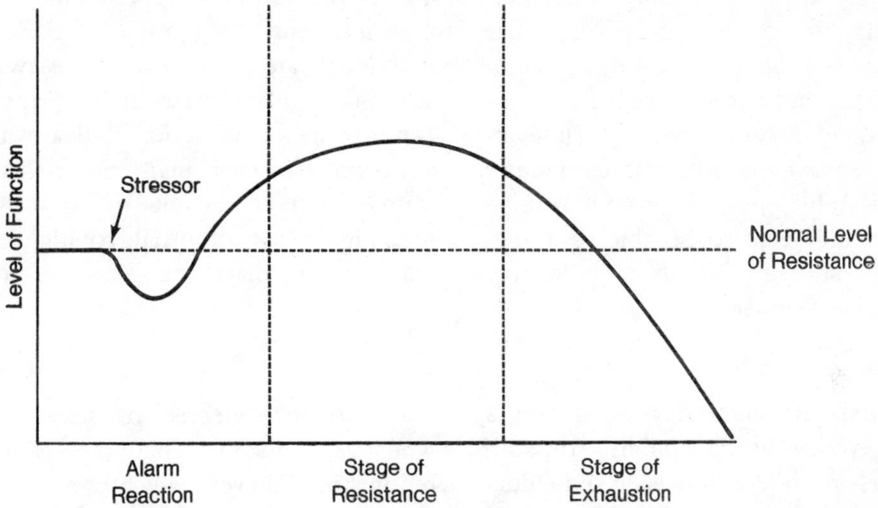

LEVELS OF STRESS

The psychophysiological stress phenomenon can be examined in detail using a "level" framework. In this model, an individual reacts to a stressor in a variety of degrees from extremely mild to extremely severe.

Level I

In day-to-day life, most people encounter events and situations which are considered nonthreatening because they are part of a usual routine. Although these situations are nonthreatening, they are stressors. In routine day-to-day situations,

---

Responses to day-to-day stress (Level I) are automatic or habitual adaptations and require a minimum of energy expenditure.

---

the individual relies on self-regulating and maintaining devices as well as problem solving to accept and adapt to stress. These responses are automatic or habitual adaptations and require a minimum of energy expenditure, such as the commute to work in heavy traffic. Such stressors trigger the sympathetic nervous system. This in turn stimulates the hypothalamus, which stimulates the adrenal medulla to increase the release of adrenal catecholamines (epinephrine and norepinephrine).[5]

One of the results of this mechanism is increased blood flow to the brain and muscles, which manifests itself in "cues" which can be perceptible to the individual involved. In this case, such cues might include an increase in energy in response to the need to accomplish tasks, an increase in ability to respond to multiple stimuli and an increase in alertness and sensitivity to the stimuli.

This process of alarm-resistance occurs

62 relatively rapidly and is practically imperceptible to the individual. Individuals responding to routine situations utilize biological, economic, educational, philosophical, psychological, social and spiritual resources in adapting to their ever-changing environments. Most individuals are comfortable in dealing with routine situations and seem to be able to anticipate crises and respond in a predictable and effective manner.

Level II

In contrast to routine day-to-day events are the ever-occurring, mildly stressful, new or less-routine events each individual experiences. These events, such as a job interview or an important social event, can be perceived as threatening. In such instances, the alarm-resistance cycle is more obvious to the individual but not prolonged.

The release of adrenal catecholamines continues to increase blood flow to vital organs. In addition to a heightened sense of awareness and greater energy, the heart rate increases; cardiac output, blood volume and blood pressure increase due to vasoconstriction; gastric secretions increase and peristalsis then decreases; resistance to mental fatigue occurs; bronchial dilation occurs; and the eyes accommodate to see at a distance. The individual experiences a slight increase in heart rate and/or palpitations; a sensation of bladder fullness and an urge to void frequently; diaphoresis; anorexia, nausea and/or abdominal distention; temporary insomnia; slight tachypnea and/or cold hands and feet.

In addition, the individual frequently experiences anxiety, fear, guilt, shame and/or frustration with the self in threatening situations. As a result of these cues individuals are more likely to be aware of stress than in the previous level and they can take deliberate action to deal with the situation. However, many times this mild state of stress can be masked by the individual's use of usual coping mechanisms to mediate the response to the stressor.

Level III

A moderate degree of stress occurs when an individual encounters a persistently stressful event which previous adaptations have not resolved, such as continued stress following continued job interviews or when a new situation, such as surgery, is perceived by the individual as potentially threatening. The individual's perception of danger precipitates emergency behaviors wherein there is a conscious or unconscious redistribution of resources within the human system in an effort to sustain stability.

This is a critical type of experience for the individual as the person balances precariously between successful and unsuccessful resolution of the problem. In Selye's terms, there is a struggle between the resistance and exhaustion stages of the GAS. During this level, the alarm-resistance phenomenon is more obvious, and a variety of changes can be observed and measured over a longer period of time. Epinephrine increases myocardial contractility, and tachycardia is evident. Epinephrine stimulates the conversion of protein, fat and glycogen to glucose, and the blood glucose level rises. Simultaneously the metabolic rate and oxygen consumption rate increases. Norepinephrine continues to stimulate peripheral vasoconstriction, and hypertension, pallor and increased blood coagulation are evident. This process also decreases the blood flow to the kidney, which leads to the secretion of renin; this combines with angiotensinogen to form angiotensin I and II; these two substances plus the vasoconstriction result in water retention.[6]

In addition to stimulating the adrenal medulla, the hypothalamus stimulates the posterior pituitary to release the antidiuretic hormone (ADH), which also results in water retention. Together with the catecholamines and corticoids, ADH release serves to retain sodium, chloride and water and to excrete potassium.[7]

The hypothalamus also stimulates the anterior pituitary, which releases increased amounts of adrenocorticotrophic hormone (ACTH). ACTH stimulates the adrenal cortex to increase the release of glucocorticoids (hydrocortisone, cortisol) and mineralocorticoids (aldosterone).[8] The former serve to alter the immune response and to increase platelet production and fibrinogen levels. The latter serve to increase blood glucose and protein catabolism, which results in the loss of intracellular potassium and negative nitrogen balance; as stated, aldosterone also causes increased sodium reabsorption. The intraorganismic response to a stressor is depicted in its entirety in Figure 2.

This complex of changes results in the following cues to the individual: tachycardia, palpitations, tremors, weakness, cool pale skin, headache, oliguria, vomiting, constipation and increased susceptibility

to thrombus formation and infections. Many people will initially complain of a loss in weight and minor changes in muscular strength.

In moderately stressful situations, individuals frequently express verbally or nonverbally a concern that they lack control in a particular situation and have

In moderately stressful situations, (Level III), individuals frequently will express verbally or nonverbally a concern that they lack control in a particular situation and have difficulty carrying out their own activities.

difficulty carrying out their own activities. They also manifest any one of a variety of behaviors including denial, aggression, swings in behavior between depression and elation, and/or restriction of interaction with others, evidenced by sleep, egocentricity or decreased verbal communication. They may wish to relieve stress by displacing their emotional levels on another person. At other times, individuals try to implement previous styles of adaptation.

Individuals whose systems successfully adapt to moderate stress express improvement in their energy and capabilities as well as in their emotional states: "I feel ready to...," "I feel less afraid," "My spirits are back to normal." These comments often confirm a health professional's estimation of their current health status.[9]

Those individuals who do not success-

64

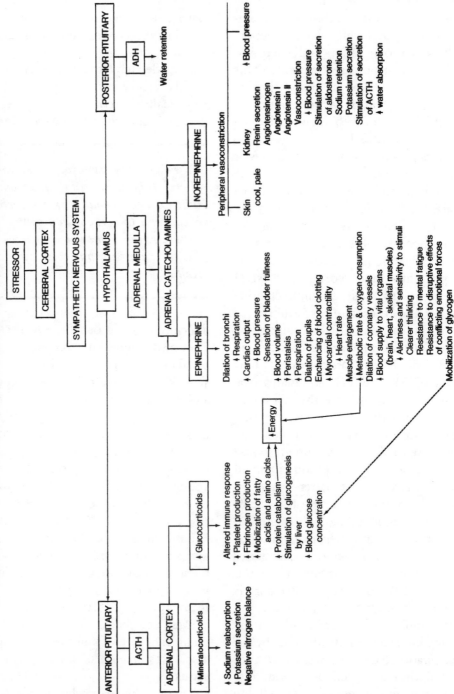

FIGURE 2. THE INTRA-ORGANISMIC RESPONSE TO A STRESSOR

fully adapt to such a stressor frequently progress to the stage of exhaustion.

Level IV

Some individuals are unable to successfully adapt to a stressful situation even with the assistance of another person. As the situation continues, these people experience a severe degree of stress, resulting in the exhaustion stage, during which they perceive events and situations as very dangerous. If individuals have made efforts to stabilize themselves and have not been successful, their reserves usually have been exhausted or the efforts used have been inadequate. "Burnout" is the word commonly used to describe this stage. Burnout may be observed in individuals with extensive, prolonged illness or a combination of severe stressors, such as the loss of a job and the loss of a close family member occurring within a short time span.

In the exhaustion stage, the body continues to receive alarm signals with little or no successful resolution. The major human systems have usually been affected alone or in combination. A person may manifest cardiac irregularities following continued tachycardia and electrolyte imbalance (hypokalemia), which could result in cardiac arrest. In other persons, these stressors will affect the contractility of the myocardium resulting in decreased output; this is observed as a decreasing irregular pulse, hypotension, dependent edema, decreasing kidney function with alteration in urinary output, syncope, mental confusion or forgetfulness, and weakness.

Persons who were anorexic in the earlier levels of stress may continue to react this way to the point of malnutrition or anorexia nervosa with catabolic effects in all physiological areas—muscle depletion, osteoporosis, blood dyscrasia—in combination with psychological problems. Continued stress can also progress to a degeneration and/or erosion of tissue in the gastrointestinal tract (ulcers, colitis). In some individuals the psychosomatic response to continued stress could result in asthma leading to status asthmaticus or pulmonary emphysema.

New stressors may be at work when the adrenocorticosteroid (levels are greatest between 4 AM and 6 AM and least between 4 PM and 6 PM for a usual nocturnal sleep pattern)[10] levels are low when adrenal cortex function is suppressed (during steroid therapy or postadrenalectomy) and when the person is less able to handle another insult such as diabetes, heart disease, an aneurysm, liver disease and/or kidney disease.

It is not unusual to find the person in a severe stress situation experiencing extreme discomfort, displeasure or purposelessness. He may be totally disorganized physically, mentally and emotionally. At this point some individuals may become paranoiac, compulsive or even phobic. They seem at times to withdraw or surrender and may be restless. In some cases these may be the cues that a neurotic or psychotic break is imminent.[11]

In most instances, stress adaptation forces, until now unidentified to the individual, are mobilized at this level. An example of a person adapting under severe stress is the terminally ill person who, although being depleted in one system,

66

In most instances of Level IV stress, stress adaptation forces, until now unidentified to the individual, are mobilized.

may rally other resources, spiritual and psychological, which allow higher levels of functioning during the course of the illness.

TYPES OF ASSISTANCE REQUIRED

Level I

Generally, individuals experiencing the routine stresses of day-to-day living require no assistance from sources outside themselves. They have adapted successfully, being able to anticipate potential crisis situations and use their own strengths to respond effectively.

Level II

Those individuals experiencing the mild degree of stress that accompanies a new event may require some assistance. Recognizing the stress experience is the first healthful step and one which these persons can usually take. In most cases these persons have the resources to deal with the stressful situation effectively but may require assistance in delineating a specific sequence of interventions through which previous stress adaptation has occurred in others. Often it helps to reflect with another person—a family member, a friend, a listener—on the question "What do you do when you get upset?" It is important that the other person—the help-

er—encourage maximum input from the stressed individual while providing support. It is realistic to expect rapid resolution of the situation.[12]

Level III

When individuals experience a moderate degree of stress and potential inability to function, assistance from a professional helper is usually required. Such professionals may be members of the clergy, counselors, nurses, physicians, psychiatrists or social workers, and the helper may require the help of another (a family member, a volunteer, a home health aide). Professionals may also institute minor therapies or treatment modalities, such as medications.

The individual being helped may require assistance for a longer period of time than persons at the previous level, but treatment should not exceed six weeks. Six weeks is identified in crisis literature as the usual time frame for the resolution of normal crises.

The assistance required may take one or several of the following forms:
- helping persons identify the stressors and the strengths they have for dealing with them;
- supporting, guiding, observing and monitoring; and
- teaching;
- doing for;
- providing an environment which facilitates coping, growth and continued develpment.

By using multiple system resources and the support and/or observation of a significant other or a health professional, the individual is able to cope. The cues which indicate adaptation as being initiated have been discussed earlier, and it is these cues which helpers must monitor. The immediate aim is to reduce stress. But the long-term goal is to allow the individuals to regain their self-maintenance capabilities and move toward their highest level of adaptation. Usually individuals learn from stress situations and use this knowledge to cope with similar future situations. Crises not resolved within six weeks are considered dangerous and require extensive professional help.

Level IV

Individuals experiencing the most severe degree of stress require the assistance of competent professionals over a prolonged period of time. This assistance may take any of the forms previously mentioned

---

A human system is a complex interdependent network that benefits most from multidimensional strategies to adapt to stress.

---

and often requires relatively constant intervention, using a broad range of modalities. Professionals in such cases should generate individualized therapeutic alternatives, designed to help the individual function once again. These therapeutic alternatives must not be separated into unidimensional categories such as biological, social or spiritual. A human system is a complex

interdependent network that benefits most from multidimensional strategies.

UNPREDICTABILITY OF STRESS RESPONSES

Stress occurs in each of our lives, and the degrees to which it affects us vary. Stressors can arise from the developmental-maturational evolution as well as from conflicting value orientations, lack of basic economic resources, psychic or physical traumas, environmental changes and extremes in rest-activity, nutritional and solitude-social interaction patterns.

What is mildly stressful for one individual may not affect another person at all and may appear to be an insurmountable obstacle to still another. In no way can one predict the reactions of individuals to a specific stress situation. The complexity of people, the diversity of experiences they encounter, and the personal, professional, financial, spiritual and interpersonal resources they do or do not have contribute to this difference in perspective.

The levels of stress discussed here are not necessarily discrete. A person can be in more than one level at a time. Indeed, people may adapt quite successfully at work, at home and in physical health, but may find a social situation extremely stressful.

UNDERSTANDING STRESS

Finally, an understanding of stress and the changes which accompany it on a cellular level and a total organism level enable individuals to understand the vari-

68 ety of interventions available to deal with it. There are three major approaches to stress:

- learning to listen to oneself and to know how one perceives stress-producing events;
- learning to alter one's response to stress; and

- learning to alter the environment if possible to reduce stress.

These interventions are available to each of us. It is the job of the professional to alert clients to these possibilities and help them choose and use the interventions when needed.

REFERENCES

1. Jones, P. "An Adaptation Model for Nursing Practice." *American Journal of Nursing* 78:11 (November 1978) p. 1900.
2. Selye, H. *The Physiology and Pathology of Exposure to Stress* (Montreal, Canada: ACTA, Inc. 1950) p. 55.
3. Ibid.
4. Ibid.
5. Guyton, A. C. *Textbook of Medical Physiology* 4th ed. illus. (Philadelphia: W.B. Saunders & Co. 1971) p. 692–700.
6. Ibid. p. 300–307, 699–700.
7. Ibid. p. 422, 421, 882.
8. Ibid. p. 886–895.
9. Naughton, R. A. and Kolditz, D. "Patients' Definitions of Recovery from Acute Illness" in Nelson, J.,

ed. *Clinical Perspectives in Nursing Research: Relevance, Suffering, Recovery* (New York: Teachers College Press 1978).
10. Zschoche, D. A., ed. *Mosby's Comprehensive Review of Critical Care* (St. Louis, Mo.: The C.V. Mosby Co. 1976) p. 287.
11. Personal communication with Sharon Scully, Ed.M. (Psychological Counseling), Counselor to the Catholic Campus Ministry at Columbia University, New York, November 15, 1978.
12. Rapoport, L. "The State of Crisis: Some Theoretical Considerations" in Parad, H., ed. *Crisis Intervention: Selected Readings* (New York: Family Service Association of America 1965) p. 25.

Stress and Holistic Medicine

Hans Selye, M.D.
President
International Institute of Stress
Montreal, Canada

IN MY WORK on stress it became particularly evident that psychological factors can often be the decisive influence both in the causation of disease and in the course taken by an established disorder. This fact is of special importance for health care providers who are in very direct control of such variables. Yet it would be an error to think that a clear distinction can always be made between physical and mental causes of stress. For example, anticipation of physical trauma can be a psychic stressor, as anyone who has ever required surgery will understand. What is really needed are principles for the management of *stress as such,* which would ensure our homeostasis on all levels.

Today's medical science, at least as we know it in the West, has only just started to explore the close interrelation of body and mind. Yet the goal of medicine should be to understand the patients as persons to establish the circumstances that precipitated their illnesses—the un-

70 derlying conflicts, hostilities, griefs—in short, the bruised nature of their emotional state. The modern physician should know as much about emotions and thoughts as about disease symptoms and drugs. This approach would appear to hold more promise of cure than anything that medicine has given us to date.

Clearly the field of stress has much to offer in this regard. The degree to which homeostasis, the basic determinant of health, is an issue of the total organism—of consciousness as well as physical existence—becomes quite apparent when one considers the following facts that emerge from stress theory:

1. That the aspects of life requiring adaptation, that is, calling forth the organic reaction and initiating the GAS (general adaptation syndrome), are not merely composed of matter, but often can be grasped only in terms of concepts or, if you will, mental states (e.g., one's "life situation"); and

2. That these nonmaterial demands can disrupt homeostasis in two ways, either by being simply beyond our power of adaptability or by causing diseases of adaptation because there is a particularly "weak link" in the structure of our organism.

This view of health and disease, then, is that they are not merely individual interactions between pathogens and human beings, and that they involve, rather, the entire spectrum of other relationships—including those with one's spouse, employer, children, neighbors, and spiritual or medical advisers. Too much considera-

Only when we shift our focus from diseased parts to the whole being can we ... understand why stress affects different people in different ways.

tion has been directed toward specific pathogens and specific disease models, and not enough toward the patient and how he or she developed the particular disease. Only when we shift our focus from diseased parts to the whole being can we learn more about what activates the adaptation syndrome at all levels within the organism and understand why stress affects different people in different ways.

The integrating concept of health as a question of body, mind, and spirit is assuming phenomenal popularity and importance even among the lay public. This holistic approach aims at enhancing our total well-being, in part through self-awareness. By learning to gauge our own innate energy, potential weaknesses and strengths, we can all benefit from this approach. True, it requires a great deal of self-discipline and willpower, but we must not lose sight of the vital awareness that in the final analysis each of us is responsible for his or her own health and well-being. Otherwise, no matter what new treatments are developed, we will continue to be plagued by stress-induced diseases.

We have always been concerned about health and have wanted to improve it as regards both the mind and the body; throughout history innumerable great thinkers have approached the problem from the points of view of theology, psychology, sociology, and, of course, particularly medicine. But whatever the approach or technique they favored, the focus has always been specialized. Only now are we really beginning to look upon health as a holistic problem. After all, we are thinking of the health of human beings as such, and we will never arrive at a satisfactory solution if all of us take different and reductionist points of view. Individually we have been successful in improving health by research limited to molecular biology, electron microscopy, pharmacology, behavioral philosophy (including religious codes), sociology, politics, economics, or any of the other specialized disciplines. But we must not look upon our particular field of expertise as the only, all-encompassing solution to our troubles and the only road to happiness. There is no point in elucidating or improving one part of the human machine if another vital part is meanwhile deteriorating and destroying the whole.

Just as wars will not be avoided by more sophisticated weaponry, so disease can never be completely eradicated merely by improvements in pharmacology, immunotherapy, or any other purely medical means.

To health care providers, the influence of occupational stress, both upon themselves and upon their patients, is of utmost concern. Yet I believe we can adjust our personal reactions to enjoy fully the eustress of success and accomplishment without suffering the distress commonly generated by frustrating friction and purposeless, aggressive behavior

against our surroundings. In order to arrive at this stage we must strive to practice a code of ethics based not on blind superstition, inspiration, or societal traditions, but on scientifically verifiable laws that govern the body's maintenance of homeostasis.

From what the laboratory and the clinical study of somatic diseases has taught me concerning stress, I have developed three general principles readily applicable to everyday living. I have summarized these precepts as follows:

1. *Find your own natural predilections and stress level.* People differ with regard to the amount and kind of work they consider worth doing to meet the exigencies of daily life and to assure their future security and happiness. In this respect, all of us are influenced by hereditary predispositions and the expectations of our society. Only through planned self-analysis can we establish what we really want; many people suffer all their lives because they are too conservative to risk a radical change and break with traditions.

2. *Altruistic egoism.* The selfish hoarding of the good will, respect, esteem, support, and love of our neighbor is the most efficient way to give vent to our pent-up energy and create enjoyable, beautiful, or useful things.

3. *"EARN thy neighbor's love."* This motto, unlike "Love thy neighbor as thyself," is compatible with our biological structure; and although it is based on altruistic egoism, it

72 could hardly be attacked as unethical. Who could blame a person who wants to assure homeostasis and happiness by accumulating the treasure of other people's benevolence? Yet this makes one virtually unassailable, for people would not attack and destroy those upon whom they depend.

What it comes down to is:
Fight for your highest attainable aim
But do not put up resistance in vain.

SUGGESTED READINGS

Coldway, E., ed. *Inner Balance: The Power of Holistic Healing* (Englewood Cliffs, N.J.: Prentice-Hall 1979).

Knowles, J. H., ed. *Doing Better and Feeling Worse: Health in the United States* (New York: W.W. Norton & Co., Inc. 1977).

Ng, L. and Davis, D. L., eds. *Strategies for Public Health* (New York: Van Nostrand Reinhold) In Press.

Selye, H. "Coping with Stress in 1979" in Dolmatch, T. B., ed. *1979 Information Please Almanac* (New York: Information Please Publishing 1979).

Selye, H. *Stress without Distress* (New York: J. B. Lippincott 1974).

Selye, H. *The Stress of Life* (New York: McGraw-Hill Book Co. 1976).

Selye, H. *Stress in Health and Disease* (Reading, Mass.: Butterworth 1976).

Selye, H. *The Stress of MY Life,* 2nd ed. (New York: Van Nostrand Reinhold 1979).

Wolf, S. and Goodell, H. *Behavioral Science in Clinical Medicine* (Springfield, Ill.: Charles C Thomas, Publisher 1976).

Part II
Stress and Life Events

Life-Cycle Stressors:
An Overview of Research

Elizabeth A. Hefferin, Dr.P.H.,
F.A.A.N.
Associate Chief
Nursing Service for Research
Veterans Administration Wadsworth
  Medical Center
Los Angeles, California

ALTHOUGH the word *stress* is commonly used in our everyday vocabulary, it is frequently used with different meanings. Conversationally, stress is used to indicate both the external causes of our bodily reaction and the reaction itself. The definitions and subject matter of stress discussed in the voluminous theoretical and research literature also tend to be somewhat inconsistent. Early treatments of the concept of stress and its related mechanisms dealt primarily with adults and their reactions to singular noxious or stressor conditions such as the threat of surgery,[1] participation in aerial combat[2] and imprisonment in a concentration camp.[3]

The medical or clinical usage of "stress" was coined by Hans Selye in the 1940s. His interest in the physiology and pathology of exposure to stress led him to review literally thousands of reports of medical research on the subject.[4] Noting that certain reaction features appeared

76 common among bodily responses to all types of stressful circumstances, he named these nonspecific reactions "stress" or the bodily "stress response," and described the mechanism of the stereotyped reaction to stress in general as the "General Adaptation Syndrome." Selye's own early experimental work focused largely on the various aspects of physiological stress,[5] and his findings concerning the activity of the adrenal glands have been critical to a large amount of later research in the area.

An overview of the research literature relating to life-cycle stressors and coping requires a brief restatement of some definitions of the more pertinent concepts. *Life cycle* refers to the various phases of human life from the perinatal period through approaching death. *Stress stimuli (stressors)* are threat or loss conditions—circumstances or situations that produce various degrees of bodily reactions which indicate that an individual is experiencing *stress* or a *state of stress*. *Stress,* then, is the set of nonspecific physiological and psychological responses of the body to any demands made on it, whether these responses are associated with pleasant or unpleasant experiences. As people proceed through Selye's General Adaptation Syndrome, they experience (1) an alarm reaction which involves marshalling the body resources, (2) a stage of resistance during which the bodily resistance to the stress response rises above normal and (3) a stage of exhaustion during which the adaptation response energy is used up or dissipated.[6] Persons have *adapted* positively to the stressor situation when their bodily alterations have ensured their safety or survival and have increased their functioning and enjoyment within their environment. They have *maladapted* when the bodily responses or alterations have resulted in internal disharmony (illness) or disharmony between them and their environment.

As has been indicated quite clearly in the preceding articles in this issue, all individuals are exposed to a variety of stressors virtually all the time throughout the course of their life spans. The authors note also that both pleasant and unpleasant stimuli may produce stress responses and that our individual perceptions of and psychophysiological reactions to these stimuli may vary quite widely. The problem seems to lie not so much in the fact that we are exposed continually to life stressors; more accurately, the problem is in the degree and duration of these stressor situations and in our variable range of personal responses and capacities to withstand and cope with such stimuli. Although most individuals have the capacity to sustain relatively high degrees of stress for short periods of time, a prolonged stress response or an overly strong stimulus can be maladaptive or destructive. The research cited in the following sections focuses on the adaptive capacities of individuals in the several phases of the life cycle.

BIRTH AND EARLY LIFE

Although a considerable amount of research has been reported on the patterns of psychophysiological growth from birth through the stages of childhood, much of what we know about the stress response patterns in infants and

At about seven months, infants display evidence of attachment behavior—crying when their mothers leave them and smiling and clinging when reunited after brief separations.

young children stems from the early work of Piaget.[7-9] Piaget's systematic studies reported that, psychologically, infants remain "adualistic" until they are between three and six months of age, i.e., that they neither distinguish between themselves and their outer world nor recognize the entry or disappearance of particular caretaking persons. Between three and six months, the biological "smiling response" becomes selective and social—a recognition of familiar people in the environment.[10] At about seven months, infants display evidence of attachment behavior—crying when their mothers leave them and smiling and clinging when reunited after brief separations. Fear of strangers and overdependence on the mother figure also occur during this period.[11,12] Piaget believes that the main intellectual progress in the first two years of life is the move from adualism to dualism through the building up of mental images of the outer world of things and people.

Numerous studies have shown that biophysiological development in infants also reflects response to stressors. In their study of diurnal sleep–waking patterns in infants observed in laboratory settings, Sostek et al. found that the constant lighting and testings resulted in the infants developing fussy crying patterns and decreased alertness.[13] When placed in the nursery setting under more normal day–night lighting controls, the infants developed sharper sleep–wake patterns and demonstrated more day and time alertness and decreased fussiness. Prematurity as a psychophysiological stressor also has been studied. Goldberg[14] cites six studies comparing preterm and full-term infant–parent pairs, each study reporting consistently different behavioral patterns between the groups. Because of the delayed physiological development and the hospital-controlled protective environment needed by the preterm infants, parents were less actively involved in their early care. Subsequent to the initiation of the usual parent–child interaction patterns (talking, touching, face-to-face cuddling, etc.), it was noted that the majority of the preterm pairs made relatively successful adaptations. This suggests that the capacity to compensate for the delay of early interactive attention is one of the features of the "parent interaction system." Goldberg concludes that the behaviors of normal infants and their parents seem to be "mutually complimentary in a way that leads to repeated social interactions enjoyed by both infants and adults," and that when the physical status of preterm infants permits the initiation of this interaction process preterm infant–parent pairs can achieve the same or similar relationships.

The effects of maternal deprivation in early life have been studied by a number of investigators. Spitz[15] and Schaffer and Callender[16] noted (1) that when hospitalized children received little mothering or other staff attentions they tended toward poor physical growth and development,

78 whereas (2) when staff were assigned to pick up the infants and provide tactile, visual and auditory attentions, rapid gains were noted both in weight and in social–emotional development. Rheingold[17] and Glasser[18] also reported a strong relationship between social stimulation and social responsiveness in studies of hospitalized infants during their sixth to eighth month of development. Robertson[19] and Bowlby,[20,21] however, point out that even short periods of maternal deprivation may have long-lasting effects. The child's prolonged crying and unsuccessful attempt to draw the mother back may lead to an active rejection of all adults, and then to apathy and possible withdrawal into a decreased state of activity. This "mourning" phase may lead to a nonrecognition or denial of the mother figure and the transfer of attachment to a substitute mother. The nature of this bonding/attachment process and the problems associated with the development of parent–child relationships have been discussed at length in Wu's article in this issue of *Family & Community Health*.

A number of other early life stressors greatly influence the later social and physical progress of the child. For example, Stein and Susser report that the achievement of sphincter control can be delayed significantly among children whose mothers work at night during the second six months of the children's lives.[22] This suggests that the mother's (or father's) social support during toilet training is essential to the early acquisition of sphincter control. Parental social support is essential also in bolstering the toddler's trust and subsequent attempts to achieve self-control and environmental mastery (autonomy). Piaget notes that children under the age of seven live in an egotistic world, perceive things in an animistic fashion, and are accepting of all explanations and rules for living and behaving. Falls, bruises and other discouragements are seen as related to rule breaking, and misinterpretations of the environment occur frequently.[23]

When hospitalization is required during this early childhood period, the child's autonomy is undermined both through the loss of parental companionship and through fears introduced by the hospital procedures.[24] The child may become regressed, watching continually for the absent mother figure—sometimes to the point of losing libidinal as well as physical self-control.[25,26] Similar findings were reported by Miller in a review of studies concerned with the fear responses among hospitalized children throughout the infancy–to–seven-year-old group.[27] Korsch points out that allowing the parent to be present is more effective in preventing the child's adverse reactions to the hospitalization experience than any other change in the hospital procedures.[28]

Through the age of seven, children continue to be critically dependent on adults, particularly those adults serving in the parental role. Forssman and Thuwe, for example, have reported that wanted children tend to adapt or cope better with the stressors of growing up than do those children whose existence depended on a denied parental request for abortion.[29] The latter children fared worse with respect to the incidence of juvenile delinquency, need for psychiatric treatment and lowered educational achievement. Studies of the parental abuse or neglect of especially debilitated children (e.g., the mentally retarded, children with cystic fibrosis, etc.) have suggested that the extra care needed by these children may stimulate feelings of parental resentment or guilt that they cannot always provide such care.[30] As Wu's paper suggests, some theorists have linked child neglect and abuse to an incompleteness or failure of the bonding process. In their review of the child abuse literature, however, Corey et al. found little consistency across the studies in identifying specific factors relating to abuse behavior.[31] They suggest that the causal factors of child neglect or abuse may more likely be found through research into the psychological motivators of the behavior.

EARLY AND LATER CHILDHOOD

Developmental psychologists agree that children mature through a succession of developmental stages, with each stage "conferring additional or transformed competencies, cognitive abilities, and moral capacities."[32] During the early childhood stages, parents impose certain behavioral rules and regulations both to protect the child's health and safety (physical survival) and to assure the child's feelings of having a rightful role in the family constellation. As children mature into school age, they experience a broadening of their social and psychological life pattern to include the development of peer relationships and the establishment of school-oriented learning patterns.

Pratt has observed that the use of the developmental style of childrearing (reasons, information, rewards, autonomy) tends to be more effective than disciplinary methods in assisting children to develop resources and capacities for coping, learning and taking care of themselves.[33] Maladaptive behaviors associated with the strongly disciplinary style of childrearing have been identified as social aggressiveness, hostility and dependency (in boys) and regressiveness, fearfulness and social withdrawal (in girls). Studies have shown that, where parents have tended to be lax or inconsistent in the use of appropriate rules or controls, their children's failure to develop adequate coping mechanisms in early life can cause subsequent maladjustment in their neurophysical development and lead to lifelong patterns of psychosomatic as well as social complications.[34] By way of example, even the lack of parental attention to their children's protein and energy nutritional needs during the first years of life can produce serious consequences in both physical growth and brain function.[35,36] The Richardson et al. study of the later school-age behaviors of severely malnourished infants found that these children were less able to pay attention in school, had poorer memories, were more easily distracted and were less outgoing and cooperative. They also tended to be more isolated and withdrawn, were less able to develop peer relationships and frequently exhibited socially unacceptable behaviors.[37]

In the healthy child through age ten, the body tends to be taken for granted.[38] Natapoff noted a strong developmental trend in children's views of health, with

80 the comments becoming more complex and thoughtful with increasing age.[39] Among first graders, the state of healthiness in self and in others tended to be based primarily on perceptual inputs related to being able to do things, eat regular food, have pink cheeks, etc. Health in this age group generally was also perceived as an all-or-nothing condition (a person could not be part healthy and part nonhealthy), as compared with an acceptance of this possibility by 74 percent of the nine year olds (fourth graders) and 84 percent of the twelve year olds (seventh graders). The oldest group tended to view health more abstractly, requiring cues for judging both physical and mental health status.

Studies show that the ways children behave when they are ill are significantly associated both with age and with their perceived sex roles. Their degrees of emotionality and rejection or acceptance of the sick role also reflect parental ideas of acceptable illness behaviors.[40,41] As Valenti's paper in this issue of FCH points out, children continually need the reassurance of reasonable limits and discipline, even during periods of illness.

In general, children are better able to cope with crisis situations when normal social support is provided.[42] When separation from their families is involved, their emotional vulnerability may increase to the point of being unable to adapt to new social or physical environments.[43] This is especially true when children must face the possibility of parental death or recurring partial loss through repeated parental hospitalizations. Cain and Staver suggest that adaptation to this possibility can be aided through the parents' main-

taining an awareness of the children's needs for sufficient information and the encouragement of outside relationships to protect against feelings of total abandonment.[44] Actively participating in the care of the sick parent also permits some mastery over this type of threatening situation. Children who themselves face possible death, as in the case of leukemia and other malignancies, also depend greatly upon the family support structure. In a study of 18 children (ages 5 to 15 years), Goggin et al. found that the older boys were more realistic than the girls about their potential limitations. The younger boys were more at risk psychologically than the younger girls, possibly because of inadequately developed ego strength and fantasy defense mechanisms.[45]

ADOLESCENCE

The individual is probably more aware of change during adolescence than during any other period in life. Adolescence is a period that confronts both the individual and the family with numerous problems and challenges. Erikson[46,47] describes the main task of adolescence as that of identity formation and identifies four primary components: (1) the physical and emotional separation from parents, (2) the acquisition of socially oriented attitudes and opinions, (3) the preparation for a working role and (4) the definition of the sexual role. Unfortunately, these major psychological adjustments are expected to take place during a time when everything else is changing—when the individual is no longer a child but not yet an adult. Adolescents are confronted almost simultaneously with rapid physiological changes, increased cognitive development, increased peer group pressures and activities, changes in family and societal attitudes and expectations—all of which serve as stressors during this phase of their development and may interfere severely with the task of identity formation.

As Reres's paper points out, emancipation from the family tends to be desired and feared by both the adolescents and their parents. Adolescents frequently find themselves expected to continue in the child role or to assume both the adult and child roles simultaneously. This mixed role expectation often leads to aggressive behaviors and to conflicts within the family structure because the adolescent is constantly pulled between the need for adult support and the desire for independence.[48] In his study of the impact of adolescent illness on parental relationships, Peterson found that adolescents noted increased concern and social interaction when they (especially females) became overtly ill.[49] Actual as well as feigned illness tended to increase parental controls and promoted more positive relationships with siblings, even though the adolescents themselves continued to be socially active.

In the search for identity, adolescents frequently attempt to submerge themselves in a peer group identity, which provides a temporary feeling of importance and belonging. The peer group serves a dual purpose—both insulating the adolescent from the adult world and building its own norms for its members. Although the group standards, values and opinions can provide a positive back-

In the search for identity, adolescents frequently attempt to submerge themselves in a peer group identity, which provides a temporary feeling of importance and belonging.

ground for testing out adolescent roles and styles for future adult life, the group pressures for untoward experiences (e.g., use of drugs, sex, etc.) may also have the negative effect of promoting a sense of alienation from the rest of society.[50,51]

Tests of mental ability show that adolescence is also the period of greatest ability to acquire and make use of knowledge. The adolescent is capable of a high degree of imaginative thinking which, although somewhat oversimplified and unoriginal, sets up the structure for adult thinking patterns and the work role.[52] Differences in cognitive skills development among male and female adolescents (e.g., verbal skills among females, quantitative and spatial skills in males) are seen as the result of interest, social expectations and earlier training, rather than as variations in the innate mental abilities.[53]

In his study of the sexual behaviors and attitudes of American adolescents, Sorenson noted that sexual relationships begin to occur in middle adolescence, and that boys have more frequent heterosexual activities than girls. Girls more often seem to hold to a single sexual relationship (serial monogamy), while boys move on to many different relationships (serial adventure).[54] Concerns about sex-typing and homosexuality also develop at this time, as do questions of contraception,

82 pregnancy, abortion and venereal disease.

Starr and Goldstein[55] reported on a 1973 study group headed by James Coleman which examined the problems of adolescence. The group recommended the school as the most appropriate institution for helping adolescents and suggested reducing the size of high schools to enable closer student–teacher relationships. Other suggestions offered by the study group included work-study programs, opportunities to assume teaching roles with younger students, and part-time placements in other nonschool settings. Hauser and Shapiro examined the experience of adolescents with school authorities in an experiment which used participant observation in small groups. Thirty adolescent students, three principals and three teachers were organized into three equal groups. Findings showed that, over a one and one-half–year period, faculty members tended to abandon or blur their usually authoritative role behaviors as a means of coping with the stressfulness of the group situations.[56]

ADULTHOOD IN THE GENERAL CONTEXT

Because adulthood begins in the late teens and continues to the end of the life cycle, it might be considered more practical to talk about stressors in relation to its usual age-group phases: early, middle and late adulthood. What cannot be denied, however, is that major changes or shifts in life circumstances very often occur at different periods for different individuals. Moreover, a particular experience which is highly threatening for one person may just as often be relatively innocuous for another—depending on how each perceives and appraises the personal effect of the experience.[57] A life change need not be particularly undesirable to induce stress.[58] In addition, certain types of stressors or life strains can occur repeatedly throughout an individual's total life period.

A number of investigators have focused on identifying which types of life situations seem to present the greatest threats to human psychophysiological stability and have developed lists of life events weighted according to the degree of experienced stress among their study populations. Perhaps the most widely known of these lists is the 43-item Social Readjustment Rating Scale (SRRS) developed by Holmes and Rahe.[59] The scale consists of a mix of pleasurable and undesirable life events identified by people as productive of bodily stress responses (e.g., marriage, new job, job loss, death of a loved one, etc.). Since its publication in 1967 the SRRS has generated considerable public and professional interest and criticism as well as an extensive body of research. For example, Rosenburg and Dohrenwend found that both ethnicity and the degree of life experience affected the rating of life events as stressors.[60] In analyzing a number of studies focusing on social class and ethnic group membership and their judgments of the magnitude of stressful life events, Askenasy et al. found that cultural judgments about this magnitude are even greater than the various reports have suggested.[61] In pretests of a more extensive list of 102 life events actually experienced in a number of populations (the PERI Life Events Scale), Dohrenwend et al. found that group differences varied more by ethnicity than by sex or social class.[62]

In order to explore what people considered potential life strains (conflicts, frustrations and threats), Pearlin and Schooler conducted extensive interviews with a sample of 2,300 persons representative of an urban population aged 18 through 65 years. Four role areas were delineated: (1) marital strains, (2) parental strains associated with teenage and young adult children, (3) strains associated with household economics and (4) overloads and dissatisfactions associated with the work role.[63] When these persons were asked how they coped with the strains experienced in these roles, three major coping styles were identified: (1) deliberate modification of the situation to eliminate the strain, (2) cognitive control or reinterpretation of the strainful experience to ward off, diminish or neutralize the stress response before it could affect the bodily systems and (3) responses to control the stress that resulted from the strainful experience. The investigators also found that persons who appeared best able to cope with the identified stressor situations were those who used a variety of responses and resources in dealing with the associated problems.

Janis and Mann report on a number of studies dealing with the stress responses of people who tend to think carefully about possible perils or emergencies before such events happen. These persons actively seek information about the potential risks of making and implementing decisions and therefore develop preliminary plans to handle the stress in case the potential crises actually occur. According to the researchers, these persons are better able to display positive adaptive or coping behaviors when making difficult decisions if their "dominant coping pattern is vigilance rather than defensive avoidance or hypervigilance."[64]

An important resource for preventing or moderating stress responses to strainful life events is that of social support. Cobb defines social support as "information leading the subject to believe that he is cared for and loved, esteemed, and a member of a network of mutual obligations."[65] In his review of over 50 studies, Cobb cites findings identifying the mechanism of social support as a moderator of acute stress situations throughout the life cycle:

1. pregnancy, birth and early life;
2. hospitalization;
3. recovery from illness;
4. depression in the face of extensive life changes;
5. employment termination;
6. bereavement;
7. aging and retirement; and
8. threat of death.

Dean and Lin point out that the variable of social support too often has been neglected as a mitigating or even preventive factor in the relationships between stressful life events and illness, and suggest that considerable empirical research needs to be done in this area.[66] In this context, Langlie suggests two of the many possible hypotheses that could be tested concerning the reasons that social support may play a positive role in the prevention of illness: (1) social norms may affect group member health behav-

84 iors and (2) social interaction may provide preventive health care information.[67]

In their original development and testing of the SRRS instrument, Holmes and Rahe reported finding positive correlations between 43 life events and the onset of illness in large samples of American medical patients.[68] A later study suggested that this cluster of events (all of which require changes in life style) was a necessary although not sufficient cause of illness, but did account in part for the time of an illness onset.[69] Other variables to be considered include a range of etiological and environmental factors, health status and behavioral patterns, age, attitudes and the life-style patterns themselves. As Rabkin and Struening point out, the relationship between life events and stress and illness is highly complex and involves a multitude of interacting phenomena.[70] While this complexity does not deny the probability that the magnitude of the life change increases the risk of becoming ill,[71] more recent studies suggest that the quantity (degree) of change appears more primary than the quality (desirability and area) of the life change.[72] The degree of stress is not without limit, however. Hough et al. have observed that after an individual has reached a peak of 700 scale units on the SRRS, further increments of life change no longer produce the same degree or increment increase in the probability of illness occurrence. This may be related to cultural variations in the way certain stressors are evaluated.[73]

The literature points out that illness, hospitalization and surgery are potent stressor experiences which present multiple threats to many people.[74,75] Not only may the individual's level of stress fluctuate widely during the course of illness and hospitalization; these experiences also may be repeated at any time during the life cycle. In exploring the preexisting correlates of hospital-related stress, Volicer and Burns noted a positive correlation between increased SRRS scores and the degree of hospital stress.[76] Recency of a previous hospitalization prior to the present admission also correlated positively with increased stress. Preoperative fear has been associated with slower recovery rates, a stress which can be

Preoperative fear has been associated with slower recovery rates, a stress which can be reduced to some degree with appropriate preoperative information.

reduced to some degree with appropriate preoperative information.[77] Because the inability to function normally is partially legitimized,[78] fluctuations in response to additional stressors during illness and hospitalization may be masked in part by the acceptance of the "patient role." Only a relatively few studies which deal with fluctuations in dependence and independence along the illness and hospitalization experience continuum have been found.[79,80]

Despite the fact that stressful life events which bring major and prolonged change into the lives of individuals have been associated with such physiological problems as gastric distress, athletic injuries[81] and coronary heart disease,[82] studies also show correlations with adverse effects on mental health after a certain amount of change has occurred. Wildman and Johnson believe that this adverse outcome depends on the nature of the change (e.g., a continuing or major physical illness or disability).[83]

Although the findings of some early investigations have raised doubts whether the relationship between stressful events and the onset of psychiatric disorders might have been a chance occurrence,[84] research in recent years has documented that these positive associations do exist for conditions ranging from psychological distress[85] to various types of psychiatric disorders.[86,87] Mueller et al. found that psychological impairment or distress was directly associated with undesirable life events, whereas neither the strength nor the degree of change associated with desirable events produced any marked distress other than increased anxiety.[88] As a result of their work with psychiatric patients, Bloch and Bloch described a clinical project focusing on the diagnostic evaluation and treatment of patients who demonstrated psychopathology following reportedly traumatic industrial injuries and their accompanying prolonged stressful life situations.[89] These investigators found that all subjects had in fact actually experienced the identified traumatic events and had been unable to cope with the resulting physical conditions.

In comparing SRRS scores for groups of nonmentally ill persons and psychiatric inpatients, Bell found that persons in the mentally ill group had experienced more stressful life events in the six months prior to hospitalization than had persons displaying wellness behaviors.[90] The study findings also showed that persons in the mentally ill group tended to use more short-term coping methods than did the nonmentally ill persons. Obtaining similar findings, Myers et al. concluded that persons who are most able to cope with the impact of life events are those "who have ready and meaningful access to others, who feel integrated into the system, and who are satisfied with their roles."[91]

This nice delineation between persons who can successfully cope with life stressors and those who cannot (thereby requiring hospitalization and formal therapy) leaves us with the question of what happens to those individuals who are treated and then released back into the community or those who can cope only partially but are not hospitalized. In a study of the posthospitalization socialization of state hospital patients, White et al. observed a distinct shift from the initial posthospital behavior of being "somewhat physically active, outwardly oriented" to that of passivity with an inward orientation. This was especially true among the male patients.[92] No immediate answer was available (1) whether this was the result of having left the therapeutic hospital environment behind or (2) whether the behavior change was an effect of the social stigma often applied to persons who have in their backgrounds an overt history of mental hospitalization. To assist persons who can cope only partially, there has been a dramatic growth in the number and types of walk-in emergency

86 psychiatric services, alcohol and drug programs, suicide prevention centers, all types of "hot lines," etc. These services are designed to deal with the range of crises associated with life stresses. Unfortunately, as Maris and Connor point out, because relatively few of these services or programs have built-in evaluation methods or measures, the degree of their relative effectiveness remains in doubt.[93] Do persons seeking crisis assistance or guidance actually develop practical coping mechanisms, are they only temporarily helped, or are they exchanging old problems for new ones which are more socially acceptable? These questions also remain unanswered and, because they apply universally to all persons throughout the life cycle, are in need of systematic study.

ADULTHOOD: EARLY PHASE

Although the stressors described in the section above can occur at any time during the life span (particularly during adulthood), some stressors have been identified as occurring more frequently during a certain period or phase of the life cycle. Between the years 18 to 30—generally called "early adulthood"—the individual begins by being young both in years and experience and gradually develops the characteristics necessary for effective functioning in the later, more mature, years of adulthood. According to Starr and Goldstein, these characteristics include (1) a sense of responsibility, (2) the control of impulses, (3) a tolerance for frustration, (4) the ability to formulate plans and implement them, (5) an

acceptance of differences in others, (6) the capacity for intimacy and (7) the ability to strive for personal growth or self-actualization.[94]

As they enter this phase of adulthood, many young persons move away from home and are involved in advanced schooling or working in new jobs. Because of the problems and insecurities associated with such life changes, a frequent coping pattern is the seeking of moral support from peers and others (including older adults). Students in graduate school, for example, experience anxieties associated with the pressures of classwork and faculty expectations, interpersonal relationships, concerns about current and future competence and control, etc. In a study focusing on student concerns about academic progress, Kjerulff and Wiggins observed that the more competent students responded to all situations with anxiety, which apparently stimulated and gave strength to their striving for mastery. The less competent students tended to blame themselves for classwork failure while blaming others for interpersonal failure.[95] Studies exploring recent life changes among college students show that higher scores were associated with symptoms of maladjustment and feelings of being under the control of others, rather than of being under self-control.[96,97] However, a study by Gersten et al. suggested that such single or multiple events, once mitigated or controlled, caused no direct problems of disturbed behavior or maladjustment.[98] Nevertheless, Mettlin and Woelfel noted that higher levels of stress can and do occur under certain circumstances (and regardless of the apparent weight or strength of the stressful event) (1) when there is discrepancy or inconsistency in the interpersonal influences, (2) when the demands or expectations of the interpersonal influences are too strong or (3) when there are too many influences to which the individual must respond at any one time.[99]

In a review of studies of stressful situations encountered by students in nursing education programs, McKay reported that most students expressed feelings of constant strain and fatigue, inequality and lack of support between faculty and students, penalties received for weakness in judgments and general feelings of social inadequacy.[100] The coping method used by most students in these studies was also that of seeking peer support. Going beyond the mere reporting of the students' feelings and behaviors, investigators in these nursing studies also reported ways in which the nursing faculty attempted to help their students. Approaches used included adjusting programs to student needs, making changes in rules and policies, providing access to group counseling and creating opportunities for student participation in program administration. These promotive faculty interventions reflect the philosophy expressed by Washburn that only those educational programs which provide opportunities for personal growth and some mastery of life experiences can produce individuals who can adapt to the problems of life.[101]

Although many young adults remain at home with parents or other relatives while exploring initial work roles or continuing their academic endeavors, many others prefer to move away from the family environment. In either case, there may be strong feelings of ambivalence between the need for continuing parental/familial support and the drive for emancipation and independence. Despite the fact that this context of ambivalence has been discussed at length in the literature, no studies were found which explored the degree or extent of the phenomenon.

In terms of initial and later vocational choices, however, a considerable amount of empirical work has been reported. Much of the early work in this area tended to focus on vocational interests or preferences as if they were independent of the individual's total personality.[102,103] Later empirical work focused on the personal and social–environmental factors associated with vocational choice, vocational achievement and job changes. Vocational preferences, for example, have been correlated with a large number of objective perceptual tests, with parental attitudes and occupations,[104,105] and personality traits.[106,107] Studies have also shown that vocational interest scales are positively related to an individual's self-ratings of ability, values, life goals, academic achievement, adventurousness, liberalism and other personal characteristics.[108–110] Interestingly, occupations and their associated activities tend to be perceived in much the same way, and with a relatively high degree of accuracy, by people of all ages: high school students, college students, college faculty, and men and women who are in the occupations.[111] Studies also support the notion that people with similar personali-

88 ties and histories tend to enter and remain in given vocations.[112,113]

In a study concerning why people change jobs, Holland and Nichols reported that people "leave fields for which they lack interest and aptitude and seek fields for which they possess interest and aptitude."[114] While this statement of findings sounds rather like an old cliché, the study tested—both objectively and subjectively—the theory that specific types of people actually search for, and then tend to remain in, those types of work environments they find particularly

---

Young adults who are more mature in personality and more definite about their vocational interests and preferences will be more likely to adjust to adult-role responsibilities than will those who are still groping for a work-interest direction.

---

congenial to their interests and talents. This suggests that those young adults who are more mature in personality and more definite about their vocational interests and preferences will be more likely to adjust to adult-role responsibilities than will those who are still groping for a work-interest direction.

Another major source of stress during this period derives from the need to develop intimate psychosocial relationships with significant others. For those persons who choose to remain single, fulfillment of this need often requires the constant initiation or renewal of single and group interpersonal contacts and relationships. For many young adults, however, the drive for interpersonal intimacy involves the choosing of a marital partner and the establishment of a personal nuclear family household. Although a number of potential and actual stressors concerning the adjustments to the necessary exchanges and reciprocities associated with marriage or conjoint living and decision making has been suggested in the literature, there seems to be little empirical information about coping with the problems related to this transitional process.

There is, however, such a large volume of research concerning the internal structure and functioning of the family unit, the kin system, careering and family economics, parenting and many other related issues that even a brief discussion would fill many book-length manuscripts. What *can* be noted in passing is that choices in marital partners, general life styles and even interpersonal relationships have been found to be significantly influenced by (1) pressures and prejudices of family and society, (2) socioeconomic status, (3) religious and cultural backgrounds, (4) personal value systems and behavioral standards and (5) personal traits, interests and expectations. These influences have been cited in the paper on stressors in young adulthood by Sexsmith in this issue of FCH.

Because the major goal of the young husband–wife pair is usually to establish their own family unit, a few studies of this area will be discussed. According to Rainwater, the number of children that a couple has is a function of the number desired and the degree to which contraception is practiced.[115] Currently the use of family planning measures generally reflects a concerted effort by husband–wife pairs (1) to prevent, delay or promote pregnancies, (2) to assure adequate intervals between pregnancies and (3) to permit only wanted births. Research suggests that the degree of mutual concern of the husband–wife pair both for each other and for making use of family planning measures may have significant short- and longer-term effects on both the parents and their offspring. As an example, a study by Nuckolls et al. found that the proportion of women having pregnancy and birth complications was significantly higher among those women who had experienced a high frequency of life changes accompanied by a low degree of social–emotional support during their pregnancies and that when social support was high, there was no increase in complications.[116] Conflict over the acceptance of pregnancy has been associated with increased length of the labor process as well as increased levels of maternal anxiety,[117] and the degree of wantedness of the pregnancy and the seeking of adequate prenatal care have been associated with increased risk of low birth weight and higher infant mortality.[118,119] Finally, Cobb cites several studies which show that wanted children tend to adapt to or cope with the stresses of growing up better than do those who began life under circumstances where the parental preference had been for abortion.[120] Wanted children fared better in

terms of the decreased incidence of juvenile delinquency and need for psychiatric treatment and were better able to adapt to the school socialization and educational achievement processes.

As has been noted earlier, there is much in the literature about parenting and about the importance of parental understanding of their children in order to reduce parental concerns and improve child functioning. The work of Thomas et al. indicates that parents can be taught to recognize individual differences in their children and to modify or adapt their childrearing patterns to best fit the needs of each type of child.[121] Parents with handicapped and chronically ill children are especially in need of such training and counseling because the potentials of these children for socialization and self-actualization vary widely and often require considerable long-term planning and professional health care.[122] Studies show that parental attitudes about having produced handicapped children also vary quite widely (regret, denial, anger, rejection) since these children may represent parental incompetence both to the parents themselves and to others.[123] Voysey reported that parental coping patterns include the projection of false reports of progress, statements of grief and the development of cynical or actual acceptance of the disabilities and related malor misbehaviors.[124] The use of such mechanisms as denial, anger and false progress reports becomes maladaptive only when they are used too frequently, in too many situations, or for too long a duration. Rejection or cynical acceptance, however,

90   can have long-lasting detrimental effects on both the children and the parents.

ADULTHOOD: MIDDLE PHASE

Many problem situations encountered by young adults (nutritional deficits, rest and sleep problems, sexual difficulties, moral–religious conflicts, self-image problems, divorce, bereavement, etc.) also can be experienced at any time during the life cycle, since these stressor events are neither predictable nor universally experienced. Moreover, other types of life circumstances including environmental settings, educational preparation, economic resources can mitigate, submerge or exacerbate life crises.

Discussions about the stages and stressors of life development are always somewhat arbitrary at best, but are even more so when discussing the age 30-to-65 phase—middle adulthood. In general, it can be said that the decisions made in young adulthood tend to give shape and direction to life during the 30s. Certain expectations have been fulfilled, certain skills have been learned and a number of achievements have been accomplished. Gratifications during the 30s and early 40s include success in a job, a marriage, a family—the fullfillment of earlier hopes and expectations. Nevertheless, new decisions and life style adjustments have to be made, disappointments and discontentments occur more frequently, ambition for success may turn into desperation, etc. The concomitant incidence of anxiety, depression and other symptomatology (psychosomatic complaints, fear reactions and other emotional reactions),

which seemed high in the 30s, may reach maximum heights during the 40s when the individual begins to sense that life is finite and that health and even interpersonal decrements are more permanent than temporary. However, as Pruett's article in this issue of FCH points out, certain types of stressors—including career and work-related stressors, changes in the family unit structure (through death, divorce, departure of the last child, etc.), physical aging and the like—do tend to occur more frequently in this period of middle adulthood.

Although a number of studies report that good work relationships can buffer some occupational stresses and their related psychological strains, research into specific occupations suggests that such other factors as personality and prior experience may be more important in the development of effective coping mechanisms. In Pinneau's study of such high-stress occupations as air-traffic controllers, for example, the degree of social support received did not materially reduce either the physiological or the psychological strains associated with the job.[125] As with other "people-workers," policemen sometimes develop symptoms of emotional exhaustion (including cynicism and suspiciousness of others) which remain unrelieved despite peer support and counseling.[126,127] Persons experiencing group isolation (e.g., groups of men in military schools quartered in Antarctica or on isolated island bases) seem to cope better if their personalities are more internally than externally oriented.[128–130] This was also found to be true among business owners or managers whose performance was followed longitudinally for several years after a hurricane.[131,132] McDonald, on the other hand, noted that rates of illness among crews of combat ships seemed to vary in relation to both the degree of peer support and the attitudes of supervisors.[133] A study of the performance of nurses in the dynamic operating room environment showed less stress perceived by the individuals involved as the length of work experience in this type of area became greater.[134]

Such stressors as job promotion and environmental change also leave their mark on employees. Froberg et al. and others have noted that work production and the numbers of physical complaints increase following promotion to greater responsibility, to more stimulating work settings, etc., and that bodily stress responses manifested themselves both physiologically and psychologically.[135] A study by Kasl et al. monitored the health status of workers in two closing industrial plants. Physical symptoms and loss of ego strength varied significantly with the several stages of threat: news of anticipated closure (highest), actual unemployment, probationary reemployment in a substitute setting and stable reemployment.[136] When the job itself is perceived as less than desirable, however, workers' feelings about involuntary job loss tend to be more positive; the loss represents the opportunity to escape from an undesirable work situation without having to make the decision to leave, and also provides the opportunity to claim unemployment benefits without negative social stigma.[137] This does not deny that the lack of social support in terms of ethnic and social ties has been shown to exacerbate the physical and mental health consequences of involuntary job loss.[138] Moreover, in the long run, economic changes associated with unemployment also tend to affect the community—not only because of the decreased buying power of the jobless individuals, but also because of their generally depressed mood and life style changes caused by the job loss factor.[139]

Because it is becoming increasingly common for individuals to move from one family form to another across the life cycle (nuclear, nuclear with children, single parent, etc.), the problem of studying the related stressors is complicated by a vast range of intervening variables: culture, religious background, socioeconomic status and many others. Each family form presents different issues and problems, including changes in roles, interaction patterns, socialization patterns and linkage with nonfamily groups and organizations. One such critical influence on stress is the factor of housing. Stress has been found to increase with the vertical location of a living unit,[140] with the trauma of noise,[141] with crowding and the concomitant lack of privacy,[142–144] with the need to use communal facilities,[145] and with the lack of physical storage space and other structural deficiencies.[146] One study noted that, where residents and their neighbors tended to share the same demographic characteristics, patterns of social interaction were promotive of feelings of well-being and that the reverse was true where neighbors had mixed or quite different demographic characteristics.[147]

92   As may be noted in Pruett's article, one of the major stressors affecting the functioning of the family is the loss of members from the family unit. Studies were cited to document the central role of mothering, the mixed feelings of concern and relief when children mature and leave home, the female and male climacteric, and the loss of a parent or a marital partner through physical separation or death. Concern about the illness of a marital partner has been described by Croog and Fitzgerald more as a general than an acute stress experience.[148] Despite the range of stressors to which the individual may be exposed, however, Singer found that current functioning is a powerful predictor of subjectively experienced change. People who are doing relatively well seem to cope better with life changes and tend to think positively about issues and problems; people who are doing less well tend to think that things are getting worse or harder to handle.[149] Burke and Weir found that feelings of well-being and ability to cope with stressors were positively related to satisfaction with the spouse's help and emotional support.[150] Loss of a spouse, however, is usually perceived as the single greatest loss that an individual can experience throughout the life cycle.[151] The combined stress associated with the complex of physical, social, financial and

Loss of a spouse is usually perceived as the single greatest loss that an individual can experience throughout the life cycle.

psychological changes that accompany the loss may also exceed the ability of the bereaved individual to cope. Widows and widowers as a group are at high risk for mental illness. A spouse's death following a short illness has been reported to create higher stress levels than a death after a prolonged illness.[152] There is some evidence, however, that opportunities for new affiliations and the carrying out of affiliative behaviors correlate positively with adjustment to the bereavement of a spouse.[153]

As noted in earlier sections of this article, stressful life events affect individuals' health behaviors as well as their relationships with other persons. Although health habits, social support and degree of psychological well-being may affect an individual's actual health status, the number and magnitude of change events appear to be more important influences.[154,155] There is now considerable evidence to suggest stress as an etiological factor in such physiological malfunctioning as thyroid disorders, cardiac pathology, gastrointestinal dysfunction, essential hypertension and a number of other physiological disorders. As a result of their extensive review of stress studies, Kagan and Levi suggest that "the theoretical basis for the observed relationship between stress and illness includes the assumption that adaptive behavior (physiological) is required to cope with psychosocial stress."[156] Moreover, as Zahn points out, when the resulting physiological problem is visible to others, better interpersonal relationships can be maintained because there is a justification of the sick role (i.e., acceptable visibility of the stress response).[157] Multidimensional stresses which result from life changes also have been shown to interfere with both subjective and objective perceptions and judgments and to contribute materially to the incidence of home, automotive and other types of accidents.[158]

ADULTHOOD: LATER PHASE

Despite the fact that there is no clear line of demarcation between any of the phases of adulthood in our society, the later phase of adulthood has been identified chronologically as beginning at age 65. Decisions relating to autonomous functions and activities, occupational changes, choice of marital partners, concerns about health, housing, leisure activities, etc., take place throughout the whole of adulthood, and many of the associated stressors have the same magnitude, frequency and impact on an individual's life style regardless of chronological age.[159] Decrements in the functioning of human organs or organ systems or in the psychosocial capacities of people can and do occur at any age, since there are as yet no empirically predictable limits related specifically to time of occurrence. What can be documented, however, is that certain major events—such as enforced retirement and loss of friends and intimate loved ones—become more likely with increasing age, and that these negative life events are perceived as more stressful than events classified as pleasant or positive.[160] Coping with the confluence of physical, emotional and social factors, factors that might otherwise sufficiently

exacerbate each other to produce functional impairment, requires the ability to reintegrate one's goals, self-image and life role. This ability to make such adjustments varies on an individual basis.

According to Brotman, 75 percent of the American population now lives to age 65, and 95 percent of those 65 years and older reside in a noninstitutional setting. Brotman further points out that the proportion of older persons has consistently increased more rapidly than that of younger persons; that the 4 percent of those 65 years and older in 1900 had increased to over 10 percent by 1975, and that projections show a continuation of this differential to at least 12 percent of the population by the year 2000.[161] A review of the gerontological literature suggests that persons living beyond age 65 generally pass through three life stages: (1) Between ages 65 and 75, most individuals continue with normal activities unless there is a specific illness. (2) Most individuals also can carry out normal activities through age 85, although many begin to show the effects of age even without an overt disease/illness condition. (3) After reaching the age of 85, however, only a relative few individuals are seen as having the ability to carry on normal activities without some major assistance, including institutionalization.[162] Aside from the variable illness or disability factor, differences between and within these stage-of-life cohort groups are often perceived as being related to such other influences as previous life style,[163] adaptation to loss of the work role,[164,165] adjustment to minor ailments and stresses,[166] openness to both feelings

94   and ideas,[167] and maintenance of social activities and contacts.[168–170]

The illnesses and disabilities of older persons are predominantly age- or time-related, and tend to be chronic rather than acute. For the most part, chronic diseases limit mobility and comfort and are the most frequent causes of institutionalization. In general, despite the problems and hazards associated with aging, the large majority of older persons remain well enough for many years to participate in a variety of activities, are reasonably secure financially, and maintain social ties with family and friends.[171, 172] Nevertheless, and regardless of their life stage, older persons with multiple losses (work role, mobility, health, vision, spouse, mental acuity, home, etc.) are at greater risk to require some form of institutional support than are those with single or few losses.[173] As Barney[174] and Sandler[175] have noted, probably the most compelling reason for institutionalization is that these persons either outlive or overwhelm their support systems. What is not known, however, is what those at risk of institutionalization actually do in order to remain in the community. Shanas[176] and others have noted that the functional status of older persons living in the community can be quite high, despite the number and severity of their chronic disabilities. Butler and Lewis believe that this high level of functioning is based on the mechanisms the individual has developed in the past to cope with stressors and is now using to deal with the stressors accompanying chronic illnesses and other losses of aging.[177]

Aguilera's article on stressors in old age lists some of the needs of older persons if they are to continue to function in the community: adequate income, suitable housing, proper and adequate nutrition, access to transportation, etc. These persons must also carry out certain responsibilities: establishing and continuing in a range of physical and social activities,[178,179] remaining flexible and adaptable in the face of societal and community changes,[180,181] seeking and accepting health care and other helping services to assure self-maintenance.[182] Access to and use of social support factors thus appear to be important determinants of whether older individuals are relatively happy and self-sustaining. Certainly there is a strong need for companionship, and most older people are interested in sex, have sexual feelings and need sexual outlets.[183,184]

As is the case with individuals of any age, the health care needs of older persons range from periodic evaluations to maintain wellness status, through the complexity of services needed for acute care, to the supportive care needed for longer-term chronic health problems. Because persons may carry into their older years the health problems of youth and early maturity, as well as being subject to health stresses related to the aging process, the number of health problems afflicting any one individual may vary greatly. Although much can be done to alleviate or control some of the effects of the aging process, the increased likelihood of multiple health problems, combined with the slower recovery time associated with aging, often leads to more frequent and prolonged hospitalizations. For older persons who continue to need at least some medical surveillance and

Where family resources are inadequate, or where no suitable family substitute is available, the [aging] person's need for continued care may require placement in a skilled nursing facility.

skilled posthospitalization nursing care, a number of new problems arise. While there are theoretical alternatives to institutionalization for many of the elderly, some form of congregate living and continued health care may become a practical necessity. Where family resources are inadequate, or where no suitable family substitute is available, the person's need for continued care may require placement in a skilled nursing facility.[185]

Over the past four decades, a very considerable amount of research has focused on the effects of institutionalization on the physical integrity and psychological well-being of chronically ill and aging adults. Many of the early studies reflected the view that institutions for the aged were "dumping grounds," and focused on the incidence of mortality as the primary variable in relocation. Farrar et al.[186] noted that the first three months after institutional placement were the most critical. Killian found that patients with psychosis, chronic brain syndrome, poor physical functioning and poor mental status were most prone to excessive mortality.[187] However, as Blenkner points out, the high mortality rate is probably related more to the illness status of the persons than to the placement itself (i.e., removal from familiar home or acute-care surroundings).[188] Research also suggests that the individual's response to the relocation event is conditioned by (1) general personality characteristics and self-concept,[189] (2) attitude toward the move,[190] (3) age, sex, medical diagnosis and overall level of functioning,[191] (4) the degree of change in the living arrangements,[192,193] (5) the degree of continued support from significant others[194,195] and (6) a number of factors inherent to the design and operation of the institutional environment.[196,197] Noelker and Harel found that the predictors of morale, life satisfaction, satisfaction with treatment and survival were the patients' subjective perceptions of the facility and their preference and options for living in the facility itself or elsewhere.[198] Schulz noted that loss of control among the institutionalized aged was at least partially responsible for depression, physical decline and early death.[199] This suggests a need for increased attention to the patients' cognitive and emotional status at application and entry periods, as well as throughout their institutional stay.

Probably the most common problem in later adulthood is depression. Concomitant with depression may be feelings of fatigue, lack of energy, low self-esteem and insomnia. Depression following bereavement has been discussed in an earlier section of this article. The dependency related to being ill, or to being ill and institutionalized, often gives rise to fear of dependence and may be expressed in irritability, an unwillingness to cooperate in treatment and a general dissatisfaction with life.[200, 201] When an illness brings into focus the probability of diminished life expectancy or impending death,

96   indirect or even direct self-destructive behavior may occur.[202,203] This may take many forms: active or passive, lethal or relatively innocuous, easily identified or obscure. Behavioral examples include alcoholism and drug abuse, hyperobesity, disregard for one's health or safety, and withdrawal from the social environment.[204] Lieberman's research on the institutionalized elderly, however, suggested that behaviors which appear to staff as uncooperative or belligerent and destructive to the patient's health may also serve a dual psychological purpose: that of being able to express anger and frustration at circumstances related to medical condition and institutionalization and of reestablishing some feelings of control and self-esteem.[205]

WHAT WE KNOW AND WHAT WE NEED TO KNOW ABOUT COPING WITH LIFE STRESSORS

In this admittedly very brief overview of research on stressors throughout the life cycle, we have seen strong evidence that the human response to stressful situations involves a number of physiological and psychological bodily stress reactions. Lazarus classifies these stress reactions into four main categories: (1) reports of disturbed affect, (2) changes in adequacy of cognitive functioning, (3) motor behaviors and (4) physiological changes.[206] The particular pattern of physical and psychological behaviors which indicates that an individual is responding to one or more stressor stimuli varies at different developmental levels and is influenced by a vast variety of demographic, personality, sociocultural and other factors.

"Coping" refers to the process by which we consciously or subconsciously organize our efforts to meet and deal with perceived threats. According to Lazarus, both the ability to perceive situations as stressful (a cognitive appraisal) and the sources of stress vary with the different developmental periods. "To the extent that fundamental resources for coping with stress change with developmental level, then the nature of coping processes will vary too depending on whether we are dealing with an infant, young child, or mature adult."[207] If we accept the theory that cognitive appraisal is necessary to respond to threatening situations, then the three-week-old infant who cries when hungry or uncomfortable is not actually coping with these stressors: the crying is reflexive rather than cognitive and is not directed toward dealing with these stimuli as threats to safety and well-being. However, the nine-month-old child who cries when mother leaves is cognitively aware that her absence constitutes the loss of a source of support that the child considers essential to his or her feelings of well-being. (In this case, crying is a mechanism used to prevent the mother from leaving or perhaps to shorten the length of her absence.) The adult who cries during the bereavement process is acutely aware that crying will not bring back the missing loved one. The crying, however, does serve to relieve some of the tension and frustration associated with the loss, so that the individual may be better able to organize internal and external resources to resume and continue personal functioning.

Despite the volume of theoretical and empirical literature concerning the perception of stressors and the quite varied stress responses which result, there appears to be little coherence either in the ways that stress is defined and measured or in the recommendations offered for improving coping styles. We still do not have a clear picture about what conditions or processes are perceived as stressful by people at different points in the life cycle, what patterns of reaction indicate the presence of physiological and psychological stress, or what people do to cope or deal with their own stress reactions. The literature suggests that adaptation to stress is a dynamic process, and that individual differences in personality and in learned behavior patterns influence strongly the ways in which people learn to be stressed. Clinical and research data suggest also that not only the identified stressor situations but also the daily microstressors (the small everyday stressors or hassles) can act cumulatively and, in the absence of positive balancing or compensatory experiences, can be potent sources of depressive and other stress reactions. Persons who fail to adapt to stressful stimuli thus may be reflecting a continuing process of previous failures to cope effectively with daily stressors, with each failure feeding back to interfere with attempts to cope with new strainful demands.

Coping and adaptive behaviors thus appear to depend on the interplay of internal psychological forces in response to external social-environmental factors. Persons who can cope with life's daily problems most of the time are those who generally feel comfortable about themselves and can interact comfortably with and show concern for other people. Some types of coping activities (use of religion, rigidity or deliberateness in decision making, joking about problems or ignoring a strainful situation) serve to reduce or short-circuit stress reactions by modifying cognitive appraisals of situations as threats. Other ways of coping include anticipatory planning or working out in advance the most effective ways to deal with the possible harms and threats in an impending (or probably impending) crisis situation, development of psychosomatic symptoms, depression and withdrawal for a time from the social world; all of these mechanisms can be positive if used for short periods of time and without any great frequency as to become habitual.

At best, what we currently know about coping with life stressors amounts to little more than bits of knowledge which are difficult to fit into a coherent framework. What information we do have suggests that the dynamics of coping in later life seem to be predicated on earlier life adjustment patterns. What we need is a descriptive analysis—not only of the social, psychological and physiological developmental changes as people progress through the life cycle, but also of how people respond to environmental stimuli, interact with other people, make adaptive or maladaptive decisions, etc., and practically on a day-by-day basis. We need to know what people perceive as inputs, what they use or reject as mediators, what outcomes result from the interplay of inputs and mediators, and why the whole process functions as it does.

Although we can infer from the literature that pleasurable stressors apparently produce less severe stress reactions than do those stressors considered undesirable

98 or threatening, we cannot yet compare the types or degrees of stress responses actually produced. Nor can we compare the responses to being challenged with those of being threatened by stressor stimuli.

Research on stress also seems to be focused toward the social, psychological or physiological aspects of the stressor stimuli and the human responses to these stimuli—a separation that is artificial, since people are composites of all of these aspects and their behaviors are reflective of this complexity. Because many of the problems cannot be investigated within a single discipline, research must be multi-level in its approach. Investigators must use multiple dimensions to identify inputs and mediators and to determine outcomes—seeking access to people's own perceptions and living experiences both through direct questioning and through validating the self-reports through observations and such other data collection methods as are determined useful and appropriate. Research also should be conducted in natural rather than laboratory settings, since people live and react to stimuli in natural environments and can in many instances select the changes which occur to them. The methodologic

The methodologic problems inherent in the study of stress suggest the need for new research designs and techniques which are more in accord with the multilevel nature and complexity of the problem.

problems inherent in the study of stress suggest the need for new research designs and techniques which are more in accord with the multilevel nature and complexity of the problem.

For people in the helping professions, however, the research to date does provide some insights and suggest some useful approaches for assisting clients. For example, a knowledge of the degree of change and stressful life events being experienced by an individual client may be used to help that person contain a present stress (e.g., illness or other crisis situation) within limits, and perhaps prevent additional stress that might otherwise be consequential. The helping professional may also be enabled to assist clients by exploring alternative and previously tested coping strategies and techniques for dealing with current and future stress situations.

REFERENCES

1. Janis, I. L. *Psychological Stress* (New York: John Wiley & Sons 1958).
2. Grinker, R. R. and Spiegel, J. P. *Men under Stress* (New York: McGraw-Hill 1945).
3. Bettelheim, B. "Individual and Mass Behavior in Extreme Situations." *Journal of Abnormal Psychology* 38:10 (1943) p. 424–466.
4. Selye, H. *The Physiology and Pathology of Exposure to Stress* (Montreal: Acta 1950).
5. Selye, H. *The Stress of Life* (New York: McGraw-Hill 1956).
6. Selye, H. "Implications of the Stress Concept." *New York State Journal of Medicine* 75:12 (October 1975) p. 2139–2145.

7. Piaget, J. *The Child's Conception of the World* (London: Routledge and Kegan Paul 1929) p. 220.

8. Piaget, J. *The Language and Thought of the Child* (London: Kegan Paul, Trench, Trubner 1932).

9. Piaget, J. *The Moral Judgement of the Child* (London: Kegan Paul, Trench, Trubner 1932).

10. Spitz, R. A. and Wolf, K. M. "The Smiling Response: A Contribution to the Ontogenesis of Social Relations." *Genetic Psychology Monographs* 34 (1946) p. 57.

11. Schaffer, H. R. "Objective Observation of Personality Development in Early Infancy." *British Journal of Medical Psychology* 29 (1958) p. 174–183.

12. Schaffer, H. R. "Activity Level as a Constitutional Determinant of Infantile Reaction to Deprivation." *Child Development* 37 (1966) p. 595.

13. Sostek, A. M., Anders, T. F. and Sostek, A. J. "Diurnal Rhythms in 2- and 8-Week-Old Infants: Sleep-Waking State Organization as a Function of Age and Stress." *Psychosomatic Medicine* 38:4 (July–August 1976) p. 250–256.

14. Goldberg, S. "Premature Birth: Consequences for the Parent-Infant Relationship." *American Scientist* 67:2 (March–April 1979) p. 214–220.

15. Spitz, R. A. "Hospitalism: A Follow-Up Report" in Eissler, R. E. ed. *The Psychoanalytic Study of the Child* (New York: International Universities Press 1946) II, p. 113–117.

16. Schaffer, H. R. and Callender, W. M. "Psychological Effects of Hospitalization in Infancy." *Journal of Pediatrics* 24 (1959) p. 528.

17. Rheingold, H. "Mental and Social Development of Institutionalized Babies." *American Journal of Orthopsychiatry* 13 (1943) p. 41–43.

18. Glasser, K. "Implications for Maternal Deprivation Research for Practice Theory in Child Welfare" (New York: Child Welfare League of America 1962).

19. Robertson, J. "Some Responses to Loss of Maternal Care." *Nursing Times* 49 (1952) p. 383.

20. Bowlby, J. *Child Care and Growth of Love* (London: Penguin Books 1953).

21. Bowlby, J. *Attachment and Loss, Vol. I* (New York: Basic Books 1969) p. 321–327.

22. Stein, Z. and Susser, M. "Social Factors in the Development of Sphincter Control." *Developmental Medical Child Neurology* 9 (1967) p. 692–706.

23. Piaget, J. *The Moral Judgement of the Child.*

24. Prugh, D. G. "Emotional Aspects of Hospitalization" in Shore, M. ed. *Red is the Color of Hurting* (Bethesda, Md.: National Institute of Mental Health 1965) p. 19–26.

25. Heinecke, C. *Brief Separation* (New York: International Universities Press 1965) p. 309–327.

26. Robertson, J. *Young Children in Hospitals* (New York: Basic Books 1958).

27. Miller, S. R. "Children's Fears: A Review of the Literature with Implications for Nursing Research and Practice." *Nursing Research* 28:4 (July–August 1979) p. 217–223.

28. Korsch, B. M. "Issues in Humanizing Care for Children." *American Journal of Public Health* 68:9 (September 1978) p. 831–832.

29. Forssman, H. and Thuwe, I. "One Hundred and Twenty Children Born after Application for Therapeutic Abortion Refused." *Acta Psychiatrica Scandia* 28:1 (1974) p. 21–29.

30. Blumberg, M. L. "Psychopathology of the Abusing Parent." *American Journal of Psychotherapy* 28:1 (1974) p. 21–29.

31. Corey, E. J. B., Miller, C. L. and Widlak, F. W. "Factors Contributing to Child Abuse." *Nursing Research* 24:4 (July–August 1975) p. 293–295.

32. Baumrind, D. "Reciprocal Rights and Responsibilities in Parent-Child Relations." *Journal of Social Issues* 34:2 (1978) p. 179–196.

33. Pratt, L. "Child-Rearing Methods and Children's Health Behavior." *Journal of Health and Social Behavior* 14:3 (1973) p. 61–69.

34. Jonas, A. D. and Jonas, D. F. "The Influence of Early Training on the Varieties of Stress Responses: An Ethological Approach." *Journal of Psychosomatic Research* 19:5–6 (1975) p. 325–335.

35. Cravioto, J., DeLicorda, E. R. and Birch, H. G. "Nutrition, Growth and Neurointegrative Development: An Experimental and Ecological Study." *Pediatrics* 38:2 (August 1966) p. 319–371.

36. Eichenwald, H. F. and Crooke-Fry, P. "Nutrition and Learning." *Science* 163 (February 14, 1969) p. 644–648.

37. Richardson, S. A. et al. "The Behavior of Children in School Who Were Severely Malnourished in the First Two Years of Life." *Journal of Health and Social Behavior* 13:3 (September 1972) p. 276–284.

38. Jessner, L. "Some Observations of Children Hospitalized During Latency" in Jessner, L. and Pavenstedt, E., eds. *Dynamic Psychopathology* (New York: Grune and Stratton 1959) p. 257–267.

39. Natapoff, J. N. "Children's Views of Health: A Developmental Study." *American Journal of Public Health* 68:10 (1978) p. 995–1000.

40. Campbell, J. D. "Illness Is a Point of View: The Development of Children's Concepts of Illness." *Child Development* 46 (1975) p. 92–100.

100

41. Campbell, J. D. "The Child in the Sick Role: Contributions of Age, Sex, Parental Status, and Parental Values." *Journal of Health and Social Behavior* 19:1 (March 1978) p. 35–51.

42. Viney, L. L. and Clarke, A. M. "Children Coping with Crisis: An Analogue Study." *British Journal of Social and Clinical Psychology* 13:3 (September 1974) p. 305–313.

43. Harding, R. K. and Looney, J. G. "Problems of Southeast Asian Children in a Refugee Camp." *American Journal of Psychiatry* 134:4 (April 1977) p. 407–411.

44. Cain, L. P. and Staver, N. "Helping Children Adapt to Parental Illness." *Social Casework* 57:9 (November 1976) p. 575–580.

45. Goggin, E. L., Lansky, S. B. and Hassanein, K. "Psychological Reactions of Children with Malignancies." *Journal of the American Academy of Child Psychiatry* 15:2 (Spring 1976) p. 314–325.

46. Erikson, E. H. *Childhood and Society* 2nd ed. (New York: W. W. Norton 1963).

47. Erikson, E. H. *Identity: Youth and Crisis* (New York: W. W. Norton 1968).

48. Nolan, N. et al. "Assessment and Health Promotion for the Adolescent" in Murray, R. and Zentner, J., eds. *Nursing Assessment and Health Promotion through the Life Span* (Englewood Cliffs, N.J.: Prentice-Hall 1975) p. 155–196.

49. Peterson, E. T. "The Impact of Adolescent Illness on Parental Relationships." *Journal of Health and Social Behavior* 13:4 (December 1972) p. 429–437.

50. Starr, B. D. and Goldstein, H. S. *Human Development and Behavior: Psychology in Nursing* (New York: Springer Publishing Co. 1975) p. 52–68.

51. Bruner, J. S. "The Uses of Immaturity" in Coelho, G. V. and Rubenstein, E. A., eds. *Social Change and Human Behavior: Mental Health Challenges of the Seventies* (Rockville, Md.: HEW, Public Health Service; Alcohol, Drug Abuse, and Mental Health Administration, National Institute of Mental Health 1976) p. 3–20.

52. Piaget, J. *The Growth of Logical Thinking from Childhood to Adolescence* (New York: Basic Books 1961).

53. Elkind, D. "Cognitive Development in Adolescence" in Adams, J. E., ed. *Understanding Adolescence* (Boston: Allyn and Bacon 1968).

54. Sorenson, R. C. *Adolescent Sexuality in Contemporary America* (New York: World 1973).

55. Starr and Goldstein. *Human Development and Behavior: Psychology in Nursing.*

56. Hauser, S. T. and Shapiro, R. L. " An Approach to the Analysis of Faculty-Student Interactions in Small Groups." *Human Relations* 29:9 (September 1976) p. 819–832.

57. Lazarus, R. S. *Psychological Stress and the Coping Process* (New York: McGraw-Hill 1966).

58. Dohrenwend, B. S. "Life Events as Stressors: A Methodological Inquiry." *Journal of Health and Social Behavior* 14:2 (June 1973) p. 167–175.

59. Holmes, T. H. and Rahe, R. H. "The Social Readjustment Rating Scale." *Journal of Psychosomatic Research* 11:4 (1967) p. 213–218.

60. Rosenburg, E. J. and Dohrenwend, B. S. "Effects of Experiences and Ethnicity on Ratings of Life Events as Stressors." *Journal of Health and Social Behavior* 16:1 (March 1975) p. 127–129.

61. Askenasy, A. R., Dohrenwend, B. P. and Dohrenwend, B. S. "Some Effects of Social Class and Ethnic Group Membership on Judgments of the Magnitude of Stressful Life Events: A Research Note." *Journal of Health and Social Behavior* 18:4 (December 1977) p. 432–439.

62. Dohrenwend, B. S. et al. "Exemplification of a Method for Scaling Life Events: The PERI Life Events Scale." *Journal of Health and Social Behavior* 19:2 (June 1978) p. 205–229.

63. Pearlin, L. I. and Schooler, C. "The Structure of Coping." *Journal of Health and Social Behavior* 19:3 (September 1978) p. 2–21.

64. Janis, I. L. and Mann, L. "Coping with Decisional Conflict." *American Scientist* 64:6 (November–December 1976) p. 657–667.

65. Cobb, S. "Social Support as a Moderator of Life Stress." *Psychosomatic Medicine* 38:5 (September–October 1976) p. 300–314.

66. Dean, A. and Lin, N. "The Stress-Buffering Role of Social Support." *Journal of Nervous and Mental Disease* 165:6 (June 1977) p. 403–417.

67. Langlie, J. K. "Social Networks, Health Beliefs, and Preventive Health Behavior." *Journal of Health and Social Behavior* 18:3 (September 1977) p. 244–260.

68. Holmes and Rahe. "The Social Readjustment Rating Scale."

69. Petrich, J. and Holmes, T. J. "Life Changes and Onset of Illness." *Medical Clinics of North America* 16:4 (July 1977) p. 825–838.

70. Rabkin, J. G. and Struening, E. L. "Life Events, Stress and Illness." *Science* 194:4269 (December 3, 1976) p. 1013–1020.

71. Pesznecker, B. L. and McNeil, B. "Relationship among Health Habits, Social Assets, Psychological Well-Being, Life Change, and Alterations in Health Status." *Nursing Research* 24:6 (November–December 1975) p. 442–447.

72. Ruch, L. O. "A Multidimensional Analysis of the

Concept of Life Change." *Journal of Health and Social Behavior* 18:1 (March 1977) p. 71–83.

73. Hough, R. L., Fairbank, D. T. and Garcia, A. M. "Problems in the Ratio Measurement of Life Stress." *Journal of Health and Social Behavior* 17:1 (March 1976) p. 70–82.

74. Aguilera, D. C. and Messick, J. M. *Crisis Intervention: Theory and Methodology* 2nd ed. (St. Louis: The C. V. Mosby Co. 1974).

75. Volicer, B. J. "Stress Factors in the Experience of Hospitalization" in Batey, M. V. ed. *Communicating Nursing Research* Vol. 8 (Boulder, Colo.: Western Interstate Commission for Higher Education, March 1977) p. 53–67.

76. Volicer, B. J. and Burns, M. W. "Preexisting Correlates of Hospital Stress." *Nursing Research* 26:6 (November–December 1977) p. 408–415.

77. Sime, A. M. "Relationship of Preoperative Fear, Type of Coping, and Information Received about Surgery to Recovery from Surgery." *Journal of Personality and Social Psychology* 34:4 (October 1976) p. 716–724.

78. Parsons, T. and Fox, R. "Illness, Therapy and the Modern American Family." *Journal of Social Issues* 32:8 (1964) p. 31–45.

79. Rothberg, J. "Dependence, Anxiety, and Surgical Recovery." *Nursing Science* 3 (August 1965) p. 243–256.

80. Derdiarian, A. and Clough, D. "Patients' Dependence and Independence Levels on the Prehospitalization-Postdischarge Continuum." *Nursing Research* 25:1 (January–February 1978) p. 27–34.

81. Bramwell, S. T. et al. "Psychosocial Factors in Athletic Injuries." *Journal of Human Stress* 1:3 (September 1975) p. 6–20.

82. Rahe, R. H. et al. "Recent Life Changes, Myocardial Infarction, and Abrupt Coronary Disease." *Archives of Internal Medicine* 133 (1974) p. 221–228.

83. Wildman, R. C. and Johnson, D. R. "Life Changes and Langner's 22-Item Mental Health Index: A Study and Partial Replication." *Journal of Health and Social Behavior* 18:2 (June 1977) p. 179–188.

84. Hudgens, R. W., Morrison, J. R. and Barchha, R. G. "Life Events and Onset of Primary Affective Disorders." *Archives of General Psychiatry* 16:2 (February 1967) p. 134–145.

85. Dohrenwend, B. S. "Social Status and Stressful Life Events." *Journal of Personality and Social Psychology* 28 (November 1973) p. 225–235.

86. Brown, G. W. "Meaning, Measurement and Stress of Life Events" in Dohrenwend, B. S. and Dohrenwend, B. P., eds. *Stressful Life Events: Their Nature and Effects* (New York: John Wiley & Sons 1974) p. 217–243.

87. Paykel, E. S. "Life Stress and Psychiatric Disorder: Applications of the Clinical Approach" in Dohrenwend, B. S. and Dohrewend, B. P. eds. *Stressful Life Events: Their Nature and Effects* (New York: John Wiley & Sons 1974) p. 135–149.

88. Mueller, D. P., Edwards, D. W. and Yarvis, R. M. "Stressful Life Events and Psychiatric Symptomatology: Change or Undesirability?" *Journal of Health and Social Behavior* 18:3 (September 1977) p. 307–317.

89. Bloch, G. R. and Bloch, N. H. "Analytic Group Psychotherapy of Post-Traumatic Psychoses." *International Journal of Group Psychotherapy* 26:1 (January 1976) p. 49–57.

90. Bell, J. M. "Stressful Life Events and Coping Methods in Mental-Illness and -Wellness Behaviors." *Nursing Research* 26:2 (March–April 1977) p. 136–141.

91. Myers, J., Lindenthal, J. J. and Pepper, M. P. "Life Events, Social Integration and Psychiatric Symptomatology." *Journal of Health and Social Behavior* 16:4 (December 1975) p. 421–427.

92. White, W. C., McAdoo, W. G. and Phillips, L. "Social Competence and Outcome of Hospitalization: A Preliminary Report." *Journal of Health and Social Behavior* 15:3 (September 1974) p. 261–266.

93. Maris, R. and Connor, H. E., Jr. "Do Crisis Services Work? A Follow-up of a Psychiatric Outpatient Sample." *Journal of Health and Social Behavior* 14:4 (December 1973) p. 311–322.

94. Starr and Goldstein. *Human Development and Behavior: Psychology in Nursing.*

95. Kjerulff, K. and Wiggins, N. H. "Graduate Student Styles for Coping with Stressful Situations." *Journal of Educational Psychology* 68:3 (June 1976) p. 247–254.

96. Gilbert, L. A. "Situational Factors and the Relationship between Locus of Control and Psychological Adjustment." *Journal of Counseling Psychology* 23:4 (July 1976) p. 302–309.

97. Crandall, J. E. and Lehman, R. E. "Relationship of Stressful Life Events to Social Interest, Locus of Control, and Psychological Adjustment." *Journal of Consulting and Clinical Psychology* 45:6 (December 1977) p. 1208.

98. Gersten, J. C. et al. "An Evaluation of the Etiologic Role of Stressful Life-Change Events in Psychological Disorders." *Journal of Health and Social Behavior* 18:3 (September 1977) p. 228–244.

99. Mettlin, C. and Woelfel, J. "Interpersonal Influences and Symptoms of Stress." *Journal of*

102

Health and Social Behavior 15:4 (December 1974) p. 311–319.

100. McKay, S. R. "A Review of Student Stress in Nursing Education Programs." *Nursing Forum* 17:4 (Spring 1979) p. 376–393.

101. Washburn, S. L. "Aggressive Behavior and Human Evolution" in Coelho, E. V. and Rubinstein, E. A. eds. *Social Changes and Human Behavior: Mental Health Challenges of the Seventies* (Rockville, Md.: HEW, Public Health Service, Alcohol, Drug and Mental Health Administration, National Institute of Mental Health 1976) p. 21–39.

102. Strong, E. K. *Vocational Interests of Men and Women* (Stanford, Calif.: Stanford University Press 1943).

103. Super, D. E. and Crites, J. O. *Appraising Vocational Fitness* revised ed. (New York: Harper & Row 1962).

104. Roe, A. and Siegelman, M. *The Origin of Interests* (Washington, D. C.: American Personnel and Guidance Association 1964).

105. Medvene, A. M. "Occupational Choice of Graduate Students in Psychology as a Function of Early Parent-Child Interactions." *Journal of Counseling Psychology* 16 (1969) p. 385–389.

106. Holland, J. L. *Manual for the Vocational Preference Inventory* (Palo Alto, Calif.: Consulting Psychologists Press 1965).

107. Holland, J. L. *The Psychology of Vocational Choice: A Theory of Personality Types and Model Environments* (Waltham, Mass.: Blaisdell 1966).

108. Holland, J. L. "Explorations of a Theory of Vocational Choice: V.A. One-Year Prediction Study" (Monrovia, N.Y.: Chronical Guidance Professional Service 1964).

109. Baird, L. L. "The Relation of Vocational Interests to Life Goals, Self-Ratings of Ability and Personality Traits, and Potential for Achievement." *Journal of Counseling Psychology* 17 (1970) p. 233–239.

110. Campbell, D. P. *Handbook for the Strong Vocational Interest Blank* (Stanford, Calif.: Stanford University Press 1971).

111. Marks, E. and Webb, S. C. "Vocational Choice and Professional Experiences as Factors in Occupational Image." *Journal of Applied Psychology* 53 (1969) p. 292–300.

112. Lacey, D. "Holland's Vocational Models: A Study of Workgroups and Need Satisfaction." *Journal of Vocational Behavior* 1 (1971) p. 105–122.

113. Holland, J. L. et al. "Applying an Occupational Classification to a Representative Sample of Work Histories." *Journal of Applied Psychology* 58 (1973) p. 34–41.

114. Holland, J. L. and Nichols, R. C. "Exploration of a Theory of Vocational Choice: III A Longitudinal Study of Change in Major Field of Study." *Personnel and Guidance Journal* 43 (1964) p. 235–242.

115. Rainwater, L. *Family Design: Marital Sexuality, Family Size and Contraception* (Chicago: Aldine 1965).

116. Nuckolls, K. B., Cassel J. and Kaplan, B. H. "Psychosocial Assets, Life Crisis and the Prognosis of Pregnancy." *American Journal of Epidemiology* 95 (1972) p. 431–441.

117. Lederman, R. P. et al. "Relationship of Psychological Factors in Pregnancy to Progress in Labor." *Nursing Research* 28:2 (March–April 1979) p. 94–97.

118. Morris, N. M., Udry, J. R. and Chase, C. L. "Reduction of Low Birth Weight Rates by Prevention of Unwanted Pregnancies." *American Journal of Public Health* 63 (1973) p. 935–938.

119. Gortmaker, S. L. "The Effects of Prenatal Care upon the Health of the Newborn." *American Journal of Public Health* 69 (1979) p. 653–657.

120. Cobb, S. "Social Support as a Moderator of Life Stress." *Psychosomatic Medicine* 38:5 (September–October 1976) p. 300–314.

121. Thomas, A., Chess, S. and Birth, H. *Temperament and the Behavior Disorders of Children* (New York: New York University Press 1968).

122. Sahin, S. T. "A New Perspective on the Family with a Special-Needs Child." *Nursing Forum* 17:4 (Spring 1979) p. 357–375.

123. Klein, C. "Coping Patterns of Parents of Deaf-Blind Children." *American Annals of the Deaf* 122:3 (June 1977) p. 310–312.

124. Voysey, M. "Impression Management by Parents with Disabled Children." *Journal of Health and Social Behavior* 13:1 (March 1972) p. 80–89.

125. Pinneau, S. R. "Effects of Social Support on Occupational Stresses and Strains." Paper presented at the 84th Annual Convention of the American Psychological Association, Washington, D.C., September 1976. Cited in Gore, S. "The Effect of Social Support in Moderating the Health Consequences of Unemployment." *Journal of Health and Social Behavior* 19:2 (June 1968) p. 157–165.

126. Maslach, C. and Jackson, S. E. "Burned-Out Cops and Their Families." *Psychology Today* 12:12 (May 1979) p. 59–62.

127. McClenahen, L. and Lofland, J. "Bearing Bad News: Tactics of the Deputy U. S. Marshal." *Sociology of Work and Occupations* 3:3 (August 1976) p. 251–272.

128. Herrman, D. J. et al. "Relationship between Personality Factors and Adaption to Stress in a Military Institution." *Psychological Reports* 40:3, Part I (June 1977) p. 831–834.

129. Taylor, A. J. and Feletti, G. I. "The Victoria Isolation Scale, Form A." *Journal of Consulting and Clinical Psychology* 44:2 (April 1976) p. 305.

130. Cooper, C. L. and Green, M. D. "Coping with Occupational Stress among Royal Air Force Personnel on Isolated Island Bases." *Psychological Reports* 39 (December 1976) p. 731–734.

131. Anderson, C. R. "Locus of Control, Coping Behaviors, and Performance in a Stress Setting: A Longitudinal Study." *Journal of Applied Psychology* 62:4 (April 1977) p. 446–451.

132. Anderson, C. R., Hellriegel, D. and Slocum, J. W. "Managerial Response to Environmentally Induced Stress." *Academy of Management Journal* 20:2 (June 1977) p. 260–272.

133. McDonald, B. W., Pugh, W. M. and Gunderson, E. K. E. "Organizational Factors and Health Status." *Journal of Health and Social Behavior* 14:4 (December 1973) p. 330–334.

134. Olsen, M. "O R Nurses' Perceptions of Stress." *AORN Journal* 25:1 (January 1977) p. 43–48.

135. Froberg, J. et al. "Conditions of Work: Psychological and Endocrine Stress Reactions." *Archives of Environmental Health* 21:6 (December 1970) p. 789–797.

136. Kasl, S., Gore, S. and Cobb, S. "The Experience of Losing a Job: Reported Changes in Health, Symptoms and Illness Behaviors." *Psychosomatic Medicine* 37 (March–April 1975) p. 106–122.

137. Little, C. B. "Technical–Professional Unemployment: Middle-Class Adaptability to Personal Crisis." *Sociological Quarterly* 17:2 (Spring 1976) p. 262–274.

138. Gore, S. "The Effect of Social Support in Moderating the Health Consequences of Unemployment." *Journal of Health and Social Behavior* 19:2 (June 1978) p. 157–165.

139. Catalano, R. and Dooley, C. D. "Economic Predictors of Depressed Mood and Stressful Life Events in a Metropolitan Community." *Journal of Health and Social Behavior* 18:3 (September 1977) p. 292–307.

140. Gillis, A. R. "High-Rise Housing and Psychological Strain." *Journal of Health and Social Behavior* 18:4 (December 1977) p. 418–431.

141. Pond, A. M. "The Influence of Housing on Health." *Marriage and Family Living* 19 (July 1957) p. 154–159.

142. Webb, S. D. and Collette, J. "Urban Ecological and Household Correlates of Stress." *American Behavioral Scientist* 18 (July–August 1975) p. 750–770.

143. Carp, F. M., Zawadski, R. T. and Shokrkon, H. "Dimensions of Urban Environmental Quality." *Environment and Behavior* 8 (1976) p. 239–264.

144. Sundstrom, E. "An Experimental Study of Crowding: Effects of Room Size, Intrusion, and Goal Blocking on Nonverbal Behavior, Self-Disclosure, and Self-Reported Stress." *Journal of Personality and Social Psychology* 32:4 (October 1975) p. 645–654.

145. Wilner, D. M. et al. *The Housing Environment and Family Life* (Baltimore: Johns Hopkins Press 1962).

146. Duvall, D. and Booth, A. "The Housing Environment and Women's Health." *Journal of Health and Social Behavior* 19:4 (December 1978) p. 410–417.

147. Hessler, R. M. et al. "Demographic Context, Social Interaction, and Perceived Health Status: Excedrin Headache #1." *Journal of Health and Social Behavior* 12:3 (September 1971) p. 191–199.

148. Croog, S. H. and Fitzgerald, E. F. "Subjective Stress and Serious Illness of a Spouse: Wives of Heart Patients." *Journal of Health and Social Behavior* 19:2 (June 1978) p. 166–178.

149. Singer, E. "Subjective Evaluations as Indicators of Change." *Journal of Health and Social Behavior* 18:1 (March 1977) p. 84–90.

150. Burke, R. J. and Weir, T. "Marital Helping Relationships: The Moderators between Stress and Well-Being." *Journal of Psychology* 95:1 (January 1977) p. 121–130.

151. Conroy, R. C. "Widows and Widowhood." *New York State Journal of Medicine* 77:3 (March 1977) p. 357–360.

152. Vachon, M. L. "Stress Reactions to Bereavement." *Essence* 1:1 (1976) p. 23–33.

153. Parkes, C. M. *Bereavement: Studies of Grief in Adult Life* (New York: International Universities Press 1972).

154. McNeil, K. and Pesznecker, B. L. "Keeping People Well Despite Life Change Crises." *Public Health Reports* 92:4 (July–August 1977) p. 343–348.

155. Mefferd, R. B. and Wieland, B. A. "Comparison of Responses to Anticipated Stress and Stress." *Psychosomatic Medicine* 28:6 (November–December 1966) p. 795–807.

156. Kagan, A. R. and Levi, L. "Health and Environment—Psychosocial Stimuli: A Review." *Social Science and Medicine* 8 (May 1974) p. 225–241.

104

157. Zahn, M. A. "Incapacity, Impotence and Invisible Impairment: Their Effects upon Interpersonal Relations." *Journal of Health and Social Behavior* 14:2 (June 1973) p. 115–123.

158. Selzer, M. L. and Vinokur, A. "Role of Life Events in Accident Causation." *Mental Health and Society* 2:1–2 (1975) p. 36–54.

159. Dohrenwend, B. S. and Dohrenwend, B. P., eds. *Stressful Life Events: Their Nature and Effects* (New York: John Wiley & Sons 1974).

160. Lowenthal, M., Thurnher, M. and Chiriboga, D. *Four Stages of Life: A Comparative Study of Women and Men Facing Transitions* (San Francisco: Jossey-Bass 1975).

161. Brotman, H. B. "Population Projections: Part I. Tomorrow's Older Population (to 2000)." *The Gerontologist* 17:3 (1977) p. 203–209.

162. Vicente, L., Wiley, J. A. and Carrington, R. A. "The Risk of Institutionalization before Death." *The Gerontologist* 19:4 (1979) p. 361–367.

163. Sidney, K. H. and Shepard, R. J. "Activity Patterns of Elderly Men and Women." *Journal of Gerontology* 32:1 (1977) p. 25–32.

164. Simpson, I. H., Back, K. W. and McKinney, J. C. "Attributes of Work, Involvement in Society, and Self-Evaluation in Retirement" in Simpson, I. H. and McKinney, J. C. eds. *Social Aspects of Aging* (Durham, N.C.: Duke University Press 1966) p. 55–74.

165. George, L. K. and Maddox, G. L. "Subjective Adaptation to Loss of the Work Role: A Longitudinal Study." *Journal of Gerontology* 32:4 (1977) p. 456–462.

166. Rabkin and Struening. "Life Events, Stress and Illness."

167. Costa, P. T. and McCrae, R. R. "Age Differences in Personality Structure: A Cluster Analytic Approach." *Journal of Gerontology* 31:5 (1976) p. 564–570.

168. Bell, T. "Relationship between Social Involvement and Feeling Old among Residents in Homes for the Aged." *Journal of Gerontology* 22:1 (1967) p. 17–22.

169. Cumming, E. "Engagement with an Old Theory." *International Journal of Psychiatry* 6 (1975) p. 187–191.

170. Williams, L. M. "A Concept of Loneliness in the Elderly." *Journal of the American Geriatrics Society* 25:4 (1978) p. 183–187.

171. HEW, National Institute of Mental Health. *Research on the Mental Health of the Aging* (Rockville, Md.: Division of Special Mental Health Programs, Center for Studies of the Mental Health of the Aging, Pub. No. ADM 77–379 1977).

172. Lohman, N. "Correlations of Life Satisfaction, Morale and Adjustment Measures." *Journal of Gerontology* 32:1 (1977) p. 73–75.

173. Burnside, I. M. "Multiple Losses in the Aged: Implications for Nursing Care." *The Gerontologist* 13:2 (1973) p. 157–162.

174. Barney, J. L. "The Prerogative of Choice in Long-Term Care." *The Gerontologist* 17:4 (1977) p. 309–314.

175. Sandler, R.B. "Long Term Care and the Single Status." *Long Term Care and Health Services Administration Quarterly* 2:4 (1978) p. 287–291.

176. Shanas, E. "The Family as a Social Support System in Old Age." *The Gerontologist* 19:2 (1979) p. 169–174.

177. Butler, R. N. and Lewis, M. L. *Aging and Mental Health* (St. Louis : The C. V. Mosby Co. 1973).

178. Trela, J. E. "Social Class and Association Membership: An Analysis of Age-Graded and Non-Age-Graded Voluntary Participation." *Journal of Gerontology* 31:2 (1976) p. 198–203.

179. MacDonald, M. L. "Environmental Programming for the Socially Isolated Aging." *The Gerontologist* 18:4 (August 1978) p. 350–354.

180. Atchley, R. C. "Selected Social and Psychological Differences between Men and Women in Later Life." *Journal of Gerontology* 31:2 (1976) p. 204–211.

181. Reid, D. W., Haas, G. and Hawkings, D. "Locus of Desired Control and Positive Self-Concept of the Elderly." *Journal of Gerontology* 32:4 (1977) p. 441–450.

182. Lamy, P. P. "Consider All Factors When Treating the Elderly." *Long Term Care and Health Services Administration Quarterly* 3:3 (September 1979) p. 194–202.

183. Roff, L. L. and Klemmack, D. L. "Sexual Activity among Older Persons: A Comparative Analysis of Appropriateness." *Research on Aging* 1:3 (September 1979) p. 389–399.

184. Botwinick, J. *Aging and Behavior* (New York: Springer Publishing Co. 1973).

185. Brody, E. M. *Long Term Care of Older People: A Practical Guide* (New York: Human Sciences Press 1977).

186. Farrar, M., Ryder, M. B. and Blenkner, M. "Social Work Responsibility in Nursing Home Care." *Social Casework* 45 (1964) p. 527–533.

187. Killian, J. "Effects of Geriatric Transfers on Mortality Rates." *Social Work* 15 (1970) p. 19–26.

188. Blenkner, M. "Environmental Change and the Aging Individual." *The Gerontologist* 7:2, Part I (1967) p. 101–105.

189. Stotsky, B. A. "A Controlled Study of Factors in the Successful Adjustment of Mental Patients to Nursing Homes." *American Journal of Psychiatry* 123 (1967) p. 1243–1251.

190. Gurel, L. et al. "Patients in Nursing Homes: Multidisciplinary Characteristics and Outcomes." *Journal of the American Medical Association* 213 (July 6, 1970) p. 73–77.

191. Pino, C. J., Rosica, L. M. and Carter, J. "The Differential Effects of Relocation on Nursing Home Patients." *The Gerontologist* 18:2 (1978) p. 167–172.

192. Sherwood, S. et al. "Pre-Institutional Factors as Predictors of Adjustment to a Long-Term Care Facility." *International Journal of Aging and Human Development* 5 (1974) p. 95–105.

193. Kavaler, F. "The Geriatric Patient Is More Than an Aged Person." *Long Term Care and Health Services Administration Quarterly* 1:2 (1977) p. 116–123.

194. Morris, J. N. "Changes in Morale Experienced by Elderly Institutional Applicants along the Institutional Path." *The Gerontologist* 15:4 (1975) p. 345–349.

195. York, J. L. and Calsyn, R. J. "Family Involvement in Nursing Homes." *The Gerontologist* 17:6 (1977) p. 500–505.

196. Bennett, R. and Nahemow, L. "Institutional Totality and Criteria of Social Adjustment in Residential Settings for the Aged." *Journal of Social Issues* 21 (1965) p. 44–78.

197. Newman, E. S., Sherman, E. and Sherman, S. R. "Residential Life Space: A Training Program Session for Administrators Using the Andragogical Approach." *Long Term Care and Health Services Administration Quarterly* 2:3 (1978) p. 231–237.

198. Noelker, L. and Harel, Z. "Predictors of Well Being and Survival among Institutionalized Aged." *The Gerontologist* 18:6 (1978) p. 562–567.

199. Schulz, R. "Effect of Control and Predictability on the Physical and Psychological Well-Being of the Institutionalized Aged." *Journal of Personality and Social Psychology* 33 (1976) p. 563–573.

200. Mishara, B. and Kastenbaum, R. "Self-Injurious Behavior and Environmental Changes in the Institutionalized Elderly." *Aging and Human Development* 4:2 (1973) p. 133–145.

201. Nelson, F. L. "Religiosity and Self-Destructive Crises in the Institutionalized Elderly." *Suicide and Life Threatening Behavior* 7:2 (1977) p. 67–74.

202. Meerloo, J. "Hidden Suicide" in Resnik, H. L., ed. *Suicidal Behaviors: Diagnosis and Management* (Boston: Little, Brown and Co. 1968).

203. Shneidman, E. S. "Orientations toward Death: A Vital Aspect of the Study of Lives" in White, R., ed. *The Study of Lives* (New York: Prentice-Hall 1963).

204. Kastenbaum, R. and Mishara, B. "Premature Death and Self-Injurious Behavior in Old Age." *Geriatrics* 26:7 (1971) p. 71–81.

205. Lieberman, M. "Adaptive Processes in Late Life" in Datan, N. and Ginsberg, L., eds. *Life Span Developmental Psychology* (New York: Academic Press 1975).

206. Lazarus. *Psychological Stress and the Coping Process.*

207. Ibid. p. 22.

Combating Myth: A Conceptual Framework for Analyzing the Stress of Motherhood

Mariann C. Lovell, R.N., M.S.N.
Instructor, School of Nursing
Wright State University
Dayton, Ohio

Dorothy L. Fiorino, R.N., M.S.N.
Assistant Director of Nurses
for General Pediatrics
Children's Medical Center
Dayton, Ohio

THE MYTH OF MOTHERHOOD: CONCEPTUAL AND THEORETICAL REVIEW

Motherhood is so entangled with mythical thinking that it is difficult to sort out myth from reality. Myths appeal to opinions and not to facts. If one happens not to agree with a particular myth, one cannot disprove it, but only disagree or, more wisely, attempt to change the focus of the argument.[1] A more effective method of dispelling myths is to analyze them over and over until the myths lose power over people's minds, feelings and behavior. However, too few people can deal with myths in this manner. Perhaps this is the reason "the mother myth" is so difficult to approach rationally. An understanding of the characteristics basic to myths can provide insights necessary for examining the manner in which mythical thinking influences the health status of mothers.

Patai, anthropologist and mythologist, defines myths as dramatic stories that form

108 a sacred charter authorizing the continuance of ancient institutions, customs, rites and beliefs. Once a myth becomes established, it rapidly becomes traditional by serving as an example to be emulated, a precedent to be repeated and thereby reaffirmed.[2] Patai explains the mutual reinforcement phenomenon between myths and sociocultural patterns: new myths create new sociocultural patterns, and conversely new customs and social situations create new myths.

Janeway's view of myths is congruent with Patai's, and she applies it to the experience of motherhood, stating that the "heightened emphasis on the mother role has been making women nervous."[1(p152)] This emphasis has led to doubts among women about their ability to be the conceptualized "good mother." One of the main problems with motherhood is that women cannot change their minds about motherhood if they find out they are not good at it. Little or no training is provided for mothering, and no preview experience is available. Doubts about motherhood are not discussed openly, so each mother assumes that she is the only person with such doubts. Each mother assumes she has missed out on some instinctive knowledge or expertise somewhere. Since she is seemingly at fault, she had best keep quiet and suffer the guilt accompanying her failures and defects. Janeway suggests that these myths shaping our thinking are best understood as tendencies, limiting factors and unexpected rigidities of feeling.[1]

Conflicting Messages

Conflicting messages inherent in myths about motherhood abound today in all areas of mass communication, professional and lay literature, magazines and newspapers, movies, television and radio. We read and hear statistics confirming the fact that more and more mothers are working outside the home, but television programs continue to portray Mom at home with an apron on, waiting for Johnnie to come home. Women's magazines are filled with advice to mothers. Self-help books by "experts" in every field (except the field of mothering itself) fill drug store and supermarket shelves. The fact that none of the "theories" found in these works agree on the preferred method of mothering and that Grandma disagrees with them all adds to the confusion of motherhood.

Mothers are torn between their inadequacies on the one hand and their innate natural affinity for mothering on the other. If a mother works outside the home, either out of necessity or desire, her tension, guilt feelings, conflicts and concerns about

Mothers are torn between their inadequacies on the one hand and their innate natural affinity for mothering on the other.

being a good mother increase. Working mothers are expected to be Supermoms as well as Superwives and Superhousekeepers while being superproductive and conscientious at their jobs.

The cold war being waged between mothers who work and those who do not work outside the home has a deep effect on the members of both groups. In short, mothers are criticized if they do and criticized if they do not—a criticism coming from experts, family members and the public in general. Most mothers do not have the powers necessary for withstanding the constant pressures bombarding the psychic structures or their bodies.[3-6]

Myth as a Means of Control

Both the power of mothers and their powerlessness remain mysteries. Adrienne Rich, poet and author, describes how the possibility of power for mothers has historically been befogged by sentimentality and mystification. The concept of the power of the mother is, first of all, to give or to withhold nourishment and warmth, to give or withhold survival itself. Nowhere does a woman possess such literal power over life and death as she does in motherhood.[3] Thus the power of the mother is both feared and dreaded by men and women alike. Because of this fear and dread, the power of the mother, especially within patriarchal societies, must be controlled.[7]

Mythical thinking is a major means of controlling mothers. In addition to this force, Bernard elaborates upon the means by which child-rearing patterns are used to control the lives of mothers. Bernard emphasizes that the method of dealing with child-rearing in this country today does not compare well with methods found elsewhere. By assigning sole responsibility of child care to the mother and then isolating her away from family and friends, demanding that she provide complete and continuous care, we are harming both mothers and children. Isolation of the mother is a new and unique child-rearing practice and, according to Bernard, is possibly the worst. She states, "It is as though we had selected the worst features of all the ways motherhood is structured around the world and combined them to produce our current design."[5(p9)]

Oppression and the Stress of Motherhood

Rich differentiates between two meanings of motherhood. One meaning encompasses the potential relationship of a woman with her child. The other meaning is the institution of motherhood which is created by patriarchal society to ensure that the potential of all women remain under male control.[3] It is the oppressive nature of motherhood as it is currently perceived that makes mothering the stressful role that it is, impairing the health of women and children in this country.

Understanding the oppression and its relationship to the stress experienced by mothers provides the key to resolving the health impairment of women in mothering roles. The most clear and comprehensive theoretical work on oppression is found in the book *Pedagogy of the Oppressed* by Freire.[8] Freire is a Brazilian educator who developed his theory of oppression while living and working with oppressed peoples, mostly peasants in Third World countries. Freire explains, "Any situation in which 'A' objectively exploits 'B' or hinders his [her] pursuit of self-affirmation as a responsible person is one of oppression."[8(p40)] Oppression is dehumanizing, both for the oppressed and for the oppressor. According to Freire, a basic element of the relationships between the oppressed and the oppressor is "prescription"—the imposition of one person's choice upon another person. Such prescription leads to conformity and adaptation to the ideas of the oppressor.[8]

110   By accepting and adapting to the reality of the oppressor, the oppressed have an impaired perception of themselves. The oppressed have a deep-seated fear of freedom because this freedom would require rejection of the image of the oppressor, and would necessitate acting with autonomy and responsibility. The internalization of the ideas and opinions of the oppressor by the oppressed leads to self-depreciation. The oppressed feel they know nothing because the oppressor knows all. Rather than strike out at the oppressor, the oppressed fight among themselves, becoming passive, alienated, unaware and dependent. Utilizing naive thinking, myths are accepted—myths that usurp decision-making power. For the oppressed, reality is perceived as a closed world with no exit. Although the situation of the oppressed is not helpless, the oppressed individual's narrow perception of the world causes feelings of powerlessness and hopelessness. Thus changing this narrow perception of reality becomes the basis for intervention.[8]

According to Freire, the situation of the oppressed is one of violence, a violence that is sweetened by false generosity since it does not allow for "humanness." Once an oppressive relationship is established, violence has already begun. Applying the concept of oppressive violence specifically to motherhood, Rich suggests that violence is the heart of maternal darkness.[3] She explains that "mother" is associated with "home," and people like to believe that home is a private place. People do not think of the penalties imposed on mothers who have tried to live their lives according to a different plan.[3]

> *The medical establishment robs mothers of the very act of natural birth. The "experts"—almost all male—tell mothers how they should behave and feel.*

The fine arts depict mothers in unnatural serenity or resignation. The medical establishment robs mothers of the very act of natural birth. The "experts"—almost all male—tell mothers how they should behave and feel. Psychoanalysts dwell on the harm that mothers do, while fostering belief in the myth that the work of motherhood suits women by nature. The power stolen from mothers and the power withheld from them in the name of "motherhood" is indeed oppressive violence.[3]

Miller refers to oppressors and oppressed as "dominants" and "subordinates." Through her book, Miller explains the manner in which women are placed into the subordinate role through societal expectations and myths. She maintains that the role of child rearing has been considered the job of the subordinate woman, and is hardly viewed as a function of importance. Miller points out that helping other human beings to develop has been cast into a lesser task category, and that this diminishment has led to "many psychological consequences for children of both sexes."[9(p40)]

Real versus Mythical Power

Although often overlooked and minimized, the responsibility inherent in mothering is not an easy one for mothers to exercise. A major part of the stress accompanying motherhood stems from the fact that a mother's thought, feelings and behaviors have lifelong effects on children. As this fact relates to the child's fantasy and developmental needs, both the real power and the mythical power of the mother become problematic.

Within the context of society's predominant sexual arrangements, Dinnerstein analyzes the results of U.S. child-rearing practices. She maintains that by having early child care provided solely by women, oppressive relationships are set up which extend throughout the entire lifetime of males and females. Both boy infants and girl infants are totally dependent on the mother and completely in her power. The future relationships of men and women never overcome this complete dependency on a woman, and the inevitable struggles to deal with her overwhelming power shapes all of adult life. As a result of the system of exclusive nurturing of infants by women, adult life is emotionally charged with unresolved infantile yearnings and conflicts.[7]

Dinnerstein believes that the confrontation between mother and child that is so necessary for the development of the child's own will is a vital but dangerous endeavor. It is here that we can observe the confrontation between power and weakness: the mother's will nurtures, stimulates and shelters the growth of the child's own will. At this point the mother has two equally dangerous options, both of which place the child in emotional jeopardy. She may crush her "opponent's" pride by dwelling on her child's early failures instead of minimizing them. This may take

the form of insisting that the child "obey" (acquiesce to) the mother's commands whatever the cost. The other option is to give way too far, thus leaving the child in possession of an empty field. The latter can take the form of a "hollow victory" for the child (for example, a monotone "O.K. Right. You win."). Dinnerstein sees this double risk of childhood as the basis for the childhood fantasy wish to "keep female will in live captivity, obediently energetic, fiercely protective of its captor's pride, ready always to vitalize his projects with its magic maternal blessing and to support them with its concrete, self-abnegating help."[7(p169)]

CONCEPTS FOR ANALYZING WOMEN'S HEALTH

The above theoretical sources suggest that motherhood, as institutionalized in today's society, imposes stressors which impair the health of women who mother. The authors propose that the use of traditional approaches to assessing the health of women using "obstetrical," "gynecological" or "pediatric" conceptual viewpoints actually obscures or reinforces these stressors. The following concepts, which can be derived from the above sources, can be used for assessing, categorizing and analyzing women's health data to determine if, indeed, this proposal is valid.

Nonmotivating pain is physical or emotional discomfort that has become chronic and so much a part of every day life that it is almost accepted as part of the human condition. This pain does not precipitate change in the individual's status, but rather leads to such behaviors

112 as the use of artificial aids, self-depreciation or self-destruction.[3,7,10,11]

A sense of powerlessness is related to nonmotivating pain, but is differentiated by a vague awareness of being subordinated to fate or chance. While nonmotivating pain does not precipitate action or change, a sense of powerlessness does precipitate some degree of action or change. However, the action or change is motivated not from within the individual, but from advice from experts, relatives or other authorities. The individual, while acting, has a sense of being weighed down by subordination to fate or chance, with little personal power to control or direct the actions or the outcomes of these actions.[4,12]

The good mother/bad mother conformity concept involves conforming behavior which is based on the myth of the "good mother," and at the same time behavior which reflects an attempt to overcome the myth of the "bad mother." Friere incorporates this concept with oppression, and in so doing unknowingly tailors it to motherhood: "Functionally, oppression is domesticating."[8] Oppressive reality socially isolates women who are mothers within the privacy of their own home, entrapping them in their ascribed role. As a result, mothers fear their own freedom, for seeking to free their own consciousness would require disarranging and investigating their ascribed role.[8,10,13]

An external source of identity results in a grossly distorted concept of self (or a lack of self-concept). An unauthentic being emerges—a being who is not "real," but a copy of others. The source of the mother's identity may be extracted from a wide range of external sources, including her husband, her mother, "experts," her neighbors and, as McBride states, all too often her children.[4]

ANALYSIS OF CLINICAL DATA

In order to determine if clinical data derived from nursing assessments of mothers provide support for this conceptual view of motherhood, the authors reviewed their records of interactions with 26 mothers, records obtained over a nine-month period. The mothers were the total populations of two groups of women who were the authors' independent clients. They joined the groups voluntarily for the purpose of exploring everyday problems in mothering. None of the mothers joined the groups with a stated "unusual" or "difficult" child-rearing or personal problem.

The analysis of the data was focused on determining if there is indeed sufficient clinical evidence to warrant systematic research on the stress of motherhood using the four concepts described above as a frame or reference.

Nonmotivating Pain

The records reflected an overwhelming degree of nonmotivating pain. All of the mothers indicated a perception of physical health that was less than optimal. Eighteen of 20 mothers who were asked about their participation in physical fitness or exercise programs reported having no established regimen. All of the mothers revealed vague

Eighteen of 20 mothers who were asked about their participation in physical fitness or exercise programs reported having no established regimen.

feelings of discomfort, not really bad enough to be classified as illness but bad enough to make them qualify their health states. One woman summed up her feelings as "I do feel tired, achy and not 'with it' most of the time, but I know this is my own fault—I am not really sick." Another mother stated, "I always feel like I'm about to come down with something, but I never actually come down with it." This woman had mentioned her complaint to her physician, who prescribed a round of drugs for "depression." She felt that she must continue to take the drugs so that she would not feel worse. In general, the use of drugs, alcohol or tobacco, excessive or inadequate food intake and the use of other forms of artificial aids were common.

Self-destructive behaviors that were exhibited included excessive weight maintenance over long periods of time, disregard for dietary restrictions which had been suggested on the basis of medical history of stroke or heart disease, smoking and spending most of the day in a nightgown and robe. Many of the mothers were able to verbally identify an awareness that their behavior patterns were not conducive to their health status, but felt guilty and overwhelmed by the struggle to overcome or minimize the behaviors. The tone was one of self-depreciation for not being able to overcome the struggle.

Sense of Powerlessness

All of the mothers expressed some concern or confusion about their parenting skills. They frequently expressed a deference to others in making decisions about child rearing, and a feeling that they rarely made the "right" decisions about parenting. These mothers were confused about conflicting advice given by grandparents, neighbors, medical personnel and often husbands. One of their major concerns was that the children "come out all right," but none of the mothers felt certain that her children could be predicted to meet her expectations of "all right" better than other children. All of the mothers in one group had attended at least two lecture series offered by the local school psychologist on "how to be a better parent." They reported frequently seeking advice from books written by "experts" on all aspects of child care.

All of the women studied saw themselves as the least important member of the family. The ways in which this was expressed reflected the overwhelming sense of powerlessness that they felt about their lives. They viewed themselves as the persons expected to "make the sacrifice"— whether by eating the squashed donut, taking the least desirable seat, watching the television program someone else chooses or doing the dirtiest job that nobody else will do. Their lack of personal goals, even when questioned directly about their own goals in life, was evident. There were some expressed fleeting desires

114 to "finish my education," "get a job," "use my education," "do something interesting with my life" or "do something for myself," but these types of goals were identified as needing to be deferred until after all of the children were in school or grown. There was generally a tendency to avoid discussing the future.

Good Mother/Bad Mother Conformity

The domestication of the women in these groups, 23 of whom were full-time mothers, was clearly evident. Conformity to the mythical "norms" of a "good mother" and attempts to overcome "bad mother" myths were expressed frequently in response to a wide variety of questions and discussion cues. When requested to list family members in order of their "importance," all of the mothers listed either their husbands or children first or second, and themselves third. In a discussion among six of the women, all made derogatory comments about mothers who are employed outside the home. All of the 26 mothers stated that they loved their children and wanted to be home with them.

The women reported that their children were the source of most of their activity during the day, but they reported very little actual personal contact or meaningful interaction between themselves and their children. Contrived busyness was pervasive, leaving little satisfying personal time or time for real family interaction. The things that keep the women so busy centered around their children's or their husband's activities, and the mothers were left with only a superficial involvement of their own in community activities or in meaningful friendships.

The women sensed that something was missing in their lives, but were uncertain about what this was and were unhappy with themselves for feeling this way. None of the women expressed a desire to explore the nature of the gender arrangements that predominate their lives, even though they could clearly identify the dramatic differences in their own lives and those of their husbands. Despite their confusion over how to be good mothers, they all viewed themselves as "good" mothers, and felt that their primary commitment in life was to their children, at least until the children were grown.

Efforts to overcome the "bad mother" myth were paradoxically evident. If anything about their home or children or

If anything about their home or children or husband was not right, the women tended to express the feeling that it was their fault.

husband was not right, the women tended to express the feeling that it was their fault: they did not keep the house as clean as it should have been, they caused or did not prevent whatever problems their children were having, they were neglecting the husband in some manner, they even failed to train the dog properly.

External Source of Identity

Some of the data cited in support of each of the preceding concepts also support the concept of external source of identity. The women studied viewed themselves as the least important members of the family. Their stated goals, even when questioned explicitly about their personal goals, were usually family goals or goals related to their children. When asked about their personal goals before motherhood, most of the women stated that they either set out to "get married and have children," or that they just assumed that some day they would get married and have a family. The mothers spoke about wanting or having an education or career before marriage, or about wanting an education or career after the children were grown. However, none of the women mentioned other forms of self-fulfillment or personal growth and satisfaction apart from their husbands or children, such as developing artistic or musical talent, reading for pleasure, or developing personally staisfying relationships outside the family.

In summary, the data obtained from these groups of mothers using nursing assessments appear to confirm the validity of the conceptual framework described above. While the degree to which each mother experienced the stress of motherhood varied widely, the data for each of the proposed concepts are significant enough to suggest that stress in the motherhood experience is not an isolated, occasional perception. The source of stress experienced by the mothers appears to stem from the socially ascribed form of mothering that is perpetuated by myth. The data summarized suggest that this myth is self-perpetuating—creating and reflecting the lack of personal motivation,

sense of power and sense of self that are needed to take steps to decrease the stress.

IMPLICATIONS FOR NURSING RESEARCH

The experience with these groups of mothers reveals that nursing research is vitally important if nurses are to fully understand the stress of motherhood and to further develop theory which can be used in providing nursing care for mothers and children. The clinical evidence suggests that the conceptual framework described above has potential empirical validity. Systematic study to confirm this empirical validity is needed as a first step in a research program designed to study the stress of motherhood.

Additional questions which need to be addressed are:

- To what extent do mothers experience nonmotivating pain, a sense of powerlessness, good mother/bad mother conformity or external source of identity?
- To what extent do these phenomena affect the well-being of women?
- What are the variables which determine the degree of stress experienced by mothers?
- How does the mother's health status affect the health of children?
- In what ways do men contribute to the stress of motherhood?
- How have nurses in the past, and how do nurses now contribute to either decreasing or increasing the stress of motherhood?
- What nursing interventions are effec-

116   tive in decreasing the stress of motherhood?

nursing care with mothers indicates that these questions can be addressed. Empirical data are available; creative systematic research is needed to provide understanding of and prediction in these areas of concern.

While these questions are stated in general abstract terms, experience in direct

REFERENCES

1. Janeway E. *Man's World: Woman's Place, A Study in Social Mythology* (New York: William Morrow and Co., Inc. 1971).
2. Patai, R. *Myth and Modern Man* (Englewood Cliffs, N.J.: Prentice-Hall, Inc. 1972).
3. Rich, A. *Of Woman Born: Motherhood as Experience and Institution* (New York: W. W. Norton & Co. 1976).
4. McBride, A. B. *The Growth and Development of Mothers* (New York: Harper and Row, Publishers 1973).
5. Bernard, J. *The Future of Motherhood* (New York: The Dial Press 1974).
6. Chodorow, N. *The Reproduction of Mothering: Psychoanalysis and the Sociology of Gender* (Berkeley: University of California Press 1978).
7. Dinnerstein, D. *The Mermaid and the Minotaur: Sexual Arrangements and Human Malaise* (New York: Harper and Row, Publishers 1976).
8. Freire, P. *Pedagogy of the Oppressed* (New York: The Seabury Press 1968).
9. Miller, J. B. *Toward a New Psychology of Women* (Boston: Beacon Press, 1977).
10. Janov, A. *The Primal Scream: Primal Therapy—The Cure for Neurosis* (New York: Dell Publishing Co. 1970).
11. Laing, R. D. *The Politics of Experience* (New York: Random House, Inc. 1967).
12. Ehrenreich, B. and English, D. *For Her Own Good: 150 Years of the Experts' Advice to Women* (Garden City, N.Y.: Anchor Press/Doubleday, 1978).
13. deBeauvoir, S. *The Second Sex* (New York: Alfred A. Knopf 1964).

Part III
The Stress of Illness

Emotional Aspects of Dialysis and Transplantation

The Reverend Albert L. Galloway, Jr.
Associate Chaplain (Service)
Indiana University Medical Center
Indianapolis, Indiana

IT WAS NOT many years ago that most kidney diseases were identified as Bright's Disease. Patients with kidney disease were advised to set their houses in order and their families counseled to make the patients comfortable and prepare for their death. Less than 20 years ago, hardly a family had not become acquainted with this disease either within the family's own ranks or its close circle of friends. In the late 1950s the twin treatment modalities of dialysis and transplantation began to emerge from concept, through tentative beginnings, to developmental programs, arriving where they are today. Now there are highly specialized teams working in complex programs, which in turn are part of regional networks interlaced across the country. Scientific data, research results, technical innovations, patient successes and failures, even kidneys are traded back and forth

120

through regional and national programs to ultimately rehabilitate the consumer—the patient with end-stage renal disease.

The state of the art of dialysis and transplantation has come a long way from those early days when a grief stricken relative, having lost a loved one to kidney disease, gifted the local hospital with a new "artificial kidney" machine. In the past, those new machines were promptly hidden away in the nearest closet because no one knew how to use them. A few bold surgeons began thumbing their noses at the rejection mechanism built into humans by developing the techniques for transplantation using the only patient population that could survive the invasion of their bodies by foreign tissue, namely, those with identical twin donors. A combination of conscience and curiosity led physicians to bring the machines and techniques out of the closet and begin offering them to a wider clientele.

The physicians of this transition period were bold, aggressive and adventurous. The patients were a rather select group, noted not only for their medical needs but also for their cooperativeness, goal orientation and ability to see a commitment through to its conclusion. This was necessary because a limited dialysis capacity mandated that "dialysis slots" not be tied up indefinitely—others were waiting in line. The commitment was to dialysis *and* transplantation, and an air of urgency surrounded the unit. If for no

other reason than habit, this aura still lingers to some degree.

Thus from a humble beginning there developed vast programs supported by government dollars and staffed by highly trained professionals and para-professionals attempting to coordinate all their efforts into a working unit. This unit delivers effective health care to as many end-stage renal disease patients as can benefit from the twin therapeutic modalities of dialysis and transplantation. Today, tens of thousands of people are acquainted with both treatment modalities, and this number is increasing. The vast growth of these programs across the country is attributable not only to improved techniques, better equipment and accumulated experience, but also to two other major developments.

One of these developments is "home dialysis" in which a patient, after a training period with a partner in the dialysis center, has the machinery and related equipment installed in his home. Supplies are delivered directly to the home, and dialysis is performed there on a regular basis. Hospital visits are limited to periodic clinic evaluations and "back-up dialysis" when complications warrant. The effect of this development has been to place large patient populations "in orbit" from the center, freeing up the main units and creating large pools of persons awaiting transplantation. It effectively removed them from easy accessibility to the supportive services that had grown up as an adjunct to the basic medical care of the center. It also doubled the number of people under stress, since for each patient involved with a home dialysis machine, there was now a partner (usually a mate, parent or sibling) sharing the stress of the patient and experiencing problems unique to himself and his role.

The other development that radically altered the character of dialysis and transplantation programs was the Social Security Administration's assumption in 1972 of responsibility for payment of 80% of the cost of treating end-stage renal disease by dialysis, transplantation or both. It is estimated that this coverage extends to as much as 90% of the general population. Dialysis populations have boomed, magnifying not only the number of patients in emotional as well as physical stress, but also extending that stress to staff and indeed institutions as well.

The literature is well stocked with articles diagnosing the stress experienced by patients in dialysis and transplantation programs. Attempts (largely unsuccessful) have been made to determine personality correlates of the "successful" dialysis patient. Researchers have examined suicidal behavior in the patient population, and even the psychological significance of urination has been explored. Observations have been made of staff and patient reactions, and various treatment and intervention approaches have been attempted. Most have had some success, especially in the particular patient populations in which they arose.

Perhaps that is the key to successful stress management—treatment programs adapted to the peculiarities of the center and its people.

THE PROGRAM

The first thing a patient might notice when entering a dialysis/transplant program is that he is committing his medical well-being not to a single physician, as has been his custom, but to a whole battery of experts, physicians and nonphysicians. He also finds himself in relationship to many other patients with varying degrees of seniority in the program. In effect, he is joining an already existing family in which he must discover, declare and maintain his own space. Like an adoptive child, entry into the family depends on the accepting attitude of the parents. Similarly, continuance in the good graces of the parents requires obedience to the rules of the home.

The patient is referred from his home community to the program by the "local medical doctor," perhaps first passing through the hands of a regional specialist. The patients first exposure to the program is through the particular nephrologist to whom he has been referred. Some go no further, being successfully treated by diet and medication and returned home. Others are considered candidates for dialysis and/or transplantation, either now or in the forseeable future, and are introduced to the rest of the team or official family. However benevolent the team may perceive itself as being, the patient often

122 views it a formidable panel of judges who hold his life in the balance.

The team members come to see the patient one by one as he attempts to rest in the strange bed in the strange hospital. Each one talks to him or examines him from his own professional point of view, attempting to understand the patient from the necessities of his own discipline for feedback to the rest of the team. The pieces are then put together to form the best possible composite picture. The patient, of course, is piecing together his own puzzle, sorting out personalities, figuring out where the pieces fit and sometimes who he must please and who is less important.

Not all teams are alike. Some teams have more members than others, and not every member sees every patient. However, the resources available to most teams for the assessment of candidates for dialysis in all transplant programs are similar.

The members of the team typically seen by patients referred to the Indiana University Medical Center, include a surgeon, nephrologist, business and social service staff, a chaplain, psychiatrist or psychologist, researcher, immunologist, and house staff. The surgeon may be the transplant or vascular surgeon who must determine if the patient can withstand the rigors of the known surgical interventions. Particular focus is on the vascular system's ability to accept blood-access surgery procedures with reasonable hope of success. The urological surgeons are also part of this group. They must determine if the urological system is intact, with particular reference to its readiness for transplantation surgery.

Sometimes corrective surgery is indicated. The nephrologist of the department of medicine has already been mentioned, and at this phase he is the primary physician for the patient and usually acts as his presentor to the committee. The business interests of the institution must be represented for the simple reason that the bill must be paid. Social service often deals with this aspect, but is also concerned with evaluating the family constellation as a functioning unit and support group, evaluating the adequacy of the home situation for potential home dialysis and interviewing the potential dialysis partner.

The chaplain, in addition to providing pastoral care, may evaluate the patient in terms of his motivation and relationships. A psychiatrist or psychologist may be used to determine the presence of underlying psychopathology that could inhibit the patient from cooperating in his own treatment program and suggest or provide therapy when indicated. Research interests may also be represented in the group. The immunologist, although a member of the department of medicine, deserves separate mention by virtue of the pivotal position played in tissue typing all patients and families as well as cadaver tissue obtained. Although often less visible, this department's mystique can prompt a unique positive regard in the patient's eyes. Finally, house staff members are also represented, not only because of their relationship to the patient, but also because the experience in the committee function and process may be important to their future professional careers.

To varying degrees patients perceive themselves being weighed in the balance by this formidable group of experts. They wonder how they will be judged. Will they measure up? What is the standard? Many have heard stories of patients judged by their social worth, their community involvement, their potential as future taxpayers and worse. Indeed, some early committees were forced to use such criteria, but quickly moved away from such judgments.

The group uses criteria based on the knowledge that the program requires a level of self-care and management unique to health care delivery and an awareness of just what is available inside the house. Hence, in piecing together its puzzle, it raised two questions: (1) Can we join the patient in *his* pursuit of health and wholeness? (2) Can the patient reasonably benefit from the therapies we have to offer? Admission (adoption) into the program rests on an affirmative reply to those questions.

THE PATIENTS

Dialysis

Patients quickly perceive the necessity of seeking approval from the team. Subterfuge abounds. Symptoms may be masked, financial resources denied, marital conflicts minimized, even literacy lied about. Anything to gain admission (adoption)! Little regard is paid to the criticism and pressure the patients will surely have to endure and the guilt they will have to bear when the deception is uncovered. And it is not a bad stratagem, for, once in the program, quitting is as difficult as joining was perceived to be.

The surgical implantation of the shunt (later, fistula) is an outer and visible sign of an inner and (almost) spiritual relationship signifying unto all the joining of this patient to this program. With the exception of the almost miraculous return of renal function, the only way one can exit from the program is through death.

Following admission into the first steps of the program conservative medical management may continue until dialysis is required. Some surgical interventions may be necessary. Certainly not all patients require all the procedures, but neither do many escape without several. Blood-access problems are common and often become a focal point of stress for the patient who sees himself accumulating a series of scars on his arms and legs. Cosmetic concerns set in and can be particularly upsetting to young women. The ugly bulge of the fistula, the care-requiring plastic loop of the shunt and the scars of previous suture lines symbolize to the patient his bondage to the machine.

And bondage is what he often feels. Once he has entered dialysis, he takes up life with his machine. Whether the patient is trained for home dialysis or managed "in-center," he now enters into a relationship with his "Machine." The machine becomes a part of him and he a part of the machine. He sees his blood flowing to it and returning to his body.

124 He knows that without it he cannot live and is grateful. He also knows that it consumes a significant portion of his waking hours (18 to 20 hours per week), and he hates it. One patient while blessing the physicians because they were "children of God doing His work," cursed the machine as a human invention. Another saw his being tied to the machine as parallel to the old Western movies he attended as a child. In these the hero would be bonded at the wrist to the villainous Indian and, each armed with a knife in the free hand, would fight to the death. It is not surprising that one patient "killed" his machine in a fit of frustration by putting a bullet through its conductivity meter. More often, nicknames such as Lurch, Igor and the Tin Vampire reveal the patients suspicion that the machine is macabre and almost human.

The artificial kidney is not a complete substitute for the real thing. Although it can take off accumulated water weight, remove unwanted chemicals and other substances and free the patient for another few days of reasonably normal life, it cannot restore wasted muscle mass, halt bone deterioration, replace lost blood cells or return sexual function. The patient may experience, in addition to his cosmetic concerns, great sadness over lost body image and function. Moreover, his need for regular dialysis and the overwhelming tiredness caused by his chronic anemia may take him out of the working pool. This can strike at the very heart of the patient's sense of identity, for most of us know ourselves by how we look and what we do. It is particularly devastating for the male whose sense of identity is intimately involved with, if not solely dependent on, his ability to function as breadwinner and as a sexual being. The problem may be slightly easier for women, because our society permits them a wider range of emotional expression, has taught them that it is acceptable to be dependent and does not define their sexual role in "performance" terminology.

Most people manage to rise to the great crises of life. The difficulties of patients on dialysis stem more from the chronicity of their situation. Over a period of time, as dependency is required and self-governance preached, as deep weariness moves in and normal activity is encouraged, erosion begins to take place. The standard of living may have to be compromised. Role reversal may occur in the family. Children may begin to show the strain by developing bad habits or bad behavior. Loss of self-esteem leads to loss of the esteem of others. Lost libido can set couples to drifting apart. Hopes for the present and dreams for the future may have to be shelved for the time being or scrapped altogether. The patient wonders if it is worth it at all and thinks about death. Some try to halt dialysis, but face massive levels of guilt when their families learn of it and massive walls of resistance from the staff which is, after all, dedicated by oath and inclination to saving lives, not losing them. A few do quit, however, and a few more commit suicide, some actively, but most by more passive means such as gross dietary or fluid indiscretions. The vast majority press on, coping by whatever mechanisms are available to them.

The chief and often principle mechanism of coping is denial. The patient attempts to live normally as if there were no disease and no limitations. After a few close calls, such as salt or water overloading, clever patients learn the technique of "creative cheating." They have, for example, a slice of pizza or ham and a big drink of forbidden liquid just before or in the early phase of dialysis knowing that these foods will be removed by the dialysis machine just before the damage can be done. Best of all, the physician will not be able to tell. This level of denial is valuable, since it works as a self-regulating reward system and contributes to the patient's sense of controlling his own life. Less creative denial, of course, leads to physical penalties and harsh staff (and sometimes fellow patient) criticism.

Some patients cope by regressing to a dependent child-like stage. They withdraw from life and many of its activities and relate to their world as invalids. Although this works for some with extremely understanding and dedicated support systems, it more often incurs the emotional withdrawal of loved ones and the negative judgment of the staff.

Another mechanism is anger. Anger is an emotional stage experienced by anyone experiencing significant loss. Some patients find their anger to be the only expression of autonomy and control in their lives, and it becomes their lifestyle. If their anger is not too violent

and if their families are sufficiently resilient, this can be an adequate adaptation. This is especially true when the staff is not threatened by the anger.

The most successful patient is the one who can perceive dialysis as a necessary part of his life and, while giving it the prominent place it requires, does not grant it priority over other life goals and aspirations. The strongly goal-oriented patient will experience ready acceptance by the staff and most likely have the smoothest course. Problems may occur when he is at a particularly low moment and cannot for a time live up to the image others have of him. He is often placed in a position of high regard and used as a source of inspiration and help for others. He relates to the staff as a peer, and staff members often find it difficult to allow him his emotional lows.

Another person under considerable stress is the partner of the home dialysis patient. This is usually the spouse or parent (sometimes a sibling or offspring), and the problems he experiences are magnifications of those experienced within the family constellation. The dialysis partner is often overlooked by family, friends and staff in their haste to support and aid the patient. As a result he often becomes the "forgotten hero" and becomes resentful and angry. Divorces have occurred and many marriages barely manage to hide the deep rifts that develop.

One partner, at fairly regular intervals, would leave her husband and call from a public phone booth 30 miles away to inform the staff so that they could make other arrangements for the patient. She

126

would assure the staff that she had taken her husband off the machine before she left, but that she could stand it no more. She was always talked out of leaving and endured until her husband eventually died. Her pattern of angry flight and a call for help may have been healthier than the actions of those who flee inwardly from the relationship.

Transplantation

The overwhelming majority of patients yearn to move from a dialysis situation to transplantation. Here the stress is focused on the event of surgery and the immediate postoperative phase when the body's rejection attempts must be met and defeated. Anxiety is high, and the intensity of the care lends itself to dramatic interpretation by the patient.

Patients often speak of successful transplantation as being "born again" in a physical as well as a spiritual sense. It holds the promise of a practically normal life, and the prevailing belief that transplantation is the largest cause of death among dialysis patients does not stay many from seizing the chance when it comes. Their hope is further inspired by the successfully functioning "graduates" they have met, heard about or seen in the transplant clinic.

The stresses of the transplant patient begin with the search in the family for a suitable donor. About 30% of the patients have someone in the family who is an acceptable match. Tension comes to these "potentials" if care is not taken to keep early negotiations confidential. Internal family pressures to donate can be crushing, and the potential for guilt can be mountainous. Careful handling of the donor/donee relationship can obviate later feelings of debt and dependency when the transplant works and guilt when it does not. Care must also be taken to prevent the donor from becoming another "forgotten hero" in the immediate postoperative phase when the drama and attention is quite naturally focused on the recipient.

Most patients require donor tissue from a cadaveric source. In earlier days, when potential donors were moved to the site of the transplant, the waiting patient often grew morose when he realized that he had a heavy investment in the death of another human being. Today, with organs being harvested at many sites and shipped nationwide, anonymity is available. The potential recipient is seldom in the hospital until the kidney has arrived and been typed and some preliminary tests performed.

Hope and optimism follow transplantation. The patient sees an end to all his troubles, and care must be taken to keep him realistically appraised without dampening his hopes. Yet a certain percentage of transplants inevitably fail, and most accept this rather well after a brief and classic grief reaction. The program provides for return to dialysis and perhaps a second chance.

More difficult to manage are the hopes that are not realized even when the transplant is successful. Function may not be all that the patient hoped for. Some dietary and medical restrictions may have to continue. Blood pressure problems may continue, bones may remain weak and sexual function may not return. The successful transplant patient may, because of medication, have problems with weight, acne and cushingoid appearance.

One woman, after an prolonged hospitalization following transplantation, decided on a second honeymoon to celebrate her new beginning. She bought a new nightgown and reserved a motel room to surprise her husband. After dinner she went to prepare herself with a shower, new perfume and her new gown. Taking a final look in the mirror before presenting herself to her waiting husband, it struck her. She was flat where she should be round, and round where she wanted to be flat. She saw stringy hair and a worse case of acne than she had had as a teenager. She sat on the edge of the tub and wept.

The months after transplantation are ones of continuing, if decreasing, anxiety over renal function. Other adjustment problems arise. There is a general period of emotional unwinding that may take several months to complete. Reentry into normal living and readjustment of the family patterns to premorbid status takes time. Since renal transplantation is a recent development, no assurance can be given the patient as to how long his new kidney can work. A little doubt always lingers. The doubt is focused on the regular clinic visits that the patient will make at ever-expanding intervals. Little solid data is available, but observations of almost 200 transplant patients who returned home suggests that a period of six months to a year for readjustment to normalcy is not unrealistic.

Treatment

Treatment modalities for the stresses of the dialysis and transplant patient vary from program to program. Various types of group processes seem to be the most successful, because they combine the resources of informed therapeutic leadership, prophylactic application and group support and pressure. One-to-one therapy, although often successful, smacks of psychotherapeutic first aid and is seldom invoked early enough to head off emotional scarring. It is not economical financially or in terms of the large numbers of patients in need. Home dialysis moved the patient population away from the center at which resources are concentrated and the support group could be assembled. The use of local community resources such as clergy and mental health workers can be less effective because of the stigma of seeking emotional help in the home community, the lack of understanding of the depth of the patient's need and the absence of a peer support group.

THE STAFF

No survey of the emotional factors surrounding a dialysis and transplantation program can be fully scanned without a comment regarding the staff. It is well recognized by such staff groups that the strains on them are legion. There is nothing in the training of physicians and nurses that expressly prepares them for long-term dependence relationships. The family for which they provide care grows larger

128 and more demanding. As they are pressed for more and more services from their patients, they are also compressed by more and more regulations. The physicians react as any human would. They are tempted to lash out in anger and, having done so, withdraw in guilt. The nurses, who spend so much time with the patients in the course of care and training, attempt to protect the patients from such angry outbursts or become possessive of them when they perceive that the physician has yielded his own possession. Members of other involved disciplines react similarly according to their nature and degree of involvement.

The people drawn to work in dialysis and transplantation are often strong willed, highly motivated, intelligent and very dedicated. They have explored frontiers and brought some order out of chaos. They have delivered hope to a group that was, only a few short years ago, hopeless. They have snatched many from the doorway of death and set them on their feet again. Yet the cost to themselves is high.

The careers of physicians in dialysis are not long, and nurses seldom stay for more than one to three years. Something must be done to extend the useful life of these very dedicated and able people. Something must be done to free them to enjoy the satisfaction of work well done. What form this would take is not clear, but evidence suggests that it must involve the staff as a group and requires leadership from someone with no more than one foot in the camp of the renal team.

SUGGESTED READINGS

Abram, H. S. and Wadlington, W. "Selection of Patients for Artificial and Transplanted Organs." *Ann Intern Med* 69:3 (September 1968) pp. 615–620.

Abram, H. S. "The Psychiatrist, the Treatment of Chronic Renal Failure, and the Prolongation of Life: I." *Am J Psychiatry* 124:10 (April 1968) pp. 45–52.

Abram, H. S. "The Psychiatrist, the Treatment of Chronic Renal Failure, and the Prolongation of Life: II." *Am J Psychiatry* 126:2 (August 1969) pp. 43–53.

Abram, H. S., Moore, G. and Westervelt, F. "Suicidal Behavior in Chronic Dialysis Patients." *Am J Psychiatry* 127:9 (March 1971) pp. 119–127.

Abram, H. S. "The Prosthetic Man." *Compr Psychiatry* 11:5 (September 1970) pp. 475–481.

Bagwell, E. "Kidney Transplantation as Viewed by the Donor." *Transplant Proc* 5:2 (June 1973) pp. 1061–1063.

Basch, S. H. "Damaged Self-Esteem and Depression in Organ Transplantation." *Transplant Proc* 5:2 (June 1973) pp. 1125–1127.

Beleil, O. M. "Landmarks in Organ Transplantation—A Historical Review by a Kidney Transplant Recipient." *Transplant Proc* 5:2 (June 1973) pp. 1031–1033.

Bergan, J. J. "Current Risks to the Kidney Transplant Donor." *Transplant Proc* 5:2 (June 1973) pp. 1131–1134.

Blackburn, W. W. "Survival With a Living–Related Donor Transplant." *Transplant Proc* 5:2 (June 1973) pp. 1093–1095.

Brock, D., Lawson, R. and Bennett, W. "Preoperative Workshops With Patients Waiting for Kidney Transplants." *Transplant Proc* 5:2 (June 1973) pp. 1059–1060.

Christopherson, L. K. and Gonda, T. A. "Patterns of Grief: End-State Renal Failure and Kidney Transplantation." *Transplant Proc* 5:2 (June 1973) pp. 1051–1057.

Craven, P. B. "Motivations of a Living–Related Kidney Donor." *Transplant Proc* 5:2 (June 1973) pp. 1071–1072.

Fox, R. C. and Swazey, J. P. *The Courage to Fail* (Chicago: University of Chicago Press 1974).

Friedman, E., Delano, B. and Butt, K. "Pragmatic Realities in Uremia Therapy." *N Engl J Med* 298:7 (February 1978) pp. 368–370.

Glassman, B. M. and Siegel, A. "Personality Correlates

of Survival in a Long-Term Hemodialysis Program." *Arch Gen Psychiatry* 22 (June 1970) pp. 566–574.

Halper, I. S. "Psychiatric Observations in a Chronic Hemodialysis Program." *Med Clin North Am* 55:1 (January 1971) pp. 177–191.

Kaplan-deNour, A. "Some Notes on the Psychological Significance of Urination." *J Nerv Ment Dis* 148:6 (1969) pp. 615–623.

Leff, B. "A Club Approach to Social Work Treatment Within a Home Dialysis Program." *Social Work in Health Care* 1:1 (Fall 1975) pp. 33–40.

McKegney, F. P. and Lange, P. "The Decision to No Longer Live on Chronic Hemodialysis." *Am J Psychiatry* 128:3 (September 1971) pp. 47–54.

Muslin, H. L. "On Acquiring a Kidney." *Am J Psychiatry* 127:9 (March 1971) pp. 105–108.

Muslin, H. L. "After The Kidney Transplant." *Curr Concepts Psychiatry* 2:2 (April 1976) pp. 2–4.

Nelson, J. B. *Human Medicine* (Minnesota: Augsburg Publishing House 1973).

Overley, T. M. "Psychiatric Problems in Renal Dialysis and Transplantation." *J Indiana State Med Assoc* (April 1971) pp. 301–302.

Short, M. J. and Wilson, W. P. "Roles of Denial in Chronic Hemodialysis" *Arch Gen Psychiatry* 20 (April 1969) pp. 433–437.

Strange, P. V. and Sumner, A. T. "Predicting Treatment Costs and Life Expectancy for End-Stage Renal Disease." *N Engl J Med* 298:7 (February 1978) pp. 372–378.

Tuckman, A. J. "Brief Psychotherapy and Hemodialysis." *Arch Gen Psychiatry* 23 (July 1970) pp. 65–69.

Warshofsky, F. *The Rebuilt Man* (New York: Thomas Y. Crowell Co. 1965).

Whitwell, B. L. "The Transplant Nurse." *Transplant Proc* 5:2 (June 1973) pp. 1129–1130.

Psychosocial Needs of Patients with Acute Respiratory Failure

Laura Jo Linn, R.N., M.N., C.C.R.N.
Critical Care Clinical Nurse Specialist
Veterans Administration Medical Center
  (Atlanta)
Decatur, Georgia

I MET MR. SNOW while working in a respiratory intensive care unit. He was a small man, about 65 years old, with clear blue eyes and, fittingly enough, snow white hair. I received a report from the night shift: "In bed four is Mr. Snow, a chronic lunger admitted last night with pneumonia. He is on the MAI at 40% with an IMV of six. His gases are adequate. You know how these lungers are, we'll never get him off the ventilator." I walked to the bedside and saw a frightened man connected to the respirator. I introduced myself and told him I would be his nurse for the day. He grasped my arm in a thin trembling hand and gave me his writing slate. Printed in crooked letters were the following words: "Please don't give up on me." At that point I became more sensitive to the psychosocial needs of patients with acute respiratory failure (ARF). Their nursing care demands more than physical care to help them meet their need for oxygen, much, much more.

132

THE PATIENTS' EMOTIONAL NEEDS

Unable to meet the basic need for oxygen, patients with ARF find themselves dependent on strangers and mechanical equipment for their lives. They are often in the stressful environment of an intensive care unit, isolated from their loved ones. They are anxious and afraid. Often they are intubated, making communication difficult, and they may be restrained. The increased level of catecholamines from stress, plus the often used sympathomimetic drugs, increases the feeling of anxiety. Often confusion occurs secondary to hypoxia and the environmental stresses. It is the role of the nurse to support such patients both physiologically and psychologically.

Anxiety is a complex unpleasant reaction to stress and the threat to one's self-concept.[1] It is associated with insecurity, helplessness and isolation.[2] Patients with ARF are experiencing a threat to their self-concept and to life itself. While trying to improve the patient's oxygenation status, the nurse also assists the patient to reduce the level of anxiety. This not only benefits the patient psychologically, but also decreases oxygen consumption at a critical time.

Interference with breathing is frequently related to deep insecurities about life, death and suffocation.[3] Initially, patients are completely dependent on the health care team. To feel secure in the team members' care, patients must trust them and their abilities to make judgments and carry out procedures. Confidence in nurses caring for the patients is of primary impor-tance since the nurses spend more time with the patients than any other member of the health care team. A feeling of trust will not only decrease anxiety but will affect acceptance of future treatment regimen. Nurses can control the environment to establish a feeling of confidence, for example, by being consistent in performing procedures. This is accomplished quite easily by following procedure manuals. Continuity of care is provided by utilizing the nursing care plan and by having the same nurse care for the patient on consecutive days. By informing patients of the daily routine in the intensive care unit, the environment becomes more predictable. Preparing the patients for procedures and telling them of changes in their therapy also increase the feeling of security.

Nurse Intervention

Nurses should approach the patients in a calm, reassuring and professional manner. During the initial treatment of ARF, explanations are kept concise. Patients are told that they are in the hospital and are being helped to breathe better. At this point, long explanations are not understood and are another source of anxiety. Touching patients and verbally reassuring them make them feel secure. Any disagreement over treatment or questions about the functioning of equipment should not be discussed near the patients.

Faced with thoughts of death, patients may express concerns about dying. Nurses should allow the patients to express these concerns and deal with them realistically. Referrals to the chaplain or psychologist may be indicated.

With improvement in condition, patients can make more decisions regarding their care, to decrease their sense of helplessness: they can choose, for example, when to have a bath, which side to turn onto or what type of juice to have with breakfast. Do not imply choice when there is none. For example, refrain from asking "I'm going to suction you now, alright?" In most situations, patients are going to be suctioned whether it is alright with them or not. Implying choice when there is none increases the feeling of helplessness. An alternate response is to express an awareness that the procedure is uncomfortable but necessary to enable them to breathe better.

Keeping the patient involved in progress and therapy, for example, by arranging meetings with patients and members of the health care team to discuss the patients' progress, decreases feelings of helplessness. Patients also feel more in control by being allowed out of bed as soon as possible to reach their belongings on the bedside table, comb their hair, feed and bathe themselves. Assessing ability to perform these tasks and allowing patients to complete them result in diminished feelings of helplessness and anxiety.

Patients in ARF are physically isolated from their families and loved ones by the confines of the intensive care unit, as well as emotionally isolated in fighting for every breath while surrounded by healthy people. Allowing families to visit and letting the patients keep small trinkets reminiscent of home at the bedside decreases the feeling of loneliness. As patients get to know the nurses, there will be less feeling of isolation. For this reason, setting aside time to sit and talk with patients reduces the feeling of loneliness. Some patients feel better when they see other patients in the intensive care unit "in the same boat." The camaraderie among patients in the intensive care unit can be a positive factor. However, nurses must be prepared for patients' distress in the event of the death of their "comrades."

Patients on Mechanical Ventilation Have Special Needs

Patients receiving mechanical ventilation have special needs. They are dependent not only on strangers to keep them alive, but also on a machine. The fear of mechanical failure or becoming dislodged from the machine is constantly present. Informing patients of the alarms and other safety features on the machine decreases the fear of dislodgement. Telling patients about the close monitoring of patients and the backup systems including oxygen and a bag-valve-mask also decreases fear.

Patients often see the ventilator as an extension of the self, and anxiety results when personnel tamper with the machine. Informing patients before changes are made on the ventilator alleviates some anxiety. Unnecessary adjustments on the ventilator should be avoided.

For patients on mechanical ventilation, the need to communicate is intensified, yet the ability to do so is compromised.[5] Therefore, nurses should provide for an alternate method of communication such as a magic slate or pencil and paper. Every effort is made to understand the patients. Often they are confused, weak, sedated and cannot make their needs known. A

134   poster board with a list of needs and feelings for patients to point to may be used. The list could include pain, bedpan, need to talk to someone (family, physician, minister, nurse), I'm afraid, etc. The inability of patients on mechanical ventilation to talk may contribute to development of stress ulcers.[6] Making communication easier may decrease the incidence of this complication, as well as alleviate anxiety and isolation.

Unable to communicate verbally, patients become more aware of nonverbal forms of communication, facial expressions and touch. The nurses' expressions while suctioning patients or assessing oxygenation status indicate to the patients how the nurses accept them. Nurses can also utilize the patient's facial expressions, position and other nonverbal cues to evaluate the patient.

Patients receiving neuromuscular blocking agents while on the ventilator are totally dependent on those around them and are unable to communicate their needs. Nurses should offer such patients verbal support and tell them that they are being constantly monitored. Nurses should know that neuromuscular blocking agents do not decrease patients' anxiety. They are aware of their environment, but cannot respond to it in the usual manner. Nurses should check to see that an antianxiety agent is ordered for patients and administer it appropriately. (The use of antianxiety agents in ARF patients is controversial; see Rhodes, M. L. "Acute Respiratory Failure in Chronic Obstructive Lung Disease,"—this issue *Critical Care Quarterly* page 9.)

Patients on the ventilator are subject to many procedures. All should be explained before they are done, using terminology the patients understand. It should not be assumed that patients remember a particular procedure; often they are confused or sedated and do not remember what procedures have been done.

Patients on mechanical ventilation are often restrained to prevent dislodgement of the endotracheal or tracheostomy tube. Particularly if patients are confused, combative or sedated, they may naturally reach for the tube to remove the noxious equipment. Every effort is made to support the patient and explain the reason for the restraints. When at the bedside, nurses can often remove the restraints without incidence. Nurses must assess the necessity of the restraints and discontinue their use as soon as possible since they are an added source of anxiety for patients.

Suctioning is an uncomfortable but necessary procedure for patients on mechanical ventilation. Patients suffer from a feeling of suffocation when being suctioned. This feeling can be prevented by preoxygenating the patients and limiting aspiration to 10 to 15 seconds.[7] Preoxygenation can be administered in several deep breaths via a bag-valve-mask delivering 100% oxygen or by sighing the patient several times on the ventilator with 100% oxygen. (One hundred-percent oxygen may be contraindicated in patients with COLD whose respiratory effort is not being controlled by a ventilator.) Counting while suctioning will remind the nurse of the time limit. Strict adherence to this procedure will make suctioning more tolerable for the patients and will prevent hypoxia and the feeling of suffocation.

Weaning patients from the ventilator requires intense psychological support. Dependent on the ventilator for life, patients are suddenly threatened with separation from the very machine keeping them alive. Often anxiety will prevent patients from enduring long periods off the ventilator.[8] Initially nurses should remain with the patients, observing their reactions to weaning. Words of encouragement plus the presence of the nurse at the bedside decrease patient anxiety.

Personality influences the response of patients to illness. The more inadequate the personality before illness, the more inadequate will be the response to illness.[3] The family and previous medical records are sources of information about patients. Such information is utilized to predict patients' responses to illness and to plan medical intervention. For example, a history of alcohol abuse would alert nurses to watch for delirium tremens and to prevent their occurrence with appropriate sedatives. If patients were receiving antipsychotic drugs at home, the physician should be informed in order to decide whether to continue them. If the patient had been hospitalized before, the nurse is able to gather valuable data and to anticipate problems and prevent their occurrence. (The use of hypnotic, tranquilizer and narcotic drugs is controversial; see Rhodes, page 9.)

Denial of the illness, refusal to accept treatment, inability to function and the use of illness to demand attention and control the environment are anticipated reactions to illness.[3] Teaching patients about the disease and treatment plus allowing some control over the environment will help patients adjust and decrease these reactions.

INDIVIDUAL PSYCHOLOGICAL NEEDS

There are many causes of respiratory failure, and each patient has individual psychological needs, many of which are related to the underlying pulmonary disease. Patients with COLD are often depressed.[3] This depression is accentuated during the hospitalization for ARF. Patients are aware that the disease is chronic and that the ordeal of ARF is a constant possibility. Patients with COLD are supported during the acute phase by verbal encouragement and are taught how to cope with a chronic illness. Patients need to have control over their environment and are often extremely regimental in the way in which they want their care given. Modifying the plan of care to meet the needs of the patients decreases feelings of helplessness.

Patients with asthma present challenging psychological needs. Although the primary factors in most cases of asthma are environmental, genetic, infectious and immunological, some nurses and physicians believe that asthma is always psychogenic.[3] As a result, patients may be treated as if the asthma is their own fault. Nurses must strive to overcome this prejudice and treat patients in an accepting manner. Having nurses give a presentation on acute asthmatic attacks may increase their knowledge and acceptance of the disease.

Nurses must also strive to overcome any prejudice they feel toward patients with

135

136 self-induced drug overdoses. Sometimes these patients in the intensive care unit are next to patients who are trying as hard as possible to get well but are failing. The contrast is difficult to accept, but every effort must be made to treat the patients in an accepting manner.

The extremely obese patient also is subject to rejection. Some feel the problem is caused by the patient. A psychologist or a psychiatric nurse clinical specialist can help the staff work through feelings regarding specific patients. Allowing the staff to verbalize their feelings helps them recognize and overcome prejudices.

ENVIRONMENTAL SOURCES OF ANXIETY FOR THE PATIENT

Respiratory diseases are anxiety provoking for the nurse.[9] There are few circumstances as frightening as a patient who is unable to get enough oxygen. If nurses are not careful, they will transmit their feelings to the patient. An understanding of ARF and a thorough knowledge of the therapy involved decrease anxiety. Nurses must be comfortable with all the equipment used in treating ARF. A hospital program for nurses on all aspects of respiratory therapy is invaluable.

The intensive care unit is another source of anxiety for patients with ARF. Placed in a strange environment, surrounded by equipment constantly beeping or buzzing, the patient finds that days run into nights. Confusion, disorientation and misperceptions, and less often delusional and hallucinatory behavior, may result.[10] These behavioral changes may be caused by sensory deprivation, sleep deprivation or sensory overload. By controlling environmental variables, nurses can decrease the stresses associated with the intensive care unit.

Sensory Deprivation

Sensory deprivation occurs when the absolute level and/or degree of structure in sensory input are reduced.[11] Symptoms of sensory deprivation include the loss of sense of time; delusions, illusions and hallucinations; restlessness; and psychotic behavior.[12] Admission to the intensive care unit increases sensory deprivation.[13] The environment drastically limits the type of sensory input. No longer do patients participate in the same degree of social interaction with friends and loved ones. They do not listen to the evening news, see the sunrise, hear the alarm clock. All of these stimuli help keep a person oriented. When sensory input is altered, confusion may result. Nurses frequently orient the patient to person, place and time. Having a clock at the bedside or wearing a wristwatch helps patients keep track of time. Dimming the lights at night and opening the window shades in the day help patients distinguish day from night.

Meaningful sensory input can be provided in several ways. By spending time talking with patients, nurses decrease sensory deprivation. Allowing family and friends to visit at scheduled times provides patients with sensory input and a time structure. A radio at the bedside increases sensory input, but it should be meaningful to patients, not merely added noise. A tape recorder with messages from loved ones may be significant to patients. As the patients' condition improve, it may be helpful to let them walk to the window periodically or even leave the intensive care unit for brief periods of time.

When patients become confused and have delusions, illusions or hallucinations, patients are reminded that they are in the hospital. They are told that what they are seeing is not real, and what is actually there is described. Patients are reassured, and nurses spend more time with them during such occurrences. Sensory deprivation has the same symptoms as other complications that are prone to develop, such as hypoxia and metabolic disturbances. Nurses must assess patients with this in mind.

Sleep Deprivation

Allowing time for patients to get adequate sleep in the intensive care unit is definitely a challenge. Monitoring vital signs and treatments, and administering medications seem endless. Particularly for pulmonary patients, suctioning and lung physiotherapy make prolonged rest impossible and often detrimental. Nursing care is planned taking the need for rest into consideration. Patients should be allowed at least two-hour blocks of uninterrupted sleep throughout the night. Frequent rest periods are planned throughout the day. By combining the taking of vital signs, pulmonary hygiene measures and medication administration, nurses can allow patients to rest. Dimming the lights at night and keeping the environment quiet are conducive to sleep. Monitoring equipment to measure heart rate and arterial pressures allows constant surveillance of

patients without disturbing them. Keen observations of respiratory rate, pattern and depth provide meaningful data. At times, however, pulmonary patients must be frequently awakened to assess mental status, and sleep must be interrupted. Nurses assess the situation and set priority needs at these times.

Sensory Overload

Sensory overload is another threat to patients in the intensive care unit. Increased levels of noise and continuous sensory input lead to anxiety. Nurses should decrease as much extraneous noise as possible. Personnel are instructed to keep voices down at night and to keep conversation patient centered. Lights should be dimmed at intervals. Much of the noise in the intensive care unit is from alarms, respirators and suction equipment, and little can be done to prevent it. However, explaining the various noises to patients is helpful. In planning the construction of intensive care units, noise control should be considered.

THE FAMILY

An acute illness of one family member places stress on the entire family unit. Family relations profoundly influence the quality and quantity of psychological support the patient receives during illness. If the family relationships are inadequate during times of health, it is unlikely that they will improve during a time of acute illness.[14] Nurses should assess family interactions and make every effort to include various members in their plan of care.

138   During the initial treatment, families should be informed of the condition of the patients as soon as possible. Brief explanations are warranted at this time. Families must be prepared for the initial visit to the patients and subsequent visits if therapy or condition has changed drastically. Particularly if patients are on a ventilator, the families should be told of the equipment surrounding the patients. Due to television, most lay people are familiar with the sight of a ventilator and tend to associate it with hopeless cases of coma.

Nurses should accompany families to the bedside during the initial visit and offer support. If patients have been intubated, the families are told that the patients are unable to speak. Often, family members stand at the bedside speechless and motionless. Initiating conversation with the patients and providing them with writing slates help maintain communication. Nurses should let the family members know that they can hold the patient's hand. Often in the maze of tubes, visitors are hesitant to touch the patient.

It may be helpful to allow family members to perform small tasks such as combing the patients' hair, rubbing their back or putting a cool cloth on their forehead. This may help family members feel less helpless and reestablish communication between the family and the patient. Nurses must determine the readiness of the family to help in any patient care activities, however.

Nurses should make every effort to allow visitors at scheduled intervals. Often in the hectic pace of the intensive care unit, families are kept waiting for visiting privileges. If visitors are kept out due to the admission of a patient or rounds by the physicians, the family should be informed. This decreases anxiety concerning who "has taken a turn for the worse" and requires immediate care.

Nurses must establish rapport with the family. They earn their trust by providing expert care to their loved ones and by keeping them informed of the patients' progress. Nurses often act as liaison between families and physicians and set up appointments for discussion of the patients' condition.

Witnessing personality changes in the patient, family members may have reacted negatively, and now that the person is acutely ill, they may feel guilty.[15] An explanation of the cause and subtlety of the personality changes may decrease this feeling of guilt. Nurses must allow family members to express their feelings. If necessary, other members of the health care team are consulted to assist the family in coping with the illness.

Assessing family interactions provides nurses with meaningful information for planning patient care. Problems may surface, such as financial insecurity, that influence patients' reactions to acute illness. Referrals to appropriate persons may result from observation of family interaction.

SUMMARY

In summary, patients with ARF have many psychosocial needs. Nurses can decrease patients' anxiety and fear, support patients on mechanical ventilation and meet the special needs of patients with different underlying pulmonary diseases. By recognizing their own anxieties and prejudices toward patients with ARF, nurses are able to provide a higher level of nursing care. By becoming involved with patients' families and including them in the plan of care, nurses can support them during a time of crisis and enable them to better support the patients. Nurses must recognize and meet the psychosocial needs of patients with ARF with the same deliberateness and skill they handle the physical needs. By receiving total patient care during the crisis, patients maintain a feeling of security and human worth.

REFERENCES

1. Aspinall, M. J. *Nursing the Open-Heart Surgery Patient* (New York: McGraw-Hill Book Co. 1973).
2. Roy, C. *Introduction to Nursing: An Adaptation Model* (Englewood Cliffs, N.J.: Prentice-Hall, Inc. 1976).
3. Kent, D. C. and Smith, J. K. "Psychological Implications of Pulmonary Disease." *Clin Notes Respiratory Dis* 16:3 (1977) p. 1.
4. Murphy, E. R. "Intensive Nursing Care in a Respiratory Unit." *Nursing Clin N Am* 3:3 (1968) p. 434.
5. Hudelson, E. H. "Mechanical Ventilation from the Patient's Point of View." *Respiratory Care* 22 (1977) p. 654.
6. Sellery, G. R. "Airway Problems in the Intensive Care Unit" in Spoerel, W. E., ed. *International Anesthesiology: Problems of the Upper Airway* (Boston: Little, Brown and Co. 1972).
7. Bendixen, H. H. et al. *Respiratory Care* (St. Louis: The C. V. Mosby Co. 1965).
8. Fitzgerald, L. and Huber, G. "Weaning the Patient from Mechanical Ventilation." *Heart and Lung* 5:2 (1976) p. 232.
9. Hargreaves, A. G. "Emotional Problems of Patients with Respiratory Disease." *Nursing Clin N Am* 3:3 (1968) p. 482.
10. Kimball, C. P. "The ICU Syndrome, A New Disease of Medical Progress." *Med Insight* 5:11 (1973) p. 9.
11. Adam, H. B., Robertson, M. H. and Cooper, G. D. "Sensory Deprivation and Personality Change." *J Nervous Mental Dis* 143:3 (1966) p. 256.
12. Hudak, C. M., Lohr, T. and Gallo, B. M. *Critical Care Nursing* 2nd ed. (New York: J. B. Lippincott Co. 1977).
13. Kealy, S. L. "Respiratory Care in Guillain-Barre Syndrome." *Am J Nursing* 77:1 (1977) p. 60.
14. Gaudinski, M. S. "Psychological Considerations with Patients on Respirators." *Aviation, Space Environmental Med* 48:1 (1977) p. 72.
15. Kudla, M. S. "The Care of the Patient with Respiratory Insufficiency." *Nursing Clin N Am* 8:1 (1973) p. 189.

Stresses and Coping Styles of Parents of Children Undergoing Open-Heart Surgery

Linda A. Lewandowski, R.N., M.S.
Pediatric Clinical Nurse Specialist
Yale New Haven Hospital
Assistant Professor
Yale University, School of Nursing
New Haven, Connecticut

PARENTS OF CHILDREN undergoing open-heart surgery face many stresses. Although having a child undergo any type of surgery is stressful for parents, open-heart surgery can be especially difficult. One reason for this is the importance of the heart; even young children recognize that the heart is vital in sustaining life.[1] Open-heart surgery is particularly stressful because it requires the heart to be stopped temporarily.[2]

THE STUDY

To study their stresses and coping styles, the author observed and interviewed 59 parents of children over a period of approximately two years who were undergoing open-heart surgery. The observations took place during the parents' first visit to their child in the intensive care unit (ICU) following surgery. The parents were not aware of being observed, but knew about the study and had given their consent to participate in it. The parents were interviewed alone the day after the child's surgery, most often while the child was still in the ICU.

The unit was a 12-bed ICU in a large West Coast medical center. The ICU consisted mostly of adult patients; most pediatric patients in the unit had undergone open-heart surgery and were being cared for in the large open main room. Immediate family members were allowed to visit at any time of the day or night for as long as they wished unless a special procedure had to be done or an emergency arose. If this occurred, the family member was requested to leave and was notified when to return. Most of the nurses in the unit encouraged parents to visit their child as often as they wished.

Coping

Coping has been defined in many different ways by many different authors. The author views Murphy and associates' positive "healthy" concept of coping as useful for nurses in looking at the behavior of patients and their families.[3] Although Murphy and associates have formulated concepts through their work with young children, the author has observed many of the same coping styles and strategies in parents.

Murphy and associates define coping as "any attempt to master a new situation that can be potentially threatening, frustrating, challenging, or gratifying."[3] They elaborate that "coping" points to a process—"the steps or sequences through which a child comes to terms with a challenge or makes use of an opportunity. Adaptation is the result."[3]

Murphy and associates refer to many other authors using "coping" in the context of "an individual's *failure* to cope with certain external difficulties or with his problems."[3] They prefer to look at coping in a more positive sense; that is, there is no such thing as "failure to cope." No matter what behavior an individual displays, that behavior is that individual's method of coping with that particular situation at that particular time.

Hamburg[4] discusses his belief that people develop and learn how to cope with the resources they have available as determined by genetic make-up and individual experiences. He adds that there is a wide range of individual differences in responses to stress, just as there are differences in individuals' thresholds of frustration.

STRESS

Stress is defined by Goldenson[5] as "a condition or situation that imposes demands for adjustment on a person." Using Murphy and associates' concept of coping in looking at this definition, it seems that stress is a situation or condition that requires an individual to cope and thereby adapt.

Many parents find even the decision to consent to their child's open-heart surgery difficult.[6] They must decide on an operation that results either in a longer and improved life for their child or may result in death.[7] The decision is even more difficult when the child appears active and healthy at the time the cardiologist recommends surgery.[6] It becomes a somewhat easier decision when the parents can see the child becoming increasingly ill.

The hospital environment may cause stress: little privacy in the hospital waiting room, a strange environment with unfamiliar people who might be crying or talking loudly, and disrupted sleeping and eating patterns.[8] Sources of stress outside the hospital also exist. Parents may worry about other children at home. A personal illness or sickness of another family member may increase a parent's stress, particularly if a family member or close friend has recently died.[8] Parents may be concerned about having to take time off from jobs. They may be a great distance from family and friends in a strange city. Personal problems between the parents occur frequently in families with chronically ill children, and those problems may be accentuated during this time. Instead of being mutually supportive, some parents cause each other even more stress.

Many times parents are not prepared for the sight that greets them when they first enter the ICU, even though they may have had much preoperative teaching including a tour of the ICU. For the first time they see their child underneath mounds of tubes, tape, and intravenous (IV) lines, and surrounded by machinery of all types. It was at this point that many parents in the author's experience were observed running from the unit, backing away from the child, or crying hysterically. The parents were frequently in high anxiety states that made it difficult to give their children the necessary support.

Many writers have described how stressful it can be for a lay person just to enter an ICU. Hay and Oken graphically describe the atmosphere a parent encounters: "A stranger entering an ICU is at once bombarded with a massive array of sensory stimuli, some emotionally neutral, but many highly charged. The atmosphere is not unlike that of a tension-charged strategic war bunker."[9] Wallace states: "As most lay people have never set foot in such a specialized and mechanized area of the hospital, the equipment alone overwhelms them."[10] Roberts agrees stating: "It is a foreign environment to the family members. Initially they feel as though they have entered forbidden territory."[11] Parfit has also described what seeing the child in the ICU may be like for parents:

> The monitoring machines and their zigzag tracings, the transfusion apparatus, the comings and goings of white-coated doctors and technicians, while in one sense reassuring the parents that everything possible is being done, nevertheless are frightening to parents who are already under stress. Bleeps, tubes, flashing red lights, and alarm bells increase their sense of awe and fear.[12]

Events such as the publicity of the Karen Ann Quinlan case,[13] the California Right to Die Bill, and other cases that have portrayed the use of ventilators and other such machinery may also concern parents. Suddenly they see this much-publicized equipment on *their* child!

Television has also exposed many of these machines to parents and may have engendered inaccurate expectations. For example, a father told the author that "on TV, the heart patterns are always the same all the way across the screen." When he was standing alone at his daughter's bedside and some static interference was displayed on the monitor screen, he was thrown into a panic.

144

During the interviews, parents often expressed shock at seeing their child with all of the equipment and tubes, and felt a lack of preparation for what they had seen. Even those who had received extensive preoperative preparation including a tour of the ICU reported shock at actually seeing their child after surgery. The parents also reported much anxiety during this time.

Besides discussing the appearance of their child, parents sometimes reported an enormous sense of relief that the surgery was at last over. Many of the parents had concerns about the outcome of the surgery. Concerns about the possible death of their child were either expressed or hinted at by almost all of those interviewed, even those who had been assured by the surgeon that this was very unlikely. Feelings of helplessness and powerlessness were expressed by many parents: "I see her lying there, but there's not a thing I can do to help her!" Callahan describes a parent as the child's "absolutely prejudiced protector who will take his side against the world."[14] Parents who are accustomed and devoted to fulfilling this protector role may feel a profound sense of loss and may feel powerless to help and protect their child who is now seemingly under the jurisdiction of machines and hospital staff.

We are all very familiar with physiologi-

SOME PARAMETERS TO ASSESS THE STRESS LEVELS OF PARENTS OF CHILDREN UNDERGOING OPEN-HEART SURGERY

1. Age
2. Sex
3. Educational level
4. Marital status
5. Socioeconomic status
6. Occupation and job security
7. Ethnic background and culture
8. Religion and its meaning to the individual
9. Insurance and financial concerns
10. Individual personality and temperament
11. Parent's past medical history, including psychiatric
12. Past experience with illness, hospitals, surgery, critical care units, death
13. Recent illness and/or death among family or friends
14. Meaning of this child to the parent
15. Age of this child
16. Other children in family (baby-sitters, time spent away, etc)
17. Meaning of the heart to the parent
18. Past experience with and/or family history of heart defects, heart disease, etc.
19. Type of cardiac defect child has

SOME PARAMETERS TO ASSESS THE STRESS LEVELS OF PARENTS OF CHILDREN UNDERGOING OPEN-HEART SURGERY (continued)

20. Type of surgery child is having and if it is a palliative or corrective measure
21. Child's first surgery, or, if not, number of times parent has experienced this previously and previous outcomes
22. Information parent has received from hospital staff or others regarding possible outcomes, survival rates, etc
23. Ambivalence and/or guilt about decision to consent to child's surgery
24. Amount and type of preoperative teaching parent has received
25. Knowledge of and relationships with other parents whose children have undergone cardiac surgery and their outcomes
26. Atmosphere of hospital waiting room and accommodations for visitors
27. Distance from home to hospital
28. Accommodations close to hospital and cost involved
29. Amount of sleep parent has gotten recently
30. Recent eating patterns and last time parent ate
31. Recent major life change events (eg, moving to a new city, recognition for a major accomplishment, new job, etc)
32. Other stressors in and out of hospital (eg, broken plumbing in the home, difficulty finding a parking place, a minor earthquake or major storm the day before, etc)
33. Amount of equipment attached to child postoperatively
34. Child's postoperative course
35. Child's postoperative appearance (eg, pale, blood on bed and child, etc)
36. Child awake or still asleep when parents first come to visit
37. Postoperative courses and outcomes of other patients in the unit
38. Amount of guilt feelings about how reacted to child in the past (eg, "I shouldn't have hollered at him," "I should have let her have that new toy," etc)
39. How strong parent's feelings of helplessness and powerlessness are
40. How strong parent's fear of child's death and how realistic this fear is
41. Attitude of nursing staff, physicians, etc (eg, supportive to parent, encouraging of parental involvement, outwardly annoyed or hostile, "mixed" messages, etc)
42. Number of different people parent must interact with and receive information from in the hospital
43. Child's ability to interact with parent (eg, intubated, restraints, amount of sedation, etc)

146 cal assessment parameters, but not with parameters that can be used to assess stress levels. (See boxed material, p. 78.) Although it is beyond the scope of this article to discuss how the parents' stress level can be affected by each parameter, in most cases the effect will be self-evident.

PARENTAL COPING STRATEGIES

Coping strategies as defined by Murphy and associates are specific behavior sequences, however simple or complex, that are used to deal with a specific challenge or problem.[3] There are as many possible varieties of coping strategies and styles as there are people and situations.[4] These strategies are developed over time and progressively modified as a person's experiences change.[4] When a strategy used successfully in the past does not work for new demands, new coping strategies must be developed if the situation is to be mastered.

Murphy and associates state that defense mechanisms may be, and often are, part of the overall coping effort of an individual. They believe defense mecha-

nisms sometimes assist in dividing a complex situation into manageable parts, through repressing the excessive threat and focusing on the one that can be mastered.[3] Jacobson agrees and lists some of these "mechanisms of defense" as projection, denial, displacement, and intellectualization.[15]

Murphy and associates believe that each individual uses his or her own individual coping strategies. They have, however, identified some strategies that children seem to have in common and use most often. Parents also use some of these coping strategies on their initial visit to their child in the ICU. (See boxed material below for additional parameters the nurse may use to assess parental coping strategies.)

Initial Immobilization

The initial reaction of many parents to seeing their child in the ICU is to stop a few feet away from the child's bed and stare at the child and the mounds of equipment. This is often a time to assess the new situation. The parents might be described as using delay to reduce the

---

SOME PARAMETERS TO ASSESS POSSIBLE COPING STRATEGIES OF PARENTS OF CHILDREN UNDERGOING OPEN-HEART SURGERY

1. Parent's perception of situation (realistic or distorted)
2. Available situational supports
   Parent's relationship with spouse
   Proximity of and relationships with other family members and friends
   Parent's relationships with hospital staff and other possible support systems (eg, clergy)
   Family's interaction with each other in the hospital
3. Ways parent has coped with stress in the past
4. Decision-making abilities at this time

SOME PARAMETERS TO ASSESS POSSIBLE COPING STRATEGIES OF PARENTS OF CHILDREN UNDERGOING OPEN-HEART SURGERY (continued)

5. Degree of dependence/independence
6. Parent's interaction with other people
7. Parent's interaction with child preoperatively
8. Parent's interaction with child in the ICU and amount of support given

   How much talks to child, tone of voice, what parent says, eye contact established

   Touching, stroking of child

   Physical proximity to bed and child

   Focus on child or on equipment and happenings in rest of unit
9. Length of stay in the ICU and visiting pattern (unless this is regulated by hospital visiting rules)
10. Types of questions parent asks and number of times asks the same question
11. Types of concerns voiced or voicing no concerns at all
12. Number of phone calls to unit from parent and type of information requested
13. Verbalizations about own anxiety levels, coping strategies, etc
14. Brief attention span or inability to focus on any one thing
15. Amount of involvement in child's care parent seems to desire and to be able to handle at that time (much influenced by degree of involvement possible depending on child's condition and on attitude of staff toward parental involvement)
16. Parent's outward physical appearance
17. Nonverbal behaviors (eg, restlessness, pacing, rocking back and forth, tightly clasped hands, rigid posture, wringing of hands, tenseness, biting of lips, fingernails, shaking, crying, etc)
18. Somatic signs and symptoms (eg, headache, gastrointestinal upset, constipation, frequent urination, backache, etc)
19. Manifestations of various coping strategies:

    Immobilization

    Visual survey

    Withdrawal (physical or emotional)

    Restructuring—focusing on a part

    Concern or preoccupation with "little things"

    Intellectualization

    Anger

    Depression

    Denial

148 initial impact of a situation.[3] Murphy and associates elaborate on this coping strategy by describing characteristics they have observed such as:

> Temporary postponement or taking time out to become clear about what was involved, to give oneself a feeling of control and security in moving into a situation slowly step by step, restricting the amount of stimulation to which one would expose oneself at any given moment, interposing delay in the form of 'I'll do it when I feel like it,' allowing time for mobilization of energy.[3]

Therefore, it would seem that the conscientious nurse who brings a parent by the arm close to the child's bed may in actuality be doing the parent a disservice. The parent may be trying to cope with the situation by waiting and gathering together resources. Seeing the child for the first time may be very frightening, and the parent may not be ready to move closer yet.

One mother in the study illustrates the need for parents to be allowed to move in as they are ready. The staff answered all of the mother's questions and respected her need to sit a few feet away from the bed of her 3-year-old son. After sitting there for about 25 minutes while the nurse was at the foot of the bed charting, she spontaneously walked to her son's bedside, leaned over, talked to him gently, and stroked his head. It would be helpful for nurses to realize that sometimes it takes time for parents to master the situation. This example illustrates the disadvantage of five to ten minutes per hour visiting privileges (how strange to think of it as a "privilege" to "allow" parents to be with their child!) for parents who need time before they are able to give the support the child needs.

Visual Survey

Murphy and colleagues describe another way of becoming familiar with a new situation as visual survey.[3] This coping strategy occurs very frequently with parents visiting their children in the ICU. There is just so much to look at, the machines, lights, other patients, staff in scrub dresses or white coats, not to mention the child and all the attachments. The parent may need to become familiar with the new environment before focusing on the child. The nurse may need to wait until the parent is able to concentrate on any explanations the nurse is giving.

Withdrawal

In some cases, parents may passively withdraw from the situation by avoiding asking about or talking to their child. A few parents manifested active withdrawal when they physically left the unit after brief one- or two-minute visits. Nurses should respect parents' needs for periods of withdrawal and be judicious in when and how they intervene.

Restructuring: Focusing on a Part

After about five minutes, one mother began to relax a little and focus her attention on the tape on her son's right leg that was securing an IV. In the next few minutes, her gaze wandered back to that piece of tape again and again. The overall situation was perhaps too much for her to cope with, and since there was not too much she could do about it, she focused on one small problem that could be remedied. By asking the nurse to loosen the tape, she seemed to mobilize some of her energy and exert some measure of control over the situation.

A Time of "Little Things"

To a busy ICU nurse, concerns like a piece of tape that appears too tight can seem trivial. After all, why should parents worry about minor things when their child is critically ill? The answer is that restructuring the situation into something the individual can deal with may be the parent's strategy for mastering the situation; by being aware of this, nurses may be more understanding of a parental response that otherwise seems inappropriate.[3] Such interventions can help parents cope with feelings of powerlessness by giving them a small measure of control over their child's care.

Often, very little things can make a profound impact on an anxious, helpless parent. During one interview, a father enthusiastically described how the nurse had asked him to help her out and how he really felt like he had been able to do something for his child. The nurse had asked the father to hand a syringe to her and then to hold the child's hand still while she drew some blood from the arterial line. From the father's perception, the episode had had an enormous impact toward relieving some of his feelings of helplessness and powerlessness.

Parfit describes the importance of parental involvement well:

Almost everyone rises to an emergency and can cope with crisis if they feel there is something they can do. So it is with parents. They are far less likely to become overwrought, hysterical, or paralyzingly depressed if they are given a job, however small, which they are helped to feel is useful.... Except in the most acute emergencies there is usually something that an anxious parent can do, whether it is just to hold a hand, act as a calming or familiar influence, or sing a well-loved and soothing nursery rhyme to a toddler.... It is far too easy for professionals in a hurry to deny parents the right to do something for their sick child.[12]

Intellectualization

Parents sometimes seem intensely interested in the equipment, and in asking about the child's heart rate, blood gas, and so on. They may be using the coping strategy of intellectualization, dealing with the situation on an intellectual level. Although Murphy and associates do not discuss this strategy, it is being presented here because it is a strategy observed to be very frequently used by parents. In the author's experience, this seems to be a strategy used most often by fathers. They may become intensely interested in the workings of a particular monitor, the incidence of congenital heart disease in the general population, the specific surgical technique, or a particular laboratory value. Patiently answering the numerous questions of anxious parents may be the most helpful approach for the nurse wishing to assist them in gaining mastery of the stressful situation. Even though the parent may not really understand the significance of an arterial Po_2 of 88 mm Hg, numbers

150

may be much easier to deal with at the time than the possibility of their child's death.

There may come a point at which this method of coping is carried to the extreme, however, and some type of intervention may be necessary. During one visit, the father of a critically ill infant used a stopwatch to time his child's ventilator. If at any time the ventilator delivered 59 rather than the desired 60 breaths per minute, he would hurriedly inform the infant's nurse in an upset voice. Another nurse who had a good relationship with the family took the father aside and talked to him. Then the father was able to admit that his real concerns were not for the

ventilator rate but his child's possible death.

SUMMARY

It is important to remember that there is really no such thing as being unable to cope; any behavior manifested by the parents is their way of coping with the situation. Having a greater awareness of the vast stresses parents of children in ICUs must face and the coping strategies they may employ will hopefully allow nurses to be more sensitive and empathic next time a family member steps through the ICU door.

REFERENCES

1. Roberts FB: The child with heart disease. *Nursing Times* 71:1080, 1972.
2. Aspinall MJ: *Nursing the Open-Heart Surgery Patient.* New York, McGraw-Hill Co, 1973, p 152.
3. Murphy LB, et al. *The Widening World of Childhood: Paths Toward Mastery.* New York, Basic Books, Inc, 1962.
4. Hamburg DA: *Competent Coping. This Question of Coping Series,* section 2, Hoffmann-La Roche, Inc, 1973, p 2.
5. Goldenson M: *The Encyclopedia of Human Behavior: Psychology, Psychiatry, and Mental Health.* Garden City, New York, Doubleday and Co, 1970, p 1263.
6. Glaser HH, Harrison GS, Lynn DB: Emotional implications of congenital heart disease in children. *Pediat* 33:367–379, 1964.
7. Barnes CM: Working with parents of children undergoing heart surgery. *Nursing Clin North Am* 4:13, 1969.

8. Kuenzi SH, Fenton MV: Crisis intervention in acute care areas. *Am J Nursing* 75:832, 1975.
9. Hay D, Oken D: The psychological stresses of intensive care nursing. *Psych Med* 34:110, 1972.
10. Wallace P: Relatives should be told about intensive care—but how much and by whom? *Can Nurse* 67:33, 1971.
11. Roberts SL: *Behavioral Concepts and the Critically Ill Patient.* Englewood Cliffs, New Jersey, Prentice-Hall 1976.
12. Parfit J: Parents and relatives. *Nursing Times* 71:1512, 1975.
13. The right to live—or die. *Time* 106:40, 1975.
14. Callahan SC: *Parenting: Principles and Politics of Parenthood.* Baltimore, Penguin Books, 1973, p 109.
15. Jacobson GF: Crisis Intervention from the Viewpoint of the Mental Health Professional. *Pastoral Psych* 21:21, 1970.

Postburn Psychological Adaptation: An Overview

Patricia Mieszala, R.N.
Psychiatric Burn Nurse Clinician
Sumner L. Koch Burn Center
Cook County Hospital
Chicago, Illinois
Consults Nationally to Burn Facilities

It was 2:30 PM one sunny Sunday afternoon. A perfect day for a ride on the lake. Nine people boarded a craft to enjoy a leisurely afternoon on the water.

Bob T.C. (aged 32) and Donna T.C. (aged 29) were a bit reluctant to go for the ride with their two children, Tommy (aged eight months) and Debbie (aged two). They were not very fond of boating and felt that perhaps with so many people aboard they wouldn't be too safe. They also didn't know the owner of the boat, who was but an acquaintance of Bob's father. However, Bob's parents convinced them that all would be fine and the experience would be fun.

After about an hour on the water a strange noise was heard from the engine area of the boat. Ted (aged 26), the owner of the boat, went to see what was causing the noise. All of a sudden, the engine exploded! There was fire everywhere! Ted, although injured, managed to extinguish the flames. The coast guard boats arrived in minutes. Five of the nine people aboard were injured and brought to the nearest burn facility by helicopter.

152 Ted, who was closest to the engine site at the time of the explosion, was the most extensively injured. He received a 50% partial- and full-thickness injury to both legs, feet, hands, chest, upper back, neck and face.

Bob, who was standing near Ted at the time of the explosion, received a 35% partial-thickness injury to both legs, arms, hands and face.

Donna was holding Tommy prior to the explosion, intending to change his diapers on the other side of the boat. However, she stopped to talk with Ted and Bob, deciding the change could wait a few more minutes. Donna was admitted to the burn center with a 20% burn injury of the face, neck, both arms and right thigh. Tommy received a 25.5% burn of the face, left hand and arm, both lower legs and feet.

Debbie was standing with her father at the time and received a 43.5% partial-thickness burn of the head, face, feet, both hands, arms and legs.

From that moment through the next several months, perhaps longer, Ted and the T.C.s would experience one of the most devastating experiences known to humans.

TIME AND AGAIN burn injuries occur to adults and children alike. The immediate impact of the injury—the initial hospitalization period, often filled with painful or uncomfortable treatment procedures, and many new faces and a new environment with which to become familiar—may be only the beginning of psychological as well as physical devastation.

What occurs within the hospital environment during the primary postburn hospitalization can either facilitate a "working through" process for patients and their families or inhibit this process, leaving much unfinished business to deal with after hospital discharge. Groups serve as reference points for humans to evaluate themselves.[1] Postburn patients rely heavily on their hospital environment and people contacts to begin to adjust to a new body image and self-concept. They begin to reestablish a sense of self-worth, which is the main goal of postburn psychosocial rehabilitation.

A careful study of a facility caring for the postburn patient often reveals what in the milieu facilitates this adjustment and what makes overall adaptation to burn injury more difficult. A burn facility that provides patients with an area for recreation away from treatment areas (or at least mobility about the area) also provides a setting for spontaneous exchange among patients and visitors. This allows patients to "test out" new behaviors in reestablishing or reenforcing their self-images. In contrast, a burn or hospital facility that isolates the patients throughout the entire hospitalization and restricts "people contact" (for what may be sound medical reasons) also unnecessarily retards patients from facing and dealing with issues in preparation for the postdischarge period.

The "where" of the burn care facility is also important in considering postburn adjustment. For example, caring for burn victims in a facility hundreds of miles from their homes makes visiting cumbersome for families and friends. This compounds the concern of the patients regarding the extra strain on their families, acting as an additional "irritant" in postburn adaptation and adjustment.

DEFINITION OF STRESS

The term *stress* can be misinterpreted. In reviewing works on the types and degrees of stress, an existing common denominator can be recognized. Stress, often thought of as a short-term stimulus easily overcome, is really a complex set of changing conditions that have a history and a future. Consequently, postburn adaptation and adjustment is not a simple, short-term situation, but a lengthy, complex process.[1] The burn team must be aware of this, so that consideration regarding the initial phases of adjustment to stress can be initiated with patients at the onset of postburn hospitalization. Varying degrees of planned support and intervention should be supplied p.r.n. throughout the patient's hospitalization.

INITIAL POSTBURN PERIOD

Following a patient's admission to a burn care facility, a complex pattern of interrelating among people begins. Unlike social situations, where one selects and controls relating patterns, newly admitted burn patients and their families are faced with a deluge of hospital staff with whom to relate.

Information, to establish patient history and develop care plans, is as important as initial resuscitation procedures. However, due to states of extreme anxiety in both patient and family, some questions asked receive incorrect, confusing or no answers at all. This initial period is an extremely important one for the patient-staff-family circle of relating, and it can be by far the most volatile.

A brief description of what is seen within each segment of the patient-staff-family circle during the immediate postburn period may reveal some of the problems to expect as well as make useful interventions more apparent.

PATIENTS

During the immediate postburn phase patients are often alert, oriented and rational, although overwhelmed with their sudden tragic situation. Their level of comprehension and understanding relative to the degree of seriousness of the injury is grossly distorted. Some patients may use denial as a mechanism to buffer the impact of being faced with a severe physical/psychological crisis. Others may exhibit what is commonly termed the "flood reaction." Although brief in duration, during this period the patient manifests concern over multiple issues in a disorganized fashion (employment, financial matters, life/death issues, family responsibilities, other patients burned in the same situation, etc.). Patients often require outside intervention and reassurance of assistance to become more realistic in giving priority to problems according to immediacy.

There are, however, extraordinary situations that result in the patient being comatose, confused, disoriented or psychotic on admission. These patients may have been electrically injured or have had a history of alcohol, drug abuse or previous psychopathology (as in victims of suicide attempt). Patients experiencing hypoxia may also manifest these reactions.

In dealing with children during the immediate postburn period, withdrawal is the most commonly seen initial response. This withdrawal can be short or long term, depending on the extent of injury and preburn history findings. Lengthy withdrawal periods, where the child appears lethargic with little or no response to painful procedures, are usually seen in extensively injured, very young children.

154   The combination of both severely traumatic physical and psychological factors must be taken into consideration in determining the cause. The application of biologic dressings or a permanent autograft appears to reduce the amount of physical discomfort for the child, who then begins to exhibit personality disturbances more actively. Initial feelings of guilt and anger are intense. Postburn children are known to interpret their primary hospitalization and all painful treatment procedures as a "punishment" for some wrong they have done. At times children will initially exhibit extreme anger and "lashing out" at the staff. This may be a preburn learned behavior in the face of past stress, a fear response, or a form of denial and unwillingness to accept their present restrictive situation. This response is most often seen in older children. Given a few weeks time, children begin to deal gradually with the reality of their hospitalization and all it entails and become more comfortable with their caretakers.

FAMILIES

The initial postburn period is a very traumatic one for primary family members and/or visitors. Due to high levels of anxiety over the burn situation itself and lack of exposure to and knowledge of burn care, family members of burn patients approach the burn facility for the first time with much hesitancy and quiet fear or complete hysteria. In either case, the relationship of the situation to the severity of injury and outcome to the outward appearance of the patient (especially if the open method of wound care is initially employed) is usually distorted and out of proportion. This is only compounded by the multitude of sensory stimuli about the family in the burn facility (equipment being used; protective gowns and masks if worn; other patients in view, especially if children and adults are cared for in the same facility; audible sounds of patients crying or screaming during dressing changes, etc.)

Family members of pediatric patients, especially parents, experience varying degrees of guilt and may or may not express this initially. Blaming one another for causing or allowing the burn situation to occur is often seen. Some family members will appear unduly cautious or inconsistent in reporting how the burn occurred. In such instances, especially if the location and appearance of the burn are suspicious, further investigation to rule out child abuse or neglect may be in order.

Unlike the burn patient who initially experiences a quiet period before reacting, family members begin by overtly reacting (sometimes overreacting) until more is known and understood.

BURN TEAM

Upon admission of a patient to the burn facility the staff moves about with speed and efficiency to initiate resuscitation procedures. Little is known about the patient; however, the attitude and approach used by individual staff members during the immediate postburn period can be perceived either as friendly, caring and calming to the patients and their families, or mysterious, frightening and intense. Patients and their families rely on verbal and nonverbal cues given by staff around them to help clarify their distorted perception of individual patients' conditions and prognoses. Unfortunately, at times patients and family members misinterpret these cues or exaggerate their meaning, which only adds to the distortions.

The feeling tone of staff members during this initial period resembles the heroism that accompanies life-saving dramatic situations. Some sadness and anger might be felt, especially surrounding the admission of a child. Sometimes staff respond in awe at the amount of tissue damage, appearance of the patient or how the accident occurred. None of these feelings, however, can interfere in providing life-saving procedures; consequently, many of these initial staff reactions must be put aside hopefully to be dealt with at a later time.

It is not unusual to approach staff members days after a patient has been admitted, asking how the patient was burned and hearing "I really don't know" as the answer. Staff members utilize protective mechanisms, as individually appropriate, to create the distance from the patient as needed to be able to perform their professional functions. However, this does not mean that they are "uncaring" about the patient. There soon exists a "forced" relationship between the staff members and the burn patient. Due to the patient's lengthy hospitalization, state of dependency and the amount of daily, direct contact with patients, close relating, especially for nursing personnel, is inevitable. Consequently, measures to "slow down" the relating process (initially and throughout the patient's hospitalization) may be employed. These measures reduce the degree of intensity in relating and allow concentration on delivering deliberate, excellent burn nursing care.

Some staff members exhibit an overzealousness to instruct patients and families of "everything" there is to know about the burn facility and postburn care. Although well intentioned, they soon learn that, since the adjustment to stress is a process, technical information must be delivered at a pace that patients and families can tolerate. Initially, greater emphasis on rapport building by delivering supportive words in addition to a minimal amount of technical information is a much wiser investment of personal, professional energy in dealing with newly admitted burn patients and their families.

INTERVIEWING

Interviewing may be useful in attempting to elicit a preburn history and provide supportive contact to patients and families during the immedite postburn period. Following are recommendations for successful interviewing.

1. Limit the initial questioning of patients and families to information absolutely essential for care purposes (preburn medical history, primary family support, present place of employment or others needing to know of patient's hospitalization etc.) until increased trust in hospital staff is established.

2. Continued interviews should be resumed and conducted in segments over the first few days postburn and throughout the patient's hospitalization as greater rapport is built among patient, family and staff. This accumulation of information allows for a greater understanding of patient behavior and support systems as well

156

as more meaningful staff interventions.

3. Be supportive during interviewing. Patients and especially family members are easily intimidated by direct questioning. Parents of children who are burned often feel that the physician and/or nurse obtaining the initial history are attempting to "accuse" them (by the tone of the interviewer's voice and his attitude) of being responsible for the child's condition. Become sensitive to the issues surrounding "wounded parenthood." Some childhood burn situations are indeed accidents!

4. The same questions and information repeatedly asked of the patient and/or family may meet with negative reaction. For some, revealing family history, details of the accident and so on, may be very difficult. Being asked for the same information from a number of different staff people can provoke anger or defensive responses. An effective communication system within the burn team can prevent redundancy in collecting the necessary patient information.

PATIENT INTERVENTION

In providing supportive contact to patients during the immediate postburn period, the following may be useful:

1. Learn the typical initial responses of the postburn patient.

2. Provide consistent one-to-one individual contact, which is most effective during this initial period for the following reasons:

   • assists in maintaining reality orientation;

   • allows the staff member to assess patient sensorium;

   • assists in counteracting the "flood response" by providing an auxiliary ego function of ordering priorities of coping;

   • encourages patients to reestablish control over their situation;

   • provides diversion to minimize pain sensation;

   • encourages appropriate ventilation of feelings (especially the intense, initial feelings of anger and guilt); and

   • allows the staff member to explore and evaluate supportive systems available to the patient.

3. Some facilities bring in Burns Recovered people to assist acute patients. In my experience, this technique is best utilized with hospitalized burn patients later in the hospitalization, when motivation decreases. Initially, patients, due to their internalized and ego-centered states, have difficulty dealing with comparatives. Instead of becoming motivated, patients may become overwhelmed at the successful rehabilitation of the visitors. Their primary concern at this time is survival, along with a multitude of other here and now issues. Their response to this approach may be one of anger or complete withdrawal.

4. Due to the number of uncertainties and fluctuating physical responses to procedures and complications that may occur during the entire postburn hospitalization, a suggestion to the patient to adopt a "one day at a time" philosophy of thinking is most helpful.

FAMILY INTERVENTION

The following can aid adaptation of the family during the immediate postburn phase.

1. Prepare family members prior to their initial visit with the patient. Many lay persons have never been exposed to the physical devastation of postburn trauma. A brief orientation to the appearance of the patient (especially if open method of treatment is employed), the sensorium level of the patient (especially if facial edema is present) and the environmental aspects (private room; intensive care unit where ventilator patients may be; mixed pediatric-adult intensive care unit, etc.) is essential. It has also been found useful to act as an alter ego to visitors about to visit the postburn patient for the first time by suggesting what to say and do when they arrive at the bedside. Many times the appearance of the patient is so overwhelming that all good intentions of verbalizing support temporarily escape the visitor. A staff escort to accompany the visitor to the bedside initially is of great value.

The final suggestion in supporting the visitor through this initial, traumatic experience is to recommend the visitor step away from the bedside after the initial contact with the patient. This initial visit should last only a few minutes in time. Visitors, often overwhelmed by the appearance of the patient, have a tendency to stand silent at the bedside and gape at the patient, feeling obligated to remain there yet very helpless. This combination of feelings causes anxiety levels to soar and is of no supportive value to the patient or visitor. A staff member "giving permission" to the visitor to leave the bedside and return when they feel stronger is a much appreciated family-staff intervention.

2. Initial focus in dealing with families should include concern for *their* response to the situation as well as factual information on the patient's condition.

3. Limit the amount of facts given to visitors during the first 24 to 48 hours. The anxiety level of visitors during this period is extremely high, and comprehension/memory levels of functioning are affected by high anxiety. The main concern of families and visitors of extremely injured patients at this time is "Will the patient live or die?" They listen and watch carefully to elicit verbal or nonverbal messages from the staff that will answer this question.

Present patient condition, with here and now treatments being given, is sufficient initial information. Other information, including items of general burn care, possible complications and treatment procedures, should be taught to visitors as soon as they seem receptive.

4. Educating and orientating primary visitors to the burn facility and to the type of burn care being given to the patients is essential in alleviating extended anxiety and assisting visitors to understand changes in treatment or patient condition. Visual aids are useful in teaching families and visitors the elements of postburn

158 care. The use of slides or a prepared "Visitors Guide" are teaching tools that can assist families during this acute, initial period.

5. Frequent supportive contacts given to primary family members and visitors reassures them of the care and concern of the entire burn team for the patient and prepares the family for the very important role they play in the patient's rehabilitation.

STAFF

Staff too may need to adapt during the immediate postburn phase. The following recommendations may aid in this process.

1. Find outlets to verbally share with one another staff feelings surrounding how the burn situation occurred and the patient's physical status.
2. Reflect on the team work executed by the staff in performing initial resuscitation procedures.
3. Knowing some of the patient's history, begin to establish a workable care plan that is realistic and pertinent to patient needs.
4. Together with other staff members, discuss possible complications that may interfere with patient prognosis.
5. Show your concern for family members. If lack of time in giving family support is an issue, turn to available resource people for assistance (social worker, nurse clinician, psychologist, clergymen, other available nursing staff, etc.).
6. Begin to realize the limitations of the profession in dealing with extremely burned patients (especially the very young and the very old) or those with multiple complications. Realize that your best in burn nursing care may be their last comfort in life.

Emergency or Constriction Phase

Some of the patient reactions seen in the emergency or "constriction"[2] phase of psychological adaptation to stress coincide with the immediate response of the postburn patient to the burn injury. The term *constriction* refers to the behavior seen within the first few weeks postburn. Patients often become very quiet and withdrawn. They verbalize little and appear depressed, uninterested in their environment or people around them. Hamburg interpreted this as humans' way of buffering the reality of their present vulnerable state, and a period in time utilized to quietly prepare themselves (psychologically) for a sudden, stressful situation that has already occurred. This withdrawal response has also been observed in victims of heart attack or other sudden traumatic experiences.

Initially Ted and Bob were treated in the intensive care unit, Tommy and Debbie in the pediatric convalescent area (although monitored as intensive care patients) and Donna in the adult convalescent area of the burn center. There was much excitement among the staff. Admitting five patients at one time was not ordinary. Much work went into the initial resuscitation of all involved, and much thought backed the decisions of where to place the patients and how to deal with their overall response to the situation and their interacting process.

Ted, a fairly quiet person, initially responded with withdrawal, eventually verbalizing his intense feelings of guilt as the owner of the craft. His personality was somewhat depressive, and he had a low pain tolerance, yet he chose to deal directly with the reality of the situation as quickly as possible.

Bob, placed next to Ted in a four-bed room in the intensive care unit, experienced a myriad of feelings during the acute postburn period. He too chose to deal with issues "head on" but found, through staff assistance, that pacing himself was much more realistic. He eventually dealt with the issues of anger and guilt: anger because this tragedy had interfered with life plans (the T.C.s had just purchased a new home) and had left him in a helpless state; and guilt because he felt responsible for making the decision to take part in the boat ride that resulted in this tragedy for his entire family. Bob was very verbal in expressing feelings, and, because of his independent, responsible nature, the forced dependency on the staff was very difficult for him to accept. Bob expressed no animosity or blame toward Ted, but rather discussed the situation openly, and they eventually became very supportive of one another.

Tommy and Debbie initially responded with fear and withdrawal, as do most pediatric patients. Their parents, due to physical injury, were unable to give them the amount and consistent support they needed. It was necessary to increase staff and extended family supportive contact. Debbie, who was more severely burned than her brother Tommy, began verbalizing and responding more during the second week postburn.

Donna, the least severely injured, initially responded to the situation in a very unrealistic, protective fashion. Her exuberance in showing concern for the other three members of her family and Ted was commendable—or so thought the staff. She visited the children and spent time in the intensive care unit with Bob and Ted,

moving about in her wheelchair. She responded with complete denial regarding the fact that, although less severely injured, she too had visible, painful open wounds. Her attitude of being the pillar of strength in this tragic situation, the model mother and wife, and the cheerful support to her family came to a staggering halt the third day postburn.

With staff assistance Donna began touching base with the real picture of having her entire family injured and in a hospital; but, more important, she began dealing with her own injury. She openly expressed anger (which was often directed at the staff) and stayed in her room. Periodically she would ask about the condition of the others, but never asked to see them. She expressed feelings of guilt, in that if she would have taken Tommy to the other side of the boat to change his diaper, neither of them would have been injured. This response lasted for two weeks and dramatically depicted a person's need to deal with one's personal reactions to stress prior to being able to provide overt support to others. It also portrayed the initial, internalized, ego-centered state, which is essential in early postburn adjustment attempts.

It is important to note that the burn team needed to focus on the fact that each of the five patients had to be treated as an individual, with individual reactions and needs, before dealing with the T.C.s as a family unit with complex interrelating patterns. Ted needed to be approached as an individual first, then a person involved in the same situation with the T.C.s, but not as an integral part of the T.C. family.

Both the extended family members of the T.C.s and Ted's family members responded to this tragedy with quiet disbelief and anger. Initially, there was little exchange among this group of varied

160 family members. Guilt and blame were unspoken feelings, while concern for survival predominated. The staff, being aware of initial family concerns, focused on relating patients' conditions, understanding initial postburn care, orienting patients to services available at the center, and being able to support the individual patients and each other in a positive fashion. In time and with staff assistance, family members of the T.C.s and those belonging to Ted were able to share with one another those feelings of anger, guilt and blame which were so intense immediately following the accident. This exchange, which provided expressed relief to various family members, was achieved within the understanding environment of staff-led family group sessions.

Foundation For Solid Communication and Support System

Initial responses and interventions during the initial postburn period are crucial to patients, families and staff. The ability to construct a solid communication and support system, useful to all, during the reactive and rehabilitative stages of adjustment relies heavily on the foundation built during the first few weeks postburn.

REACTIVE PHASE

Following the initial postburn period is the reactive phase of postburn adjustment. During this phase the patient's condition becomes a vivid reality to all.

Patients

As patients begin to deal with the reality of the here and now, they begin to overtly express feelings. They actively respond to painful procedures such as tubbings, debridement, dressing changes and exercise programs. Affect readily fluctuates, impulse control is poor and thinking is often unrealistic. Patients begin to react to the appearance of wounds and question the outcome of skin grafting procedures.

Patients now become more actively involved with their environment. They begin to see other patients around them as individuals and not reflections of themselves. They often compare overall conditions and begin making statements as "I'm sure lucky I wasn't burned as badly as Mr. N."

In a burn facility utilizing ward areas, patients now group together to establish a share system that is most useful in coping with daily stress.

Regressive behavior is often seen in patients experiencing long-term hospitalization. In burn patients, behavior such as thumbsucking, bedwetting and whining are frequently seen in older children and adults. By definition, regression is a reversion to childlike behavior which gives "good feelings." Good feelings are few and far between for postburn patients, so they often develop temporary behavior to meet some of this need. If behavior does not interfere with physical/functional treatment and progress, it should be dealt with as a temporary necessity that will be given up once more appropriate outlets are possible.

Overt hostility and anger can continue to be expressed throughout the reactive phase of adjustment. Patients are still uncertain about the final outcome of appearance and functioning. They are still experiencing pain and discomfort to some degree. The "why me?" questioning or active bargaining with the staff to postpone a dressing change are examples of anger expressions and are often difficult to deal with.

Patients often exhibit "magical thinking," which is an early form of a coping attempt. For example, patients in pain may refuse to exercise to maintain function. They indicate that they will exercise when they get home and the pain ceases. In reality, due to progressively tightening contractures, pain becomes more intense when exercises are postponed.

Some of this magical thinking is directed toward the medical/nursing staff; patients may believe that physicians and nurses know how to take pain away and make a patient comfortable. It can be very anger provoking for some patients to realize that in postburn care this is not always possible. Staff members must focus on all the issues, direct and indirect, which cause hostility and anger in the postburn patient and must view the overt expression of anger as useful to the patient's adjustment and not as a personal attack.

Autonomy and control issues are prevalent. There is a definite conflict felt by some patients who are reluctant to give up the dependency that occurs during their intensive care period, even though they have a strong need to resume their independent status. Sometimes in an effort to gain back some control over themselves and their environment, patients make unrealistic requests (wanting to ambulate too soon after a grafting procedure) or gain control through negative behavior (refusing necessary procedures or exercise). The staff members who recognize the patient's need for control facilitate this need by providing areas and issues where patients can exercise control.

Nightmares often occur, especially with fire victims or those intentionally burned by another individual. Hostility, blame and anger are often behind this mental reworking of the burn situation. Patients often fear that these nightmares will continue "forever" and fear telling others about them. Discussing these situations with patients and letting them know that most burn patients having such nightmares report that they are temporary and seem to cease once the patients feel certain of successful recovery is comforting.

Sporadically, the patient experiences short-term periods of depression which may or may not include crying, but will not interfere with treatment or other physical functions. These should be viewed and accepted by staff and family members as natural responses to the painful reality of a tragic situation and necessary stepping stones toward postburn adjustment.

This is also a period in which patients begin to reactivate concern for family members and initiate planning to reestablish life roles altered by hospitalization.

Families

Following the initial postburn period, family members group together and actively support one another. Good rapport and well-established communication with the staff reassures the family that the patient is receiving the best of care. It even becomes a bit easier for them to accept relatively minor setbacks as non-life-threatening complications come about.

As time goes by, family members well prepared by the staff for an unavoidable loss will be better able to accept the death of a loved one. Time has offered the

162 opportunity to strengthen family support to one another.

Family members feel less helpless during this period, since they are now able to do concrete activities to "help" the patient. The staff can facilitate family assistance in caring for the patient, providing guidelines for the family to follow so their "helping ways"do not interfere with patient progress or staff functioning. Remember that the safest policy is to have the family work with the staff, not instead of the staff.

In some instances, once family members see that the patient is beyond the life-threatening stage, they visit less frequently or not at all. The staff may need to remind the family of the patient's need for support and diversion throughout the long hospitalization.

When a very complex family system exists, there may be occasional disputes among family members during visiting times. The family may need to be reminded that the patient's needs in the hospital setting are the priority and that additional stress caused by family members arguing around the patient merely adds to the already existing stress situation.

Some family members, unable to deal with their personal guilt response to the situation, or feeling angry and discouraged by the long-term hospitalization and demands being placed on them by the patient, respond with anger toward the staff. They may find fault with everything and everyone in the hospital setting. Taking interest in assisting the visitor to verbalize the real cause of the frustration and various ways to deal with it is often a useful approach.

Focus for families during this period may preclude patients' concern about "How are things going to be after discharge?" They may be concerned and ask questions pertinent to their role in physically caring for the patient, as well as those pertaining to psychosocial situations (What should I do if my child doesn't want to take a bath in the tub where he was burned? How should I prepare my younger children to accept their father's changed appearance? etc.).

Realize that, after discharge, family members will be the primary caretakers and the ones available to assist the patient in the transition from hospital to home. It is essential to afford them as much time as necessary to prepare for this role. Answering questions related to this before the patient is ready for discharge is not uncommon.

Staff

During this phase, staff members are faced with a multitude of challenging situations from both patients and families. Maintaining a consistency in communication among staff members assists greatly in dealing with almost any problem or difficult situation that arises. The possibility that one may have certain negative feelings about individual patients and family members is a reality. Basing patient and family approaches and interventions on these negative feelings is disaster!

It is during this period too that sudden, severe complications leading to the demise of a patient (who everyone felt would do well) can cause much sadness and questioning among the staff. Patients whose survival has been unprecedented (with regard to extent of injury) may do well during the immediate postburn phase only to die weeks later from sepsis or pneumonia. Several of these situations simultaneously occurring in a larger burn facility can be very devastating to staff morale. Team spirit, verbal outlets and staff members reinforcing each other can assist individuals and the group during these times when personal and professional limitations are so very apparent.

Staff members are faced with the "degree of involvement" issue with patients during this lengthy reactive period. The patient is more responsive and more demanding of staff attention and support. Nursing personnel, faced with 24-hour patient contact (with patients hospitalized a few weeks to two to four months) experience a long-term forced relating situation and must choose the level of interacting, with patient and personal, professional interest in mind.

Routine procedures, such as lengthy dressing changes or tubbings, can become physically wearing on the staff, leading to low tolerance levels of patients reactive behavior. Supervisory personnel must be acutely aware of individual workload and assignments and provide intervention as appropriate to avoid negative staff-patient situations.

"Busy times" for staff during this period easily cause family questions to be regarded as unimportant or interfering. Family members avoided by the staff will establish their own means of getting questions answered which will cost far more staff time in the end. Considering family members as an active part of the burn team instead of "outsiders" assists in meeting their needs when expressed as well as those established in our care plans.

Dealing with patients' expressions of pain is one of the most difficult nursing issues in caring for the postburn patient. Due to possible smoke inhalation or the long-term hospitalization anticipated, narcotic medications are administered infrequently and in small doses. Throughout the hospitalization the postburn patient experiences varied degrees of pain paralleled with varied degrees of anxiety. In doing pain-provoking procedures it is a common feeling among staff that they are the "cause" of the pain. Burn team members must look toward a greater understanding of pain as it is perceived by individual patients according to physical, psychological and cultural bases and interpreted and expressed quite individually.

Gathering information related to the above and providing information to the patient relative to the reality of his pain experience is essential. This includes informing patients that they will have pain, how intense it might be and how long it might last.[3] Utilize, if possible, what patients perceive as being useful in relieving pain and assist patients in understanding that the cause and control of pain rests with them and not the staff. Suggest what patients can do for themselves to relieve the intensity of pain (relaxation techniques, distraction, positioning, etc.). For burn nurses, dealing with patients' pain becomes an art. Realizing that the availability and presence of a concerned staff member to answer questions and allay fears can at times be more effective than administering analgesics is truly a professional accomplishment.

164 Following the initial period, Bob and Donna continued verbalizing their feelings and concerns to the staff. Bob, being very intelligent and an attorney by profession, had many questions regarding the physical aspects of his injury and those of the rest of his family. He dealt with psychosocial issues with some hesitancy; however, participation in a twice weekly scheduled patient group session led by several staff members assisted him in realizing that others had been dealing with similar issues. He began sharing feelings and concerns, especially relevant to his less-than-expected ability to cope with pain, feelings of helplessness and anger surrounding the forced dependency caused by the accident. He expressed guilt feelings surrounding the extent of Debbie's injury, because he was directly caring for her at the time of the accident. The children were brought to him as often as he requested until he was able to visit them in a wheelchair.

Donna, sufficiently dealing with issues involving her own injury and experience, slowly began to resume concern for her three family members. She continued to respond to pain with varied degrees of anger, but found self-conducted relaxation exercises to be of great assistance. When feeling stronger, she would ask to have the children brought to her room, and eventually began visiting the children and her husband on her own for longer time periods. Donna began focusing on some positive aspects of the hospitalization, which included attending patient group sessions with her husband. These sessions fostered an open sharing of feelings which had been difficult for both to do prior to the accident. Respecting their individual needs to discuss concerns privately, both Donna and Bob were seen individually by members of the psychology team throughout the hospitalization.

Tommy and Debbie continued to respond actively to pain but were easily distracted (with appropriate play stimulation) following procedures. They responded favorably to added attention supplied daily by hospital-provided elderly volunteers called Foster Grandparents. In time, Debbie began talking about the burn accident and her injuries. A stuffed rag doll from home kept her company in bed during the entire hospitalization. Due to having both hands burned she was temporarily unable to draw pictures, so the storytelling method was used to assist her in venting some of the fears and anger she was feeling. She eventually began playing with other children on the ward and especially enjoyed going to the playroom each day.

A musical mobile was hung over Tommy's crib and brightly colored plastic blocks provided him with play stimulation. The staff found that holding Tommy periodically, especially during mealtime, was apparently comforting to him. This became an integral part of his nursing care plan. Both children responded favorably to visits with Donna and Bob. Natural grandparents visited consistently and were well received.

Ted, more withdrawn preburn due to other minor physical disabilities, continued to experience difficulty in relating to staff members. His family and fiancé visited consistently. The staff, in dealing supportively with the family, identified the patient's fiancé as the person Ted related to most comfortably. She was encouraged to assist Ted in dealing with the varied issues of postburn injury. The invitation to join the patient group meetings was extended (without pressure) to Ted, who chose not to participate. Additional supportive intervention was provided through various staff members identified by Ted as being helpful to him. Although Ted had a low pain tolerance, he chose to deal with pain in a "quiet suffering" manner because this made him feel like a "stronger" person.

Family members of all concerned continued to provide consistent support, visiting regularly and becoming as active in patient care as permitted. They scheduled visiting days for everyone within their groups so that no one would become exhausted in having to visit daily. They were organized within their groups and assisted each other in coping with minor difficulties or stress periods that came about. They consulted staff members when questions arose and were open to suggestions on patient needs.

Various family members of the T.C.s began planning for patients' discharge without realizing that all would not be discharged at the same time. It was recommended that a meeting of Bob, Donna, their parents and select members of the staff take place to assist in formulating predischarge plans. Since home for the T.C.s was a considerable distance from the burn facility, much needed to be discussed relative to Donna and Tommy being discharged before Debbie and Bob. Rehabilitation and postdischarge concerns became a reality for Bob and Donna's parents much sooner than for the T.C.s themselves. Adequate time for family members to prepare was essential, and staff assistance was provided accordingly.

REHABILITATION PHASE

The final phase of postburn adjustment is often referred to as the rehabilitation phase. It is hoped that, time permitting, this phase begins in the hospital prior to discharge, making the transitional period from hospital to home much smoother. Individual members of all three segments of our circle (patient, family and staff) begin to see the final result of injury as it becomes vividly apparent. Limitations in function can be realistically evaluated and appropriate treatment prescribed. Scar formation may or may not be apparent. All are ready to plunge into concrete discharge planning.

Patients

Psychologically speaking, patients now focus on functional disabilities and appearance. They begin to mentally work on new self-concepts and are often seen testing out new behavior in the relative safety of the hospital. They become actively interested in obtaining information and support from staff members and recovered burn patients regarding the transition from hospital to home. Information on how people, once home from the hospital, dealt with exercise programs, people's questions regarding the accident, wearing pressure garments and so on, is useful to the person who anticipates these situations. Anxiety rises once more when the patient begins to deal with issues of reassuming responsibility for self-care, social reintegration and reestablishing previous family roles.

Postburn patients repeatedly voice frustration and anger in that outside of those who cared for or visited them while in the hospital, no one will ever know all they have been through. They are quite correct, and it is often useful to discuss this with them. Although people will ask many questions, much of the time, genuine understanding and feeling tone will not be transmitted. An adjacent issue involves how to respond to "nosey" neighbors who

166 really are not concerned and merely provoke the patient by asking about the burn situation, hospital procedures and so on. Reminding patients that, although the victims of a dramatic, tragic situation, they need not discuss issues in detail with everyone and can choose to verbally indicate this to various individuals is useful.

Specific assistance must be given to patients who have young children or younger siblings at home who have not as yet seen the patient with altered appearance and/or scar formation. Negative reactions are common from children on initial exposure to the patient. Discussing this with the patient, exploring their fantasies of what will occur and helping them to prepare for dealing with the situation in the best interest of the patient and young child is recommended. In some burn facilities family members are invited to bring young children in for a specially arranged visit with the patient, prior to discharge, in order to have additional staff support in dealing with the situation.

Separation from the hospital, burn team members and other patients is most difficult for many patients. Although rejoicing that this perilous postburn period is ended and they now can resume "living," a conflicting feeling of sadness and anger exists in having to leave this safe environment of understanding, caring people. Many patients return to the burn facility to visit other inpatients for a brief period after discharge in an attempt to relieve some of the antagonistic feelings. Others find sufficient support in maintaining postdischarge clinic appointments, especially if the clinic is conducted in or near the burn facility by members of the burn team who were involved in the primary inpatient care.

Families

Families are mainly concerned about "doing the right thing" for patients once discharged home. Staff discharge instructions regarding wound care, diet or medications should be clear and concise. Giving each patient family a sheet of written instructions to take home as a handy reference is useful, especially to family members experiencing anxiety feelings similar to those of the patient. At times, in their zealousness to do everything possible for the patient once home, they tend to lose sight of the patient's need to reestablish independence. They may be too quick to assist when the patient appears to be performing activities slower or less accurately due to physical disability. In discussing issues with families before discharge, this is an item of major importance. Allowing a patient time to achieve a function or complete an activity which was simple and taken for granted before the injury helps to build self-esteem.

Reassuring the family that they can call on the burn team in case there appear to be problems with respect to physical care or psychosocial adjustment once the patient is home is a comforting cushion. It is often a frightening thought for the family to realize that just a few family members must now replace the entire burn team in being primary caretakers!

Staff

Staff members, during the rehabilitation period, experience a multitude of feelings.

Their initial responsibilities in dealing with patients throughout the various periods of physical recovery and psychological adjustment have been completed. Now, as the patients resume a more independent status, staff members continue to offer support that is comparatively less intense. There is a feeling of accomplishment and a sense of joy to see a successful recovery and discharge home of a severely injured postburn patient despite some of the visible subsequent disfigurement.

At the same time there is often sadness felt at facing the separation from a long-term patient regardless of the many problems faced during the hospitalization. Some of the sadness felt by the staff may be due to reflections on the quality of life possible for a patient leaving the hospital with severe disfigurement. Sometimes staff may feel anger in seeing a severely burned and recovered child being taken home by parents, who, in their opinion, provided less than optimal support for the child during the hospitalization. Return visits to the care facility by the patients and their families is motivating and reinforces staff morale. Being able to see the severely injured postburn victim alive, functional and to some extent adjusted makes all the difficult aspects of being a member of the burn team worthwhile.

Prior to discharge, Donna had many questions regarding how to help Debbie deal with the fact that Mom and Tommy were going home before Debbie and Dad. Other concerns were focused on dealing with reestablishing a family system once all four of them were home. Donna had complete range of motion and no apparent functional disabilities. She had dealt exten-sively in counseling with appearance issues and questions relative to her relationship with Bob as husband and wife. Donna feared the possibility of intense rejection from Bob because of her minor changes in appearance.

Donna felt she had much work to do to help herself and her family members continue to work on the adjustment process. Discussion regarding issues specific to Debbie's overall response to the situation took place. Once home, it was suggested to include Debbie as much as possible as mother's helper in the care of Tommy. Children Debbie's age frequently feel responsible for negative situations in the family. Showing Debbie that Mom and Dad are not angrily blaming her and need her help in Tommy's care will dispell some of this fantasy. This behavior will also assist Debbie in accepting Tommy as a new family member.

Bob continued on in the hospital for two weeks after Donna and Tommy were discharged. He felt that Donna would have sufficient assistance from the grandparents to manage the house and care for Tommy until his return. However, Bob's hands were severely burned. Close to the time of discharge, he began to face the reality that continued assistance from the grandparents would be required, at least until he was able to do things more independently.

Other issues were of importance to Bob, such as those related to answering people's questions about his accident and injury. He expressed anger at the thought that people who really did not care would probably inquire the most and he would have difficulty responding to them. During patient group sessions, the role-reversal role-playing technique was used to help Bob in understanding and dealing with this concern. At discharge Bob was prepared to

168   pace himself in reestablishing his lifestyle roles as they were before the burn. He focused on the positive aspects of hospitalization, one of which was the fact that, through contact with the staff in daily care and participating in patient group sessions, he learned to openly express feelings and concerns he never felt comfortable in doing before the burn. He felt that this would definitely enhance his life and reduce the amount of tension and stress he had constantly experienced before the burn.

One last recommendation made to the T.C. family involved their move into a new home which was being planned prior to the accident. It was suggested that they remain in the original home for a short time before moving, so as to experience the new home as a positive situation detached from the accident and all the difficult adjustment that followed.

Ted remained in the hospital the longest. His inability to openly express feelings and concerns to the staff or other patients continued. This was accepted by the staff and patient group and did not have a negative effect on the quality of supportive contact that they were able to offer him during the final weeks of his hospital stay. Ted worked well with his exercise program and continued to use the support of his fiancé in dealing with crucial issues of rehabilitation. His family visited consistently and offered him the quiet support that he found to be useful. Postburn psychosocial rehabilitation would be a long road for Ted to travel, but the care and concern of the burn team gave him a firm start.

Family members of Ted and the T.C.s anxiously awaited their homecoming. Preparations were being made, and family members consulted the burn team whenever questions arose. Family sessions, where family members shared thoughts on what things would be like when the patients returned home, were held. This enabled members to voice anticipated behavior and responses. It also allowed staff members to help bring about an awareness within the group of some of the patients' needs during this transitional period.

The staff dealt with the patients and their family members during the final phase of hospitalization in a supportive and appropriate fashion, according to the needs expressed. They respected the uniqueness, individuality and level of coping of each of the five patients. When all patients were finally discharged, the staff reflected on the entire situation with all its complexities and felt an eagerness to share with one another the feelings that accompany a "job well done." Their teamwork was complete, with staff, patient and family participation. They looked forward to seeing the T.C.s and Ted when they returned to the postburn clinic and hoped that all would continue to do well.

It is usually during the rehabilitation and postdischarge period that patients can finally express feelings of gratitude unclouded by all the intense, complex combination of feelings felt throughout the hospitalization. Many patients return to the same facility for further reconstructive surgery or care, but for now, as they often express, "The initial battle is ended. The worst is over!" Psychosocially, for many, the real life battle has just begun.

REFERENCES

1. Coelho, G., Hamburg, D. and Adams, J. *Coping and Adaptation* (New York: Basic Books Inc. 1974).
2. Hamburg, D., Hamburg, B. and deGoza, S. "Adaptive Problems and Mechanisms in Severely Burned Patients." *Arch Gen Psychol* 17 (1953) p. 277.
3. McCaffery, M. "Patients in Pain." *Nursing 73* (June 1973).

SUGGESTED READINGS

Andreasen, N. and Norris, A. "Long-Term Adjustment and Adaptation Mechanisms in Severely Burned Adults." *J Nerv Ment Dis* 154:5 (1972) p. 352.

Andreasen, N., Noyes, R. and Hartford, C.E. "Factors Influencing Adjustment of Burn Patients During Hospitalization." *Psychosom Med* 34:6 (1972) p. 517.

Andreasen, N. et al. "Management of Emotional Reactions in Seriously Burned Adults." *N Engl J Med* 286 (1972) p. 65.

Bernstein, N. *Emotional Care of the Facially Burned and Disfigured* (Boston: Little Brown & Co. 1976).

Davidson, S. and Noyes, R. "Psychiatric Nursing Consultation on a Burn Unit." *Am J Nursing* 73 (July–December 1973) p. 1715–1718.

Fagerhaugh S.Y. "Pain Expression and Control on a Burn Care Unit." *Nursing Outlook* 22:10 (October 1974) p. 645–650.

Holter, J. and Friedman, S. "Etiology and Management of Severely Burned Children." *Am J Dis Child* 118 (November 1969) p. 680–686.

McBride, A. "The Anger-Depression-Guilt Go-Round." *Am J Nursing* 73:6 (June 1973) p. 104–109.

Mieszala, P. "Burn Conferences-Supportive Mechanism for Burn Nurses." *Burn Team* (June 1977).

Mieszala, P. "Regression, the Burn Patient, and the Nurse." *Burn Team* 2:2 (1975).

Mieszala, P. and Hartmann, R. "Burn Prevention—Group Teaching for Victims." *Supervisor Nurse* 7:6 (1976) p. 66–69.

Mieszala, P. and Hartmann, R. "Dealing with Burn Patients' Hostility." *Burn Team* 2:2 (1976) p. 416–422.

Mieszala, P. "Psychological Parameters of Burn Patient Care." *Practical Approaches to Burn Management* (Deerfield, Illinois: Flint Laboratories, Division of Travenol Labs, Inc. 1977) p. 62–67.

Noyes, R., Andreasen, N. and Hartford, C. "The Psychological Reaction to Severe Burns." *Psychosomatics* 12 (1971) p. 416.

Quinby, S. and Bernstein, N. "Identity Problems and the Adaptation of Nurses to Severely Burned Children." *Am J Psychol* 128:1 (July–December 1971) p. 58–68.

Rubin, M. "Balm for Burned Children." *Am J Nursing* 66:2 (January–June 1966) p. 297–302.

Seligman, R., Carroll, S. and MacMillan, B. G. "Emotional Responses of Burned Children in a Pediatric Intensive Care Unit." *Psychol Med* 3:1 (January 1972) p. 59–65.

Woodward, J. "Emotional Disturbances of Burned Children." *Br Med J* 1:18 (April 1959) p. 1009–1013.

Woodward, J. "Parental Visiting of Children with Burns." *Br Med J* 2 (1962) p. 1656–1657.

Part IV
Self-Regulation of Stress

Stress and Health: A Survey of Self-Regulation Modalities

Doris Cook Sutterley, R.N., M.S.N.
Assistant Professor of Nursing
and Nursing Consultant
La Salle College
Philadelphia, Pennsylvania

IF STRESS is the spice of life as Selye says, Why is it implicated as a contributing factor in all of the major causes of death and disability? Why does stress cause so much distress? And why has the health care system not been more effective in treating the stress-related disorders?

Stress and its effects on the health of individuals are the prime focus of concern for many health care providers. Stress is certainly not new. It has always been an integral component of life. Recognition of the role and impact of stress in our lives is new.

Selye, the pioneer of stress theory and research on the General Adaptation Syndrome, defines stress as the "nonspecific response of the body to any demand made upon it."[1]

Others have defined stress from the perspective of psychodynamic theory, behavioral or learning theory, developmental theory, biological, sociological or ethological theories. Each of these theories contributes to the knowledge of stress. For the health care provider it is essential to recognize stress as a subjective state that is

174 highly individual—not only in cognition and perception but also in the physiological indices of stress. This holistic definition of stress encompasses many of the theoretical views currently used.

Stress is a dynamic state within the individual that results from

- *any demand to adapt or change,* such as normative maturational crises, transition periods, illnesses, disabilities or losses, changes in social status, changes in occupations, unemployment or accumulation of situational life-change events
- *a perceived threat* to personal health, safety or life, self-esteem, self-confidence, belief systems or values, war, annihilation, natural disasters or environmental hazards
- *a challenge to one's ability to cope or perform,* such as lack of confidence, fear of failure, inadequate preparation for job or task at hand, lack of skills or lack of experience, unrealistic expectations of self by others or the desire to surpass one's record in physical or athletic or artistic pursuits
- *unmet needs* for approval, acceptance, affection, love, recognition, reward, success, power, material needs (food, clothing, shelter), health care, self-actualization or creative expressions.

The definition of stress will guide one's therapeutic approach and choice of coping strategies.

STRESS AND THE HEALTH CARE SYSTEM

There is increasing evidence to suggest a relationship between "undue stress" and the onset of major health problems.[2] A study of the major causes of death indicates a shift in disease patterns. (See Table 1.) In the early 1900s the infectious diseases of children and young adults were the leading causes of death. In 1972 the chronic, stress-related diseases of adulthood were the leading causes of death. The increasing evidence of diseases that appear more related to lifestyle, standards of living and personal health practices creates quite a dilemma for the traditionally oriented caregiver. Knowles emphasizes that the medical profession has reached the point of diminishing returns in efforts to cure or ameliorate illness that is most often the result of "personal misbehavior and environmental conditions."[3]

The improvement of the world population's health over the last two centuries resulted less from medical advances than from improved sanitation, better food and birth control practices.[4] Despite dramatic advances in surgical technique, pharmacological intervention in infectious disease, and assessment and monitoring technology, the contribution of medical care to overall "health care" is proportionately small.

The limitations of modern medicine are particularly evident in the management of persons with heart disease. Cassell points out that nutrition, level of physical activity, cigarette smoking and psychosocial stress combined with other factors are so interrelated in the etiology of heart disease that it is fair to say that lifestyle precipitates the disease process.[5] Can traditional disease-oriented practice eliminate "lifestyle" as the causative agent? "Even if present surgical techniques were perfected, the value of new or repaired heart in the body of a

TABLE 1
Changes in Leading Causes of Death in the United States in the 20th Century

Early 1900s

The death rate was about 28 deaths/1,000 people annually.

Leading causes of death:

Pneumonia
Tuberculosis
Typhoid fever
Various dysenteries

The high mortality rate and specific pattern of disease could be traced to urban social conditions brought on by the industrial revolution which led to massive shifts of rural population into crowded cities with poor sanitation and generalized poverty.

The number of deaths caused by tuberculosis fell rapidly and steadily during the first half of the century (from 200 deaths/100,000 people in 1900 to 20/100,000 in 1950) *before* antituberculosis drugs became available (most likely the result of improved living conditions, better nutrition, population control and less crowding).

Likewise, typhoid fever was rare by the time immunization was available. Improvement has been attributed to the introduction of good sanitation, chlorination of water supply and improved personal hygiene.

1972

The 1972 death rate was about 9 deaths/1,000 people annually.

Leading causes of death:

Cardiovascular problems (coronary heart disease, stroke, hypertension)
Cancer
Accidents
Pulmonary conditions (pneumonia, emphysema)
Diabetes
Cirrhosis of the liver
Suicides and homicides

This new pattern of disease can be attributed to the stresses brought on by affluence and modern technological society.

Source: Cassell, E.J. *The Healer's Art* (Philadelphia: J.B. Lippincott Co. 1976).

---

patient whose lifestyle remained otherwise unchanged would not be very high."[6]

The staggering increase in death and disability due to stress-related disorders calls for new approaches. These alternative approaches can be combined with traditional approaches when a disease has reached an advanced stage, or they can be used to promote and maintain health.

Stress is a dynamic state within the individual that results from:
- *any demand to adapt or change*
- *a perceived threat*
- *a challenge to one's ability to cope or perform*
- *unmet needs.*

MANIFESTATIONS OF STRESS

According to Travis,[7] a disease progresses in a series of seven stages. (See Figure 1.) By recognizing the manifestations of stress, it is possible to intervene early and to avoid excessive stress or "overstress" that results in neurophysiological alterations which are precursors to disease development.

The manifestations of stress are indica-

By recognizing the manifestations of stress, it is possible to intervene early and to avoid excessive stress that results in neurophysiological alterations which are precursors to disease development.

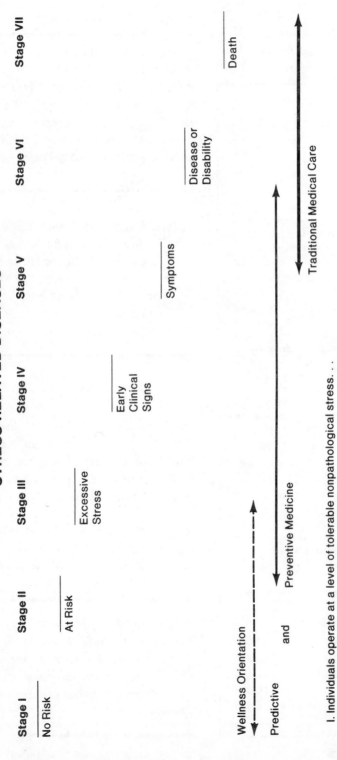

FIGURE 1. STAGES OF DEVELOPMENT IN THE STRESS-RELATED DISEASES

Stage I	Stage II	Stage III	Stage IV	Stage V	Stage VI	Stage VII
No Risk	At Risk	Excessive Stress	Early Clinical Signs	Symptoms	Disease or Disability	Death

Wellness Orientation

Predictive   and   Preventive Medicine

Traditional Medical Care

I. Individuals operate at a level of tolerable nonpathological stress. . .
II. A baseline of tolerable stress is escalated to a level of excessive stress. . .
III. Prolonged and persistent high stress levels produce alteration in neurophysiological functioning.
IV. This creates the preconditions for the development of stress-related disorders. Early identification of risk factors makes it possible to view stages II and III prior to the clinical signs of a disorder to initiate preventive techniques.
V.
VI. The onset and advancement of stress-related diseases—the area of traditional medical care.
VII.

Source: Pelletier, K. *Mind as Healer, Mind as Slayer* (New York: Dell Publishing Co. 1977) p. 314.

tions of the psychophysiological stress response which Selye described as a general, nonspecific response to all stress. However, the individual's specific response to stress is unique and highly personalized because of the interplay of such factors as genetic potential, organ vulnerability, general state of health and fitness as well as background and previous experience in dealing with stress.

Manifestations of stress cover a wide range of behaviors. These behaviors have been grouped together in Figure 2 to suggest levels of stress progressing from that which is minimal to the extreme, which is death. Some of these behaviors include:

- overeating or lack of appetite;
- excessive smoking or drinking;
- irritability-insomnia;
- chronic fatigue-depression;
- rapid, uncontrolled speech; specific mannerisms;
- sweating;
- muscle tension-spasms-pain;
- numerous physical complaints or disorders;
- any and all symptoms characteristic of the stress-related illnesses.

STRESSORS

Stress as a response must be considered apart from the "stressors," those internal or external factors that trigger the stress reaction in the individual. A stressor is anything that places a demand upon the individual for change, adaptation or readjustment. Stressors which are inherent in

experience require organism self-regulation.

The accelerated pace of living is closely related to the marked increase in stress-related disorders. The well-known study of Holmes and Rahe[8] in 1970 resulted in the life change index which they labeled the Social Readjustment Rating Scale. Numerical values were assigned to 43 common events which are typical in peoples' lives, such as changing jobs, getting married, giving birth to a child and relocating. Their systematized method of correlating life events with the onset of illness demonstrates that neurophysiological imbalance can be precipitated by normal life events perceived as stressful. Such an imbalance may lead to the onset of any of the stress-related disorders. Continued research on this scale has confirmed its validity in predicting that stressful life events, occurring in rapid succession, within a specific time frame, are related to the onset of psychological or physical disorders.

Evidence now supports the theory that stress has two major physiological effects: "1) (the) disruption of a particular neurophysiological or organ system in and of itself; and 2) (the) suppression of normal immunological functions, leading to increased susceptibility to viral or aberrant cell disorders."[9] Certainly, it is impossible to choose a lifestyle free from exposure to the stressors of air or water pollutants, noise pollution, radiation and unnatural illumination levels. All are believed to cause stress in that they all call for psychophysiological adaptation and readjustment. Any foreign or toxic substance taken into the body demands a change or alteration in function to correct the imbal-

FIGURE 2. STRESS LEVELS

0: Atarexy	I: Minimal	II: Mild	III: Moderate	IV: Severe	V: Panic
	Comfortable-relaxed state	Day-to-day stresses Nonthreatening Predictable, routine situations	Intermediate stress New or threatening experience A persistently stressful event	Adaptive behaviors fail	Totally disorganized: mentally, physically, emotionally
	Day dreaming	Senses alerted for increased activity Increased learning Adapts readily No after-effects	Perception narrowed, attention decreased Nonproductive–excessive activity Loss of control Behavior changes, mood swings, anxiety Sleep disturbance Physical symptoms: headaches, palpitations	Exhaustion Depression Confusion Anxiety, insomnia Emotional instability Projection–blame Anger–aggression Physical breakdown Symptom formation illness and disease state Burnout	Events: situations seen as dangerous, overpowering Reaching complete exhaustion Psychotic break Cardiac arrest
Drug or hypnotic induced state Hypometabolism Deep meditation	Light meditation Passive concentration				

COPING STRATEGIES

Striving to Maintain equilibrium—steady-state

GOAL—Allow individual to regain self-maintenance capabilities & move toward highest level of adaptation to avoid → severe stress

Potential Inability to Function

⟶ Use of Adaptive Coping Mechanisms ⟶

Coping Mechanisms Fail ⟶
Professional assistance necessary

Crisis intervention – emergency treatment

ance it creates. These toxic substances produce the same stress response as fear, anger or frustration produces. The human organism deals with multiple stressors simultaneously in its own way. However, for purposes of study stressors can be grouped into two categories: (1) biophysical and chemical and (2) psychosocial-cultural.

Biophysical-Chemical Stressors

The stress response is elicited by biophysical-chemical stressors. (See Figure 3.) Such stressors overtax the human organism's self-regulating processes. But the stress response in any individual cannot be explained by a simple stimulus-response or cause-effect model. Not all biophysical-chemical stressors produce the same response or degree of response in individuals. As a result, nursing practice has persistently emphasized *individual* expression of illness or distress at the same time that it has recognized identifiable patterns or symptoms of stress. Selye's initial concern with the concept of stress began with his observations that all persons suffering from diverse diseases had common signs and symptoms, such as general malaise, loss of appetite, lack of energy and muscle strength and a drawn facial expression. These degrees of "just being sick" are an expression of the organism's self-regulation efforts in the face of extreme stressors.

Paradoxically, the very substances most often used to relieve stress are themselves stressors. For example, the coffee and cigarette break or the extra drink before dinner are often used to "promote relaxation." Drugs and medication are foreign

substances that must be considered potential stressors even when taken to relieve the symptoms of stress. Nurses are quite used to monitoring and dealing with the toxic reactions called side effects that clients experience. Often other drugs are used to deal with the toxic effects of the initial prescription. This might be termed the domino theory approach to managing stress.

There certainly are many stress-related situations in which the use of medication is justified, particularly on a short-term basis. It is the extreme dependence on external substances such as drugs rather than the use of internal resources that is deleterious in dealing with chronic stress.

In fact, pharmacological firms consistently caution against the overuse of substances to manage stress-related disorders.

Excess food can also be considered a stressor since any substance that is not used nutritionally by the organism becomes yet another toxin or foreign substance to be processed and eliminated. Obesity and poor nutrition are national health problems.[10] Paradoxically, overeating is often a manifestation of the organism's attempts to deal with stress.

Proper nutrition can be a strong force in bolstering the organism's resources. For many this means revising the American's diet to include more of the whole, fresh, natural foods and decreasing the amount of prepared or processed foods. This would reduce some of the nutritional problems resulting from excessive amounts of refined carbohydrates, salt, fats and oils in the diet.[11] The increased intake of excessive amounts of animal protein combined with the reduced intake

180

FIGURE 3. MULTIPLE SOURCES OF STRESS: BIOPHYSICAL–CHEMICAL, PSYCHOSOCIAL–CULTURAL

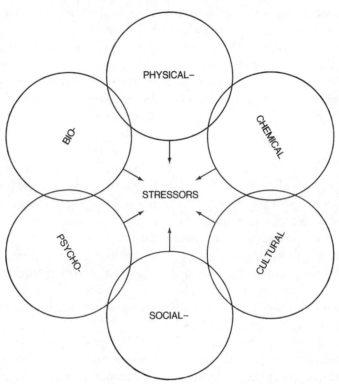

Bio-physical-chemical stressors: excessive heat, cold or pressure; illness, fatigue, exhaustion; uncontrolled loud noise, radiation and illumination levels; bacterial, viral, parasitic invaders; illness and chronic pain; all toxic substances: poisons, drugs, medications, nicotine and alcohol; chemical additives in food, excess food and excess food substances (i.e., caffeine, salt, refined carbohydrates, fats and animal protein); lack of exercise and physical activity, immobilization, inadequate sleep, rest, relaxation and periods of recovery.

Psycho-social-cultural: negative feelings—states of hostility, anger, frustration, resentment, hopelessness, helplessness, powerlessness, loneliness, depression, negative self-image, dissatisfaction with self, unable to accept failure, unrealistic expectations of self and others, unresolved personal conflict, role conflict, role ambiguity, high-pressured lifestyle, cultural mores, expectations, values, rate of change, sensory overload or sensory deprivation, pace of living, crowding, economics, unemployment and cost of living.

of protein from natural grains or natural fiber foods has been linked to the growing incidence of bowel cancer and chronic intestinal diseases such as diverticulitis. Although the relationships are well established, the mechanisms are not understood.[12] People who overeat and underexercise as a result of stress may compound

the negative effects of both these behaviors.

Regular vigorous exercise or physical activity not only reduces stress but allows the release of toxic products.[13] Evidence suggests that inactivity and immobilization can be major stressors.

Exercise and physical activity can reduce

the effects of stress by strengthening the heart, lungs and muscles; increasing energy and stamina; and improving the absorption and utilization of food by replacing intramuscular fat with lean muscle. Nurses have traditionally used physical activity as a therapeutic modality with clients in psychiatric settings. Physical activity has proven effective in reducing stress, relieving depression and promoting more restful sleep. This condition also leads to more effective utilization of calories.

Psychosocial-Cultural Stressors

Much of today's stress overload is attributed to our advanced technological society, our rapidly changing, accelerated pace of living. Increased mobility and constant change have a cumulative effect on society's members as Holmes and Rahe have discovered in their research.[14] Major social changes, such as changing laws on abortion, discrimination, homosexuality or employment practices, may cause stress in individuals.

When an individual is in a work situation that is incompatible with his personal philosophy, job dissatisfaction results and can be a major source of stress. Much of the stress research has been done in the work setting because time-pressured activity is highly stress inducing. When a worker's production is valued more for its

---

Much of today's stress overload is attributed to our advanced technological society, our rapidly changing, accelerated pace of living.

---

quantity and production speed than its quality, personal values and the values of the work setting come into conflict.

Preoccupation with time in the work setting can carry over into one's personal life. Individuals may feel guilty when they do not spend leisure or free time productively. This robs leisure time of its ability to relax, refresh and restore the individual.

Nursing assessments often include data on the patterns of living. An extensive body of research is available to coronary care nurses working with clients who are often categorized personality type A or B. This research indicates for instance that negative, angry and hostile feelings and the manner in which the individual deals with them have a profound physiological effect—they produce the stress response that lowers resistance to disease by suppressing the normal immune response. (See "Selected Bibliography on Stress.")

A great deal of stress arises from a philosophy of living that is unrealistic, from a belief system that is problematic for the individual.

Stress lies in the perception of events, not in events themselves. Stress is internal; it is the individual's response to life events. An individual's stress response may reflect dissatisfaction with self—the inability to accept failure; a negative self-image; or a sense of alienation, a hopelessness and powerlessness.

To seek relief from the negative effects of stress it is necessary to gain insight into mistaken beliefs along with their emotional consequences and physical ramifications.

Many of the diverse and seemingly

182 unrelated factors just reviewed share the ability to create a stress state. However, each individual's response to any of these stressors is highly specific, depending upon the individual's constitutional makeup or inner conditioning, previous experience with stress, and learned behaviors (or outer conditioning as Selye terms it).[15] Individual responses also depend on the unique circumstances, primarily one's state of physical and mental health.

Nursing research has identified specific factors for hospitalized patients, their families and the nursing staff. (See Appendix A.)

STRESS AND SELF-REGULATION

Nurses cannot force clients to manage their own stress-related illnesses. A growing body of literature on noncompliance demonstrates this fact. The human organism cannot control or eliminate stress. It can only, as an active open system, engage in a process of self-regulation.

Self-regulation is a more appropriate term for the management of stress, since it can be both positive and negative. Whether stress leads to disease or increased energy and achievement depends upon how the individual responds to the demands. Selye calls stress that is challenging and that satisfies a need for novelty and high sensation "eustress," meaning good stress. He calls stress that is damaging "distress."[16] Both are the body's response to any demand made upon it. Both use up adaptive energy.

Learning to live with stress requires self-appraisal, introspection and a recognition of one's own manifestation of stress. This is no small task for many who are not able to identify muscle tension in themselves, or for others who may fail to recognize stress when it manifests itself as fatigue or depression.

A client often needs assistance in recognizing the pressure or the untoward effects of stress before attempting to identify the sources of distress and choosing an appropriate course of action.

APPROACHES TO STRESS REDUCTION

The multitude of techniques used to regulate stress can be categorized under four major headings that attempt to:

1. *Alter the environmental circumstances to reduce unnecessary stress.* This may mean changing jobs or location or rearranging priorities. For example, the number of social or service demands upon a working mother may be unrealistic and stress producing. If she cannot refuse unreasonable requests for her time and involvement without feeling guilty, she may need assertiveness training.

2. *Attempt to change one's own behavior or belief.* One's response to a stress-producing situation can be changed by examining one's belief system for faulty perceptions that may require modification. Is it necessary, for example, to do the dishes before going to bed every night or to clean the house before going to work if this conflicts with other demands of a higher priority?

If individuals cannot or do not wish to change certain life events, they may have to alter their perception of those life events as being stressful. Many high-pressured executives and business tycoons choose to remain in a high-stress environment but attempt to change their responses to and perceptions of stress.

3. *Lower physiological arousal to stress* by employing techniques that have proven to be effective in countering the effects of prolonged, chronic stress.

An illness or stress-related disorder may be a very positive experience with an opportunity for learning. Many crisis situations require change and offer the potential for personal growth.

By calling attention to unhealthy practices or conditions that have created an imbalance or a disharmony in the individual, some health problems or stress reactions can be a positive force in one's life.

4. *Enhance one's resistance and immunity* to stress through high-level wellness, achieved with proper nutrition, exercise, rest and relaxation with a positive attitude toward life and a developing spiritual awareness.

Once the alternatives are known, the individual, whether a client, patient or provider, must make the choice and accept the responsibility for a lifestyle that results in personal distress or poor health. Appendix B can be an aid in identifying manifestations of stress and appropriate coping strategies.

There are various techniques for developing skills in reducing the effects of stress. All of these techniques are self-

---

All techniques for reducing the effects of stress are self-regulatory; no technique works unless people are motivated and choose to practice what they have learned.

---

regulatory; no technique works unless people are motivated and choose to practice what they have learned.

No one technique is a panacea for stress relief. The concept of stress is too complex and individualized for one approach. Each technique has value for some people but not for everyone. The secret lies in finding the technique that is most effective for individuals trying to regulate their own stress reactions. (See Figure 4.)

Nutrition and physical activity are being given prime consideration in all holistic health practices that attempt to promote optimum wellness as a defense against disease and the negative effects of stress. In some of his earlier studies Selye found that "stress, perhaps the most nonspecific reaction form of living organisms, can be both the cause and the consequence of malnutrition."[17] Although the cause and effects of stress are very difficult to delineate, recent studies reveal a great deal about the intricate interactions between nutrition and stress in the development and treatment of disease.

A healthy diet not only contains the necessary foods from the basic four food groups, but it also includes good amounts of natural foods that are free from the carbohydrate and salt excesses believed to create further stress on the body. The debate over vitamin supplements during stress continues, and many studies have indicated that there is a relationship between emotional stress and destruction of vitamin C in the body.[18]

Exercise and physical activity are integral parts of health maintenance. Regular exercise is essential to maintain an optimum level of wellness. Current

184

FIGURE 4. VARIOUS APPROACHES USED IN SELF-REGULATION OF STRESS

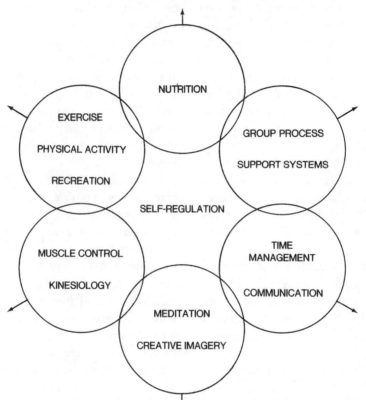

Nutrition: return to proper nutrition—more natural foods, less processed food with additives, vitamin replacement, herbal therapy and controlled fasting.

Exercise, Physical Activity, Recreation: regular physical fitness program: running, jumping, jogging, swimming, skating, skiing, cycling, Tai-Chi and yoga. Diversional activities, hobbies or special interests, gardening, fishing, boating and dancing.

Muscle Control, Kinesiology: bioenergetics (awareness through movement), functional integration, acupressure, Shiatsu, massage, progressive relaxation, dance therapy, sauna, whirlpool, biofeedback, Touch for Health, Therapeutic Touch and Alexander Technique.

Meditation, Creative Imagery: Zen, Buddhism, Sufi, Yoga, relaxation response, transcendental, clinical and standardized meditation, use of laughter—humor-fantasy, autohypnosis, guided imagery for pain control and healing, relaxation and healing using color, sound and smell.

Communication, Time Management: values clarification, sensitivity training, assertiveness training; planning, establishing priorities, overcoming, procrastination and barriers to change.

Group Process, Support Systems: Personal growth groups, psychodrama, transcendental analysis, self-help groups as peer support systems (weight control, smoking, alcohol, drug addiction, child abuse, patient recovery groups), family, social and religious support groups and professional service groups.

research supports the value of regular use of sustained physical activity to maintain full physical functioning well into the later years.

The major emphasis now in physical activity programs is aerobic exercise. Proponents of aerobic exercise claim that it strengthens the heart, lungs and muscles throughout the body and improves circulation.[19] Studies have indicated that regular sustained activity such as that used in aerobic exercise reduces blood pressure and decreases the heart rate. Paffenbargar's epidemiological study of some 17,000 men over a ten-year period revealed that people who exercise regularly have fewer heart attacks than those who do not exercise regularly.[20] It was estimated that people who expended less than 2,000 calories a week in physical activity had a 64 percent higher risk of heart attack than their more active counterparts. However, not everyone should participate in rigorous exercise. Rigorous exercise can be as harmful as a sedentary life.

Any physical activity even in modest doses improves the absorption and utilization of food, reduces nervous tension and depression, and produces conditions more conducive to sleep. Regular exercise may contribute to improved appearance and self-image, possibly because it replaces intramuscular fat with lean muscle, leading to more efficient utilization of calories.

The success of any regular sustained activity program depends upon selecting an activity that individuals truly enjoy and are willing to adopt as part of their lifestyle.

Rigorous sustained activities that increase the demand on the heart and promote more efficient functioning of the body include bicycling, running or jogging, skiing, swimming, vigorous skating or jumping rope, all considered good forms of aerobic exercise.

Other activities, although not in the category of aerobic exercise, can equally benefit the more sedentary person not in condition for more rigorous activity. A brisk uninterrupted walk, disco dancing or a regular game of tennis may be equally beneficial. Regular exercise builds strength and stamina and promotes better utilization of food. All this contributes to a level of health that will withstand the stress of modern living and eliminate some of the unhealthy practices that contribute to that stress.

Kinesiology and the Somatic Approaches

Kinesiology, the scientific study of movement, applies the organizing principles of anatomy, physiology and physics to the mechanisms of movement. It includes many modalities, one of which is bioenergetics, a series of exercises designed to bring about natural healing based upon bringing into harmony the natural environment and body rhythms. Lowen[21] and Shealy[22] use different approaches in their practices, which involve the testing and measuring of muscles. Based on these measurements they use various techniques and exercises to change tension and muscular-skeletal postures or alignments to bring about a harmony and balance conducive to promoting natural healing. This also applies to Feldenkrais's Functional Integration technique which uses a series of structured exercises to redirect the brain's habitual patterns of response to the movement in the gravitational field.[23] This method trains the brain to use more natural and efficient paths for mobility and the deployment of body energy.

Various forms of yoga may be considered kinesthetic modalities, although they also involve elements of meditative practices.

Acupressure

Acupressure, a close relative of acupuncture, is a method of reducing stress and

186 tension by reestablishing the harmony and balance of the flow of electromagnetic energy. It alters certain metabolic and circulatory processes by stimulation with finger pressure on certain points of the body. Many of the pressure points which are stimulated to relieve pain and tense muscles are often far removed from the area they affect because they are related to the meridians that crisscross the body and act as channels which transmit the flow of energy. These meridians are not directly related to human nervous systems although some are in close proximity to some of the nerves.

Acupressure is considered to be almost as effective as acupuncture and in some situations even more effective. The real value and significance in this lesser known technique is that an individual can use it for self-regulation of chronic aches and pains and muscle tension. Chan's simple book can be used by the lay person as well as any health care professional wishing to learn the technique.[24] Frank Warren from the New York Center for Pain Control also published a book of pictures locating the specific pressure points for self-use in particular problems.[25] There are many other variations in these techniques, such as Shiatsu, the Japanese finger pressure therapy, and Thie's Touch for Health, a combination of acupressure, massage and chiropractic techniques used to restore natural energies.[26]

Self-help books such as those above do not offer background theory or provide the professional practitioner with enough knowledge to appreciate the eastern philosophy of healing that has evolved from centuries of experience. The subtleties and finesse in practice can only be obtained from courses and an apprenticeship with a skilled practitioner. Once mastered, these techniques can become additional tools for the clinical practitioner to use in routine nursing care.

When an appropriate or most effective point for relieving a particular problem has been isolated, a person can be taught to use the technique thus providing a new sense of control or the ability to self-regulate recurring tension or pain.

Kurland, a neurologist and psychiatrist, has become so convinced that autoacupressure can eliminate or reduce most headaches without the use of drugs that he uses it in his own practice.[27] He has written a book for the lay public on how to use this technique because headaches seem to be the major reason for the phenomenal use of drugs in this country. (Acetylsalicylic acid, found in most analgesics, is produced in the United States at a rate of 80,000 to 100,000 pounds a day.) He claims that autoacupressure is effective even in excruciating migraine headache and has none of the side effects of strong medication.

The major points for the two main classifications of headaches are listed in Table 2, but the book is necessary for pictures of the pressure point locations and information on how to rule out that very small percentage of headaches that could be associated with a particular disease state such as brain tumor or epilepsy.

Reflexology

Reflexology is concentrated massage of the soles of the feet and works on essentially the same principles as acupressure.

TABLE 2

Acupressure Points for Headache Relief

Pressure Points

Group I—Common Type Headache—Vascular or muscle contraction (migraine, tension or pressure headaches) 4 pairs of points

Main Points (press simultaneously)

1. *Tai Yang*—side of head—one finger breadth from bony ridge at outer corner of the eyes
2. *Feng Chih*—two points under and against base of skull—in small muscular grooves at back of neck

Accessory Points

1. *Ho Ku*—between thumb and index finger (probe inward toward main body of hand)
2. *Lieh Chuch*—each wrist above styloid process—the sensitive point

Group II—Sinus Headaches—allergies, infection 4 pairs of para nasal sinus cavities

1. Frontal sinuses—above the eyes, root of the nose
   Yu Yao—center of eyebrows—directly above pupil of the eyes when looking forward
2. Maxillary sinuses—bony ridge below eyes
   Szu Pai—pressure against bony ridge
3. Sphenoid and ethmoid sinuses
   Yin Tang—just above bridge of nose (middle of flattened triangle). Use this point last; relieves nasal congestion.

Technique

Press hard with thumb nail, with thumb bent and hard enough to hurt but not hard enough to break the skin.

Press each point 15–30 sec. or rhythmic off-and-on pressure (check time with a time piece).

Press both points simultaneously.

Repeat if necessary.

Source: Kurland, H.D. *Quick Headache Relief Without Drugs* (New York: N.Y. Ballantine Books 1977).

By applying pressure and stimulating nerve endings in the soles of the feet, pain in corresponding organs can be relieved. The major purpose of this zone therapy is "to relax nerve tension, increase circulation in the blood and lymphatic systems, and get the body into top form so that it will have power to throw off any accumulated poisons.[28]

Therapeutic Touch

Therapeutic Touch is a nursing modality using the meditative state to enter the energy field of the client and to passively visualize or free the flow of energy from practitioner to recipient with the intent to support or promote healing.[29] Simply stated, it is an act of reaching out to aid others by permitting the energy flow of the practitioner to the receiver to create a state of harmony and balance that is necessary to self-healing. (More has been written about this technique in "The Yin and Yang of Clinical Practice" by Gretchen Randolph in this book.)

Massage

Massage has long been used as a therapeutic modality. At one time it was a basic nursing skill. Its virtues are being lauded again. Because of the number of stressed or tired muscles in the back of a bedridden patient, a back massage can help relieve tension in the entire body. It provides a passive form of exercise and the physical contact opens up another channel for communication—tactile communication.

Massage has great value in reducing muscular spasm and in achieving greater

188   flexibility and relaxation. Aside from its physical therapeutic use, it can be a means of reaching the mind. Massage when properly given can become a modality for unifying, coordinating and integrating the body, which means integrating the mind as well. Most people do not identify with their bodies. "From the chin up is identity; the area below is simply the vehicle that moves this identity through the world."[30] Yet it is important to experience and enjoy the sensation of being part of the body.

Progressive Relaxation

Progressive relaxation is a method of reducing stress based on the relationship between muscle tension and psychological tension. Jacobson has done extensive fundamental and applied research on the mind-muscle relationship and systemati-

---

Progressive relaxation is a method of reducing stress based on the relationship between muscle tension and psychological tension.

---

cally documented the powerful effects on muscles of such higher mental activities as imagination, attention and awareness.[31] His thesis is that anxiety and relaxation are mutually exclusive. Therefore, anxiety does not and cannot exist when the muscles are truly relaxed.

This method is based upon the individual's ability to learn to recognize the feeling of relaxation as contrasted to tension. The exercise consists of a routine for systematically tensing and immediately

relaxing all 14 major muscle groups in the body while being instructed to pay close attention to how it feels.

The original program, which was 60 one-hour sessions, was highly effective in reducing anxiety. Wolpe modified this technique to 20-minute sessions that are very intense and that require concentrated effort which probably accounts for the high dropout rate for the one technique that has proven to be most successful.

Current research still supports the original premise that even severely anxious individuals can benefit from progressive relaxation. Paul Lehrer of Rutgers Medical School found that "after progressive relaxation, individuals evidenced both reduced physiological arousal and relief from feelings of inner turmoil."[32]

Jacobson noted excellent results from progressive relaxation in treating patients with diseases such as mucous colitis, spastic esophagus, chronic insomnia, compulsive neurosis, mild phobias, neurasthenia, easy fatigability, anxiety neurosis, cardiac neurosis, compulsive tic, depression, hyperthyroidism, hypochondria, generalized spastic paresis, stuttering and stammering. "It appears that simple, deep muscle relaxation even without programmed mental activity or psychophysiological programming can lead to significant improvement in autonomic nervous system function and control of many of the psychosomatic or psychophysiological illnesses."[33]

One of the major benefits of practicing this technique is more than just learning to tense and then release tension from the muscles. It is a sensitivity program which increases one's ability to sense the presence of tension in muscles.

Mounting tension in muscles is often the first indication that stress is increasing. If practiced regularly for several weeks progressive relaxation can produce a conditioned response to the word relax. With practice, this conditioned response can be easily elicited to neutralize the effects of mounting stress.

Some nurses have found this technique more effective in reaching a state of deep relaxation than the more mental approach through meditative practices. Realizing that they are action oriented, many nurses find it exceedingly difficult to sit still in a completely relaxed state for 15 or 20 minutes.

The simple steps of the techniques are outlined in Appendix C. However, before attempting to teach others, additional reading and certainly some practice with the technique are necessary to acquire a proper sense of timing and a perception of the state of complete relaxation.

This technique has proven to be very effective in a psychiatric setting with patients prior to their group therapy sessions. Nurses claim that patients who undergo progressive relaxation are less tense and are ready to talk more spontaneously and interact more freely than those who do not participate in the exercise.

Carrington claims that a deep sense of relaxation achieved either by meditation or progressive relaxation is a good adjunct to psychotherapy because patients who are relaxed are calmer and more at ease in talking out problems.[34]

Since it involves becoming aware of bodily processes and bodily controls, progressive relaxation might be considered as a rudimentary form of biofeedback.

Biofeedback

Biofeedback is the use of a mechanical device for self-regulation. It is the "interacting with the interior self."[35] Any neurological or other biological function that can be monitored and amplified by electronic instrumentation and fed back to the person through any of the five senses can be regulated by the individual.

Every physiological change is accompanied by an appropriate change in the mental and/or emotional state; conversely, every change in mental state is accompanied by a change in the physiological state.

A meditative state of deep relaxation is conducive to the establishment of volun-

---

A meditative state of deep relaxation is conducive to the establishment of voluntary control by allowing the individual to become aware of subliminal imagery, fantasies and sensations.

---

tary control by allowing the individual to become aware of subliminal imagery, fantasies and sensations. While meditative and other deep relaxation techniques are based on overall response, biofeedback can focus on a particular area or part of the body so that a particular physiological function can be controlled, e.g., blood pressure or migraine headache. Biofeedback is being used by nurse practitioners. (See the chapter "The Yin and Yang of Clinical Practice" by Gretchen Randolph, in this book.)

Meditative Approaches

The physiological responses in meditation are the opposite in almost all respects

189

190   to Cannon's flight or fight response, a state of hypermetabolism. Meditation produces a pattern of response characterized by inhibition of the sympathetic nervous system; thus it becomes an antidote for alleviating the effects of prolonged chronic stress by producing a state of hypometabolism. Wallace's and Benson's research has supported the popular belief of regular meditators that meditation is more refreshing and energy restoring than sleep.[36]

Although there are many forms of meditation with differing goals and focus, many of them have the same effect. Carrington groups the various techniques into either religious or practical forms of meditation. Contrary to the religious practices, practical meditation is essentially nonstriving and is relatively goal-less.

The popularity of meditation accelerated after Benson published the results of his extensive research on Transcendental Meditators at the Harvard laboratory for physiological studies.[37] The results demonstrated the reduction in oxygen consumption and blood lactate levels following periods of meditation. Benson concluded that this was a natural integrated physiological response to stress in that it mimicked the parasympathetic rebound, that state of recovery following the alarm reaction in short-term, acute stress. He claims that this normal physiological response can be found in all cultures and all times. Our current lifestyle and pace of living interferes with the natural utilization of this "innate human capacity" as a protective mechanism against overstress.

Benson identified the basic elements of meditation, stripped it of any religious or cultic overtones and called it the "relaxation response." During the relaxation response the individual sits quietly with eyes closed, repeating a single sound while disregarding extraneous thoughts. By fixing attention on a single task for a protracted period of time the meditator is able to overcome the mind's usual habit of flitting from one thought to another. Focused attention on a single object or word is necessary to quiet the mind, to allow images to run through it without letting any one become distracting. With continued practice and experimentation individuals can gradually increase their ability to regulate attention and reduce or rectify the mind's overwhelming tendency to generate incessant activity and distractions.

Benson's technique is basically very simple and can be used as an introduction to the practice of meditation, encouraging the meditator to experiment and explore variations that are less rigid and more tuned to one's own needs. The four basic elements in his technique are essentially the same in all of the relaxation techniques, even hypnosis. (See Appendix D.) While the technique can be learned from his basic book, many people find actual demonstration and practice, combined with the use of videotape or film loop showing how to go through the exercise, far more effective.

The main advantage of this technique for the health care provider is its simplicity. The provider simply takes the client through the experience and provides feedback until the client is comfortable and satisfied with this particular technique. However, not everyone is able to sit still and focus attention long enough to experience the satisfying feeling that becomes the motivation for regular meditation.

Some clinical practitioners are using relaxation response to prepare patients for surgery. Patients choose to learn the technique and are encouraged to elicit the relaxation response both before and after surgery. Pre- and postsurgically, nurses at the Kaiser-Permanente Medical Center in Walnut Creek, California, are using "hypnotic tapes" which suggest to the patients that their discomfort will be minimal.[38] Patients who listen to the tapes require less analgesic medication after surgery and leave the hospital on an average one day earlier than patients who do not use the tapes.

Nurses are also using relaxation response as part of cardiac rehabilitation programs and as an adjunct to the medical regime for hypertensive patients. The use of the relaxation response has led to the reduction of dosage of the prescribed antihypertensive medication, and in some cases to elimination of the medication. Considerable research has been done on the beneficial effects of meditation in reducing blood pressure.

Autohypnosis, autogenic training and some of the creative imagery techniques which call upon the mysterious functioning of the human mind continue to elude researchers in the biomedical science. The beneficial effects of such techniques are clearly observable, yet the mechanisms by which they operate are still unknown.

Hypnosis

Hypnotic suggestion by itself is not used extensively in either medical or psychological therapy to induce and sustain relaxation. However, it is often used in conjunction with other therapeutic modalities as a form of systematic desensitization in dealing with fear and phobias and in breaking unhealthy habits such as smoking. Autohypnosis alone is not a definitive intervention in dealing with a problem. Rather it is a tool used to reduce stress and to allow the client to achieve a state of relaxation that renders the self receptive to suggestion for dealing with the problem. (Use of hypnosis in nursing is explained in "Stress Management through Hypnosis," by Thomas J. Daley and Eric L. Greenspun in this book.)

Hypnosis is not new to nursing practice. It has always been a basic but unrecognized component of natural childbirth practices. It has also been used as a form of anesthesia in some minor dental or surgical procedures.

Autogenic Training

According to Schultz and Luthe who developed the technique, autogenic training is directly related to hypnosis.[39] Other researchers believe that credit should be given to Coué and Jacobson as well. Schultz believed that self-normalization or self-regulation could be achieved from a specific state created in autogenic training, which is the exact opposite of the physiological alterations induced by stress. The shift into this "autogenic state" is encouraged by conditions that reduce sensations. Regular, brief sessions of passive concentration on physiologically adapted stimuli would gradually balance the physiology of the autonomic nervous system of the body by reducing other extraneous stimuli.

192   Proponents of autogenic training devised six exercises which have become
standard in current techniques for stabili-
zation or autoregulation of circulation,
respiration and neuromuscular activity.
(See Appendix E.) The first category of
exercises is self-suggestion phrases about
relaxation. The second is single-focus
mental concentration (as in yogic meditation) exercises ending with meditation or
abstract qualities of universal consciousness.[40]

This technique is often used in conjunction with biofeedback for focus on the
specific physiological aspect of muscle
tension while interspersed with general
suggestions for relaxation. Other therapists
encourage the use of imagery or memory
of the physical state of heaviness, warmth
and relaxation.

Various practitioners of holistic health
used this technique widely and have
published guidebooks for its use. Shealy
emphasizes the use of autogenic training
and claims that most patients take from
three to six months to go through the six
phases in the standardized technique. By
this time an individual is able with 20 or 30
seconds of concentration on these six
phases to experience the bodily feelings of
warmth and heaviness—a resting mass. It
is desirable for the individual to develop
the sensation that the body is totally numb
or even absent as if the mind were floating
up above it, providing the sensation that
the body is asleep while the mind is
awake.[41]

As with all the other relaxation techniques it is necessary to caution the individual against a sudden interruption of the
exercise while learning to achieve the
tranquil state. An abrupt termination could

*As the benefits of continued use of au-
togenic training become evident,
many individuals are willing and
ready to dispense with the use of
drugs or medications for relaxation
and pain relief.*

be undesirable and could leave one in an
irritable or more disturbed state.

With continued practice it should be
possible to induce this state of relaxation
in almost any environment without interference. As the benefits of continued use
become evident, many individuals are willing and ready to dispense with the use of
drugs or medications for relaxation and
pain relief. The fundamental aim is to train
certain mental processes to operate in such
a way that finally a very brief passive
concentration on a formula will accomplish the intended physiological change
almost instantly.

Visualization and Creative Imagery

Visualization exercises often follow the
physical relaxation techniques such as
autogenic training. The purpose of the
training and exercises is to discover by
means of imagery the dynamics of the
mind and to understand the symbolic
discourse between body and mind. It is
well known that where the mind focuses,
the emotions and the physiology are likely
to follow.

There is increasing evidence that mental
phenomena can have a profound positive
or negative impact upon an individual's
entire psychophysiology. The research
being done by Simonton and Simonton in

the treatment of cancer shows dramatic examples of the healing effects of creative imagery or visualization.[42]

The Simontons' technique of combining visualization with radiation and chemotherapy in the treatment of cancer demonstrates their belief that a person's "belief systems limit an individual's perception of reality and possibility...." The Simontons, through a relaxation process, encourage patients to create positive images of an enjoyable scene and to see themselves enjoying the activity in the scene. They then instruct the patients to visualize their cancer, for example, as a vegetable or as an animal, and to visualize their treatment and how it is working to shrink or remove the cancer. Results with patients who are able to learn and practice the technique successfully have been positive. The Simontons are continuing to research the mechanisms involved in this technique which combines traditional treatment modalities with holistic ones.[43]

Group Approaches

There has been a proliferation of group approaches available for dealing with psychosocial-cultural as well as physical stressors. The group approach in this country was originally used with tuberculosis patients who were learning to adjust to the social-emotional as well as the physical aspects of their illness.[44] Group approaches including the primary family as the group have long been used in the treatment of social-cognitive-emotional disorders.

Being in a group with individuals who share similar problems often has a releasing or freeing effect for the individual,

particularly after the ventilation of feelings takes place in the group. Group members provide support and feedback to each other throughout the process while the leader acts as a guide, model or a facilitator to the group process. Group approaches can assist individuals with problems such as chronic pain, alcoholism, drug abuse, overeating and child abuse. There are also personal growth groups, encounter groups, consciousness-raising women's groups, parenting groups and assertiveness training groups which promote more effective ways of living. (The theory, process and outcomes of assertiveness training are described more fully in the chapter "Assertiveness: Freeing the Nurse to Practice" by Gloria Ferraro Donnelly in this book.)

BEYOND NIGHTINGALE'S MODEL

Each of the self-regulation modalities discussed fits well within Nightingale's concept of the nursing goal, to put the body in the best condition for nature to act upon it. Nightingale recognized the potential of the human organism to heal itself, given the chance. She viewed the nurse as a facilitator in this process. Nurses must reach beyond Nightingale's model and promote mind-body-spirit integration to tap self-healing potentials.

Healing takes time, commitment and self-investment. Practicing nurses can experiment with self-regulation modalities in their own lives and consider their use with clients, since "each must find his innate stress level and live accordingly.... The secret is not to live less intensely—but more intelligently"[45] says Selye.

194   REFERENCES

1. Selye, H. *Stress without Distress* (Philadelphia: J. B. Lippincott/Signet 1975) p. 14.
2. Pelletier, K. *Mind as Healer, Mind as Slayer* (New York: Dell Publishing Co. 1977) p. 158.
3. Knowles, J. *Doing Better-Feeling Worse: Health in the United States* (New York: W. W. Norton Co. 1978).
4. McKeown, T. "Determinants of Health." *Human Nature* 1:4 (April 1978) p. 60-67.
5. Cassell, E. "The Limits of Modern Medicine." *Wall Street Journal* (August 2, 1977). Excerpted from Cassell, E. *The Healer's Art* (Philadelphia: J. B. Lippincott Co. 1976).
6. Cassell. "The Limits of Modern Medicine."
7. Pelletier. *Mind as Healer, Mind as Slayer.* p. 317.
8. Holmes, H. and Rahe, R. "The Social Readjustment Rating Scale." *Journal of Psychosomatic Research* 2:4 (April 1967) p. 213-218.
9. Pelletier. *Mind as Healer, Mind as Slayer.* p. 158.
10. Stauth, C. "Nutrition for Life." *New Age* 4:7 (December 1978) p. 46-61.
11. Ballentine, R. *Diet and Nutrition: A Holistic Approach* (Honesdale, Pa.: Himalayan International Institute 1978).
12. Burkitt, D. "The Link between Low-Fiber Diet and Disease." *Human Nature* 1:12 (December 1978) p. 34-41.
13. Stewart, S. "Recommendations for Physical Exercise: Guidelines for Aerobic Exercises." *Wellness Workbook* (Mill Valley, Calif.: Wellness Resource Center-Copyright 1977 J. Travis), p. 39-41.
14. Rahe, R. "Life Change and Illness Studies: Past History and Future Directions." *Journal of Human Stress* 4:1 (March 1978) p. 3-15.
15. Selye. *Stress without Distress.* pp. 34-37.
16. Ibid. p. 18.
17. Selye, H. "On Just Being Sick." *Nutrition Today* (Spring 1970) p. 2-10.
18. Hodges, R. "The Effects of Stress on Ascorbic Acid Metabolism in Man." *Nutrition Today* (Spring 1970) p. 11-12.
19. Cooper, K. *The New Aerobics* (New York: Bantam Books 1970).
20. Zohman, L. *Beyond Diet ... Exercise Your Way to Fitness and Health* (CPC International Inc. 1974).
21. Lowen, A. *Bioenergetics* (London: Collier Macmillan Ltd. 1967).

22. Shealy, N. *Ninety Days to Self-Health* (Calif.: Celestial Arts 1976).
23. Lande, N. *Mindstyles-Lifestyles* (Los Angeles: Price/Stern/Sloan Publishers 1976) p. 174.
24. Chan, P. *Finger Acupressure* (Los Angeles: Price/Stern/Sloan Publishers 1974).
25. Warren, F. *Freedom from Pain through Acupressure* (New York: Frederick Fell Publishers 1976).
26. Thie, J. *Touch for Health* (Calif.: DeVorss & Co. Publishers 1973).
27. Kurland, H. D. *Quick Headache Relief without Drugs* (New York: Ballantine Books 1977).
28. Lande. *Mindstyles-Lifestyles.* p. 182.
29. Kreiger, D. "Therapeutic Touch: The Imprimatur of Nursing." *American Journal of Nursing* 75:5 (May 1975) p. 784-787.
30. Lande. *Mindstyles-Lifestyles.* p. 186.
31. Brown, B. *Stress and the Art of Biofeedback* (New York: Harper & Row, Publishers 1977) p. 43-46.
32. Woolfolk, R. and Richardson, F. *Stress, Sanity and Survival* (New York: Monarch Press 1978) p. 180.
33. Shealy. *Ninety Days to Self-Health.* p. 43.
34. Carrington, P. *Freedom in Meditation* (New York: Anchor Press/Doubleday 1977).
35. Brown, B. *New Mind, New Body* (New York: Bantam Books 1974) p. 1.
36. Wallace, R. and Benson, H. "The Physiology of Meditation." *Scientific American* (February 1972) p. 84-90.
37. Benson, H. *The Relaxation Response* (New York: William Morrow & Co. 1976) p. 65-66.
38. Personal Communication with Regina Sullivan, R.N., Chief Recovery Room Nurse, Kaiser-Permanente Medical Center. Tapes for professionals are available by contacting Bruce Lewis, Kaiser-Permanente Medical Center, 1425 S. Main, Walnut Creek, California 94596.
39. Shealy. *Ninety Days to Self-Health.* p. 44.
40. Brown. *Stress and the Art of Biofeedback.* p. 46-47.
41. Shealy. *Ninety Days to Self-Health.* p. 45.
42. Pelletier. *Mind as Healer, Mind as Slayer.* p. 253-262.
43. The Simontons' literature and tapes are available from Cancer Counseling and Research Center, Suite 710, 1300 Summit Avenue, Fort Worth, Texas 76104.
44. Alexander, F. and Selesnick, S. *The History of Psychiatry* (New York: Harper & Row, Publishers 1966) p. 334.
45. A well-known quote of Dr. Hans Selye.

Appendices
Stress and Health

Guide for Identifying Potential "Stressors" in an Acute Care Setting

Nursing research has identified specific stress factors for hospitalized patients, their families and the nursing staff. A summary of the findings of a few selected studies is as follows:

I. Volicer, B., Isenberg, M., and Burns, M. "Medical-Surgical Differences in Hospital Stress Factors" *Journal of Human Stress,* vol. 3, no. 2 (June, 1977).

Factor	Med.	Surg.
1. Unfamiliarity of surroundings	3	3
2. Loss of independence	4	1
3. Separation from spouse		
4. Financial problems		
5. Isolation from other people		
6. Lack of information	1	4
7. Threat of severe illness	2	2
8. Separation from family		
9. Problems with medications.		

A Hospital Stress Rating Scale—by Volicer, with (49) discrete items was published in *Nursing '80,* vol. 10, no. 8, August 1980.

II. Hoffman, M., Donckers, S., and Hauser, M. "The Effect of Nursing Intervention on Stress Factors Perceived by Patients in a Coronary Care Unit" *Heart and Lung,* vol. 7, no. 5 (September–October, 1978).

Stresses caused by:
The illness
- Pain
- Relief of pain
- Uncomfortable procedures

The nursing staff
- Nurse concern
- Nurse willing to listen
- Nurse understand
- Staff teaching
- Able to communicate
- Confidence in nurses

The setting
- Roommate versus private room
- Visiting regulations
- Staying in bed
- Lose track of time
- Lose track of date
- Having sleep interrupted
- Use of bedpan/urinal
- Nurse giving bath
- Noise in unit
- Light in room

198   APPENDIX A cont'd

Personal concerns
- Change in lifestyle
- Home situation
- Financial matters
- Fear

The implications of this study are clear: If nurses are aware of what is stressful for patients they *can* intervene effectively to relieve stress." (page 809)

III. Noble, M.S. "Communication in the ICU: Therapeutic or Disturbing" *Nursing Outlook*, vol. 27, no. 3 (March 1979).
"In summary, findings from this study suggest that the most disturbing stimuli in an ICU are staff communications."

IV. Huckabay, L. and Jagla, B. "Nurses' Stress Factors in the Intensive Care Unit" *Journal of Nursing Administration*, vol. 9, no. 2 (February 1979) p. 21.
1. Workload and amount of physical work
2. Death of a patient
3. Communication problems between staff and nursing office
4. Communication problems between staff and physicians
5. Meeting the needs of the family
6. Numerous pieces of equipment and their failure
7. Noise level in the ICU
8. Physical setup of the ICU
9. Number of rapid decisions that must be made in the ICU
10. Amount of knowledge needed to work in the ICU
11. Physical injury to the nurse
12. Communication problems between staff members
13. Meeting the psychological needs of the patient
14. Communication problem between staff and other departments in the hospital
15. Cardiac arrest
16. Patient teaching

Implications: "Nursing educators and nursing administrators can make changes and adjustments to lessen these stressors." (page 21)

Begin a log or diary to assist you in your self-assessment and personal growth.

I. List your manifestations of stress (subjective feeling states, behavior changes, physiological changes)

Continue to add to this list as you become aware of these changes.

II. Try to identify your "stressors"— those factors or situations that stimulate this stress response. The source of stress is not always obvious.

When you are feeling "stressed" try to identify the kind of tension you feel (anger, frustration, anxiety, apprehension, nervousness, dread, terror, etc.) and note the circumstances.

Study these notes periodically (or share them with a counselor) and look for trends and connections between certain kinds of situations and feeling states. The "cause" often then becomes obvious.

Note what you were thinking and feeling under stress and *record* your *response*. Identify your coping strategies. Were your responses appropriate? Were they effective in reducing stress?

III. Give some consideration to the following questions:

1. How often do you feel tense, anxious or irritable?
2. How often do you eat, drink or smoke to relieve tension?
3. Do you feel that you have more to do than you can accomplish each day? Does it bother you?
4. Do you enjoy what you are doing? Do you find your daily tasks a source of pleasure and satisfaction?
5. Do you find time to relax regularly each day?
6. Do you have difficulty sleeping? How often?
7. How would you rate your general state of health at present?
8. Do you consider your present weight to be a problem?
9. Do you eat a balanced diet of wholesome foods?
10. Do you exercise on a regular basis?
11. Do you believe you are getting adequate exercise and do you enjoy it?
12. Do you believe you are physically

200

fit? (Is your resting pulse rate below 80/min?)

13. What events in your life are stressful to you?

14. Do you have someone with whom you can share your concerns, someone who is nurturing and supportive?

IV. What steps do you plan to take to try to cope more effectively with your stress?

- What unnecessary stresses can you avoid?
- Do you need to reestablish your priorities?
- How do you plan to alter those faulty perceptions that create stress for you?
- Do you plan to relax regularly to modify your stress response?

- What can you do to enhance your resistance to stress?

V. Goals:

- Begin by selecting your goals (What do I want out of life?).
- Rank them in terms most important and realistic.
- Break goals down into objectives and activities for achieving these objectives.

VI. For each specific objective list:

- The criteria by which you will measure your progress.
- Record each time you have succeeded in changing your previous maladaptive response to stress.
- *Reward Yourself!*
- Remember, meaningful self-directed change is possible, but it takes *time*.

Jacobson believed that eliminating tension from the muscles would lead to complete mental relaxation. This modification of his original method involves tensing and relaxing 14 rather than 39 separate muscle groups.

Set the stage. Create optimum environment for training:

1. Quiet—no distractions.
2. Comfortable position—couch or reclining chair (all muscles must be supported).
3. Loose clothing—no shoes, glasses, contact lenses.

The following instructions are given on a tape for home use after the client has been taught to tense and relax each muscle group in the order given below. (Remember instructions—Do not tense muscles until signal is given TENSE. Then release tension—immediately, completely, all at once—when signal is given to RELAX).

Each muscle group is tensed (30 sec.) and relaxed twice (40–60 sec.). Produce tension in ONLY one target region at a time. Avoid retensing muscle groups after they have become relaxed.

1. Rt/lf *hand* and *forearm* (dominant side first): make a very tight fist. Tense then Relax.
2. Rt/lf *upper arm*–deltoid: press elbow down into armrest toward body, upper arm toward ribs. Tense then Relax.
3. Lf *hand and forearm:* make a very tight fist. Tense then Relax.
4. Lf *upper arm*-deltoid: press elbow down into armrest toward body, upper arm toward ribs. Tense then Relax.
5. *Forehead:* raise eyebrows or make deep frown. Tense then Relax.
6. *Middle face:* wrinkle nose; shut eyes tightly. Tense then Relax.
7. *Jaws:* clench teeth; pull back corners

Sources: Bernstein, D. and Borkovec, T. *Progressive Relaxation Training: A Manual for the Helping Professions* (with record) (Chicago: Research Press 1973).

Jacobson, E. *Progressive Relaxation* (Chicago: University of Chicago Press 1938).

Jacobson, E. *Anxiety and Tension Control* (Philadelphia: J.B. Lippincott 1964).

Woolfolk R. L. and Richardson, F. *Stress, Sanity and Survival* (New York: Monarch, A Sovereign Book 1978).

APPENDIX C cont'd

of mouth, tongue against roof of mouth. Tense then Relax.

8. *Neck:* pull chin toward chest while pulling head back with rear neck muscles. Tense then Relax.

9. *Shoulders and upper back:* pull shoulder blades together, shrug shoulders, try to touch ears. Tense then Relax.

10. *Stomach and abdomen:* make stomach hard, pull inward and down. Tense then Relax.

11. Rt/lf *thigh:* bend knee forward with back thigh muscles while bending in opposite direction with top muscles. Tense then Relax

12. Rt/lf *calf-foot:* bend foot toward shin, curl toes. Tense then Relax.

13. Lf/rt *thigh:* bend knee forward with back thigh muscles while bending in opposite direction with top muscles. Tense then Relax.

14. Lf/rt *calf-foot:* bend foot toward shin, curl toes. Tense then Relax.

Mentally explore each region for any remaining tension. Terminate exercise with instructions to remain calm and relaxed and feel refreshed as if waking from a nap.

For maximum benefits repeat the exercise twice a day for several weeks. Relaxation is a skill that requires practice.

Then: short cuts can be used through *recall* and *conditioned relaxation* depending upon your ability to: (1) recognize tension in muscles and (2) remember what it *feels* like to release tension from these muscles.

Regular and frequent pairing of the word RELAX with *feelings* of deep relaxation will condition you to relax simply by using the word, which will lower your level of arousal to stress.

It may require 30 minutes initially to complete exercise. Once acquired, it can be used any time in any position for self-regulation of stress.

Consult the sources noted on page 201 for underlying theory and further comprehension of the subject.

Four Basic Elements

1. A quiet environment (to turn off external stimuli).
2. A comfortable position (sitting or kneeling with back straight; no tight clothing).
3. An object to dwell upon (repetition of a word or sound, such as ONE, a mental device such as attending to one's breathing).
4. A PASSIVE attitude (Let It Happen—an emptying of thoughts and distractions).

Relaxation response is a form of meditation—a state of concentration (by focusing on an object one cancels out all distractions associated with everyday life).

Relaxation response is NOT:

    a loss of control
    a loss of consciousness
    a state of sleep
    a state of drowsiness

Use once or twice a day 15–20 min. With *regular* practice the following results are possible for many.

During Meditation

1. A decrease in the rate of metabolism—hypometabolism, a restful state with decrease in heart and respiratory rate.
2. A marked decrease in the body's oxygen consumption.
3. A decrease in blood pressure.
4. A decrease in muscle tension.

Carry-Over from Meditation

Research continues to support the regular meditators' claims of lasting psychophysiological changes such as:

1. Lower arousal response to stress—less anxiety.
2. Better coping ability.
3. A new found acceptance of self, more tolerant of own weakness or limitations.
4. Improved learning ability with better retention and recall.
5. A sense of calm, of being collected, a more quiet philosophical attitude.

Consult sources below for underlying theory and further comprehension of the subject.

Sources: Benson, H. *The Relaxation Response* (New York: William Morrow 1976).

    Carrington, P. *Freedom in Meditation* (New York: Anchor Press Doubleday 1977).

Autogenic training was an exact, clearly defined method for self-hypnosis, developed by Drs. Schultz and Luthe in the 1930s. Basically the technique consists of a series of standard exercises for the purpose of directing physiological changes through the focus of attention. This can*not* be done by the force of will.

Visualization and imagination are used to create the desired change and then a *passive* attitude is adopted to "let it happen." As Coulé has said, the power of the imagination is far greater than that of the will.

Prerequisites—A regular time and a quiet place to practice. A comfortable position, sitting or lying down, eyes gently closed and quiet, relax the body.

Relaxation Phrases—"I feel quite quiet.... My feet feel heavy and relaxed.... (repeat for each body part) My whole body feels quiet, heavy, comfortable and relaxed." After repeating for one or two minutes go on to:

Warmth Phrases—Concentrate in a passive way, visualize ... and let it happen, "I am quiet and relaxed.... My arms and hands are heavy and warm.... My hands are warm...." After repeating for one or two minutes go on to:

Reverie Phrases—"My whole body feels quiet, comfortable and relaxed.... My mind is calm and quiet.... I feel an inward quietness." Continue using phrases allowing attention and thoughts to remain turned inward, then conclude with:

Activation Phrases—"I feel life and energy flowing through my legs, hips, solar plexus, chest, arms and hands, neck, head and face.... The energy makes me feel light and alive." As the body is reactivated stretch and take a deep breath.

6 Basic Phrases are:
Exercise
1. "Right arm very heavy."
   My arms and legs are heavy.
2. "Right hand warm."
   My arms and legs are warm.
3. "Pulse calm and strong."
   My heartbeat is calm, regular.
4. "Breath, calm and regular."
   It breathes me.

206   APPENDIX E cont'd

   5. "Solar plexus glowing warm."
      My abdomen is warm.
   6. "Forehead pleasantly cool."
      My forehead is cool.

Each exercise is repeated as often as necessary until the experience is internalized; the various states must be *felt* by the individual. Frequent and regular repetition is necessary, but not for more than two brief sessions every day.

Always end with proper activation phrases for a deliberate, self-directed termination of the session. Rosa suggests flexing the arms and hands, deep breath and eyes open with a return of energy to all body parts.

The purpose of these exercises is to train certain mental processes to operate in such a way that finally a brief passive concentration on a formula will trigger the intended physiological change almost instantly.

Consult these other sources for variations in techniques, for underlying theory and for further comprehension of the subject.

Sources:

Brown, B. *Stress and the Art of Biofeedback* (New York: Harper & Row, Publishers 1977).

Rosa, K. R. You and AT: Autogenic Training The Revolutionary Way to Relaxation and Inner Peace (New York: Saturday Review Press/E.P. Dutton, Co., Inc. 1976).

Shealy, C. N. *90 Days to Self-Help* (New York: Bantam Books, 1977).

Woolfolk, R., et al. *Stress, Sanity and Survival* (New York: Monarch Press 1978).

Health Education for the Public: Stress and Stress Management

Sharon E. Shaw, R.N., M.S.N.
Adjunct Assistant Professor and
   Coordinator
Health Resource Center
School of Nursing
Georgetown University
Washington, D.C.

RISING MEDICAL COSTS, unchanging morbidity and mortality statistics and the consumer movement have resulted in general public dissatisfaction with the traditional health care delivery system. The public is looking for additional information and skills to enable them to manage their health state and health care costs better. As a result of this movement toward greater self-care management, many self-help groups have been started over the past decade.[1]

Health professionals, spurred on by increased consumer and federal interest, are devoting more efforts to health education. In general, their programs, such as smoking cessation or ostomy clubs, teach persons specific skills needed to manage chronic health habits or illnesses and to become better patients or medical reporters.[2,3] Few, however, have aimed at putting people in the pivotal position of controlling their own lives and health. Georgetown University (GTU) has implemented

207

208 such a program to educate the public in stress management.

CONCEPT FOR PUBLIC HEALTH EDUCATION

In the early 1970s several faculty members at GTU School of Nursing developed an overall conceptual approach to health education for the public based on Orem's self-care concept of nursing and Bowen's theory of relationship systems.[4-7] These initial courses were designed to assist individuals to (1) exercise their rights and responsibilities in health and health-related decisions and (2) take action to maintain a level of health which allows them to engage in meaningful activities congruent with their life goals. Thus the program has been aimed at the process or value level of the individual rather than simply at the content or skills level. This program has focused on developing the intellectual and emotional skills needed by participants to assume increased responsibility for their health.

Initial Program

The initial broad-based program ran for 14 to 16 sessions and covered many content areas in health. These developmentally designed courses expanded upon traditional content in health education, such as risk factors, signs and symptoms, to include self-assessment skills, decision-making skills and the development of emotional objectivity about self. Individuals were thus assisted to determine criteria for themselves in health matters. These courses were interdisciplinary and, as such, presented many different points of view on

a variety of topics. Throughout each course the nurse coordinator served to facilitate individual self-processing by the use of many case studies. These case studies reinforced a holistic approach to health promotion and disease prevention and illustrated the many options available to the individual.

Current Program

While this course was well received and evaluations indicated increased knowledge about self in health, it was difficult to present such a broad curriculum and assist participants in the specific content areas affecting them most. Consequently, in the winter of 1978 GTU decided to present health education courses in eight specific content areas. The content areas presented use the same conceptual framework, that is, a focus on process for self with the course content serving as a vehicle to increase responsibility in health matters.

STRESS AND STRESS MANAGEMENT

One of the eight new courses is a course in stress management. Stress is defined as "the body's nonspecific response to any demand made upon it that requires it to adjust to an entirely new situation."[8] Stress has become a household word of the 1970s, perhaps because the only constant in today's complex society is increasing change.[9]

Many consumers and health care professionals view stress as but another germ in a unicausal view of disease. With this view, it is difficult for people to perceive the control they can exert on their health.

But stress has also come to occupy a pivotal position in the new holistic health movement. Work by Holmes and Rahe,[10] literature on biofeedback[11] and Benson's work with the relaxation response[12] all point to the potential of individuals to influence their health. Viewed from the holistic perspective, stress as a subject can

---

Many consumers and health care professionals view stress as but another germ in a unicausal view of disease. With this view, it is difficult for people to perceive the control they can exert on their health.

---

be readily presented as part of the concept of equilibrium for the individual. There is a unique blending of mind and body in response to stressors.

The public was ready for a course in stress management. Aware of the lack of medical technologies available to them on the subject, people have sensed that "stress was their own problem to solve not just their Doctor's responsibility."[13]

A nine-week course was designed to present basic content in stress and stress management while pushing individuals to process this information as it relates to themselves, their values and their life goals. The content moves from concrete to abstract during each session and during the course as a whole. With the help of case studies, participants look at a new way of thinking about themselves and health. Simultaneously participants are challenged to look at the long-term, strategic perspective while skills or tactics to deal with the short-term are learned. This

long-term perspective is fostered by providing information on the most up-to-date scientific findings and introducing uncertainty and decision making for self in the areas which lack definitive scientific knowledge. In this way, individuals are assisted to determine their own criteria.

The topics covered are:

- physiology of stress;
- stressors and their impact;
- benefits of stress;
- implications of stress;
- strategic and tactical methods of stress reduction; and
- predicting stress times for you.

Individuals are taught to monitor their own physiological parameters (vital signs and "body and head talk") and to keep records on themselves as they go. Throughout the course attention is given to the individual's strengths and the potential he has to work with. Individual coaching is additionally available to provide support.

ASSUMPTIONS UNDERLYING HEALTH EDUCATION IN STRESS AND STRESS MANAGEMENT

The following assumptions are the running themes in every session with the specific content serving as a vehicle to integrate the themes into the course:

- Assumption one: The more emotionally mature the individual, the better able that person is to deal quickly and with less distress with changing life situations.
- Assumption two: There are many issues which appear to be stressful no matter what the person's emotional

210

level, but the more emotionally mature individual will bounce back faster.

- Assumption three: Acute stress is less harmful to the individual than chronic, unresolved stress, and the most potent unresolved stress in the human organism is that of relationships with important others.
- Assumption four: For individuals at any level of emotional maturity chronic, unresolved issues will be a running theme; that is, they will show up in many day-to-day situations in a variety of forms.
- Assumption five: The more emotionally mature the individual, the more able the person is to develop approaches to life which do not become cyclic, producing more distress.[14]

These assumptions help persons get in touch with the chronic issues for themselves while providing them with the tactics and skills to handle the acute issues.

While stress is defined as the response of the individual to stressors, persons more often put effort into changing the stressful situation rather than into changing their part in the situation. Biofeedback provides one means to focus on self and to become aware of a person's normal running level of reactivity. While this and other tech-

---

While stress is defined as the response of the individual to stressors, persons more often put effort into changing the stressful situation rather than into changing their part in the situation.

---

niques are excellent, they are short term and tactical; that is, they do not address the core issue for the individual.

Developing a new way of thinking does not occur in one course. Rather, it occurs developmentally over time with this course as a beginning. GTU instructors recommend Bowen as the strategic approach but provide information on others.[15] Participants also come up with frameworks and approaches helpful to them.

NURSING AND HEALTH EDUCATION

Self-care is more than health education. It attempts to help people become increasingly aware of their rights and responsibilities to health, going far beyond just telling them what the health professional thinks they should know. If persons are going to be increasingly involved in their own care, "health professionals must acknowledge people's integrity in making health decisions and their ability to perform successfully in their own behalf."[16]

John Knowles of the Rockefeller Foundation has stated that the next major advance in the health of the nation will come not from increasing medical technology, but from what individuals can do for themselves.[17] Nursing as "the one profession now doing the most consumer health education in the United States"[18] is in a unique position to assist persons to become more responsible self-care agents and to begin to improve the health state of the nation. The challenge to nurses is to focus on the individuals—their rights and their responsibilities for self—and not to overpromise from a cause-and-effect per-spective. Health education in stress and stress management is an excellent way for nurses to meet this challenge.

REFERENCES

1. Katz, A. H. and Bender, E. I. *The Strength in Us: Self-Help Groups in the Modern World* (New York: New Viewpoints Division of Franklin Watts 1976).

2. Sehnert, K. *How to be Your Own Doctor Sometimes* (New York: Grosset and Dunlap 1975).

3. Vickery, D. M. and Fries, J. F. *Take Care of Yourself: The Consumer's Guide to Medical Care* (Reading, Mass.: Addison-Wesley Co. 1976).

4. Orem, D. *Nursing: Concepts of Practice* (New York: McGraw-Hill Book Co. 1971).

5. National Development Conference Group. *Concept Formalization in Nursing* (Boston: Little, Brown and Co. 1973).

6. Bowen, M. *Family Theory and Clinical Practice* (New York: Jason Aronson Publishers 1978).

7. Nowakowski, L. "Health Education: Learner Needs and Evaluation" (unpublished paper 1978). Available through the author, Sharon Shaw, Georgetown University, Washington, D.C.

8. Selye, H. *The Stress of Life* (New York: McGraw-Hill Book Co. 1956) p. 54.

9. Toffler, A. *Future Shock* (New York: Random House 1970)

10. Holmes, T. H. and Rahe, R. H. "The Social Readjustment Rating Scale." *Journal of Psychosomatic Research* 11:8 (1967) p. 213–218.

11. Brown, B. B. *Stress and the Art of Biofeedback* (New York: Harper & Row, Publishers 1976).

12. Benson, H. *The Relaxation Response* (New York: William Morrow & Co. 1975).

13. McGuade, W. "Doing Something About Stress." *Fortune* (May 1973) p. 251.

14. Nowakowski. "Health Education: Learner Needs and Evaluation."

15. Bowen. *Family Theory and Clinical Practice.*

16. Levin, L. *Self-Care: Lay Initiatives in Health* (New York: Prodist 1976).

17. Kramer, B. "Wiser Ways of Living: Not Dramatic Cures Seen as Key to Health." *Wall Street Journal* Lvi:3 (March 22, 1976).

18. Somers, A. *Preventive Medicine U.S.A.: Health Promotion and Consumer Health Education* (New York: Prodist 1976) p. 48.

The Yin and Yang of Clinical Practice

Gretchen Randolph, R.N., M.S.
Doctoral Candidate
New York University
New York, New York
Vice President, Member of Board of Trustees
Nurse Healers Professional Associates
  Cooperative
Portchester, New York

THE CHINESE philosophical concepts of yin and yang are particularly illustrative of the polarities existing in the American health care system. The Chinese believe that all of life consists of a dynamic balance between opposites. These contrasts are present in all of human existence. Life, in this philosophy, is a constant interaction between these complementary forces.[1]

According to Chinese thought, the yin principle is characterized by the intuitive, sensitive, subtle, mothering, nurturing aspects of human nature. Interventions of a yin nature include hypnosis, massage, biofeedback, and nutritional counseling, and would fall within the realm of the health model.

Yang, on the other hand, represents the masculine side of human nature. Adjectives descriptive of the yang principle include aggressive, intrusive, logical, scientific, organized and powerful. Interventions of a yang nature, such as surgical,

214 and radiation and pharmacological treatments, would fall within the realm of the current, commonly practiced medical model.

Yin and yang are complementary and integral to each other, as separate as they are incomplete, and together they make up the totality.[2] (See Figure 1.) The American health care system appears to be in a period of transition from yang to yin, as consumers and practitioners realize that medical-model interventions are self-limited in the amelioration of the stress-related illnesses so prevalent today.

THE HISTORY OF YIN AND YANG IN HEALTH CARE

A brief look at the history of health care can give a perspective on the relative positions of yin and yang in earlier systems.

FIGURE 1.   THE YIN AND YANG OF CLINICAL PRACTICE

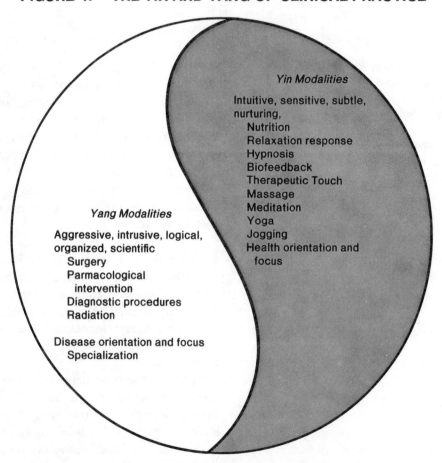

Yin Modalities

Intuitive, sensitive, subtle, nurturing,
Nutrition
Relaxation response
Hypnosis
Biofeedback
Therapeutic Touch
Massage
Meditation
Yoga
Jogging
Health orientation and
focus

Yang Modalities

Aggressive, intrusive, logical, organized, scientific
Surgery
Parmacological
intervention
Diagnostic procedures
Radiation

Disease orientation and focus
Specialization

Suppression of Yin

Nurses represent the yin aspect of our healing culture. During the Middle Ages, nursing care was provided by the independent female peasant healer. Then, as now, a struggle between the sexes existed. Evidence suggests that female healers were often identified as witches and burned at the stake because their presence threatened the (male) physicians and politicians of that time. For example, in 1322, the faculty of medicine of the University of Paris brought Jacoba Felicie to trial on charges of illegal health care practice. The primary accusations brought against her were that "she would cure her patients of internal illness and wounds or of external abscesses. She would visit the sick assiduously and continue to examine the urine in the manner of physicians, feel the pulse, and touch the body and limbs." Six witnesses affirmed that Felicie had cured them even after numerous physicians had given up. These testimonies were used against her, because the charge was not that she was incompetent, but that "as a woman she had dared to cure at all!"[3]

During the 13th and 14th centuries, the European medical profession became firmly established and female healers were largely suppressed. This was unfortunate, because the female healer treated patients by relying on her senses rather than on the faith and philosophy that were part of medical training at that time.[4] The female healers believed in trial and error and had an inquiring attitude toward natural phenomena.

Medical knowledge in the 13th century was limited and would have benefited greatly from the information peasant healers handed down through the centuries, mother to daughter, concerning herbs, dietary changes and working with human nature through natural modalities.

Through the centuries, our culture continued to move toward the yang aspect. Nineteenth century hospitals were badly in need of yin to improve atrocious sanitary conditions. It was during the early part of the 19th century that aristocratic women like Florence Nightingale decided to work to improve foul conditions and create a health-nurturing environment.[5]

Nightingale believed that the major purpose of nursing was to put patients in the best condition for nature to act upon them. In contrast, the nursing system, particularly in America, became increasingly entranced by the technology of the medical-model orientation with its disease-centered emphasis.

Emergence of Alternative Yin Methods

The nursing profession is at a critical point now because of the emergence of so many alternative means of health care, such as acupressure, biofeedback, Therapeutic Touch, kinesiology, meditation, relaxation training, hypnosis, family therapy, nutritional counseling, energy ex-

Nursing has gone through a period of half-hearted devotion to the yang orientation, but the profession never totally abandoned its dedication to the more subtle, human elements in health care.

216 change and massage, all of which facilitate patient self-help and healer–healee interaction. Nurses have a natural ability to work in nonintrusive modalities. These modalities are easily integrated into their previous training, which, like these new techniques, emphasizes the yin aspects of healing and human interaction. Nursing has gone through a period of half-hearted devotion to the yang orientation, with its emphasis on the scientific, mechanistic, organizational and masculine aspects, but the profession never totally abandoned its dedication to the more subtle, human elements in health care.

Nurses' Yin Orientation

Nurses have not assumed their optimally effective role in the yang-oriented system because the nursing model does not include the use of tools—the chemicals, machines, radiation or scalpels—to perform health care. Their tools for patient care have been primarily themselves. They have had extensive experience in dealing with the more subtle aspects—the yin—of what makes people ill. Nurses need to continue to refine and research their intuitive perception of illness and to tap their fund of knowledge about what makes people ill.

Most nurses have seen patients who seemed beyond saving but who did not die. Perhaps those patients had a certain mental attitude which prevented their death. Sometimes nurses can sense which patients are going to die quickly and which patients will go into remission or move through a quiet, constructive death process. Many nurses have experienced a sudden, inexplicable feeling that something was wrong with a certain patient, even when medical tests could not diagnose the problem. These are the kinds of intuition, coming from a collective unconscious, that nurses are becoming aware of and starting to consciously utilize. Nurses, by not going into medicine or other technology-based professions, have made a choice to do intuitive, yin-oriented healing, with emphasis on interpersonal human contact. Nurses' intuitions and perceptions—their own selves—are their strengths.

The work of Simonton and Simonton demonstrates the importance of mental attitudes. The Simontons are working with cancer patients to alter their resistance to disease through imagery. They believe that if patients feel helpless or hopeless they will spark more symptoms of cancer; if terminal, these patients will have a faster, more difficult death. Patients who can change their attitudes are not helpless or hopeless.[6] These are the people whose cancer goes into remission. Nursing, as a profession, can take advantage of a power lesson here. They can change their attitudes, like the Simontons' cancer patients, and emphasize the solid, nonintrusive strength that lies in their profession and in themselves. In this way nurses can free themselves from the cancer of helplessness and hopelessness that often paralyzes their profession. The following descriptions of Therapeutic Touch and biofeedback illustrate how nursing and the yin modalities are complementary to each other and to health care.

THERAPEUTIC TOUCH

Therapeutic Touch, a yin modality involving a controlled interchange of energy between a healthy person and a patient bolsters the patient's recuperative process. Underlying this technique is the belief that illness is a manifestation of a blockage of energy in the body.[7] A commonly used term in Therapeutic Touch is "energy channel," that is, a channeling of environmental energy through the practitioner to the client. The energy channel or meridian is an imaginary direction in the body through which energy flows in predetermined patterns.

Therapeutic Touch is a derivative of laying-on-of-hands, but it differs in that it requires the practitioner to be in a meditative state. This meditation is characterized by a focused concentration on the patient coupled with the intent to heal. In the process of doing Therapeutic Touch, the nurse becomes quiet and aware of sensory changes as the hands move at two-to-six-inch intervals around the client/patient's body. The practitioner then places the hands where the changes in the energy field were perceived and remains in a meditative state. This process usually continues for 20 minutes. Patients receiving Therapeutic Touch experience a "relaxed state with an abundance of large-amplitude alpha activity. A change in a patient's hemoglobin has also been documented.[8]

This is not a new phenomenon. Laying-on-of-hands was recorded in caves of prehistoric cave dwellers and in Ancient Greece. Therapeutic Touch as a technique with which to teach and research this phenomenon was developed by Dr. Dolores Krieger, professor of New York University.[9]

A study of Krieger's brain waves with the electroencephalogram (EEG) reveals that she alters her brain waves to a fast synchronous beta wave when meditating for Therapeutic Touch. Other practitioners' studies so far have not shown the same high-frequency beta as Krieger; however, they do show a predominance of alpha wave.[10] Two explanations suggested are that these practitioners may obtain the healing state from individual styles, or may be less experienced than Krieger.

Practitioners subjectively describe the Therapeutic Touch meditative state as "blanking one's mind," having no extraneous thoughts present, passively visualizing a flow of energy through the practitioner to the patient, combined with an intense feeling of concern/love for the patient and an openness to the environmental energies.

Therapeutic Touch as a Nursing Process

Therapeutic Touch is a nursing process and is conceptually based on Rogers's theory of the synergistic human, the theory

---

Therapeutic Touch is based on the theory that humans are "energy fields." It is the interaction between the practitioner's and the patient's energy fields that makes therapeutic touch possible.

---

218   that humans are "energy fields."[11] It is the interaction between the practitioner's and patient's energy fields that makes Therapeutic Touch possible.

Individual beings are interconnected patterns of energy. The human energy field worked with in Therapeutic Touch is thought to be present throughout the body and up to six inches outside the skin.

Therapeutic Touch practitioners, through specific training, learn to feel changes within the area surrounding the body. By altering their concentration, they can feel where changes in the field occur. This first stage of going around the patient's body is called the assessment stage. Actually, Therapeutic Touch is a misnomer, chosen during the early stages of development before Krieger learned that one does not have to touch the client's body to establish the areas of imbalance; one needs only to move closely above the skin or light clothing.

During the second stage, the treatment stage, Therapeutic Touch practitioners alter their mental state again and attempt to move energy down the body, smoothing the surrounding field. The areas of difference are often located just above the diseased site. For instance, an infection such as appendicitis might be noted over the lower right side of the abdomen. Even so, beginning practitioners must be aware that frequently with deferred pain (cardiac-right arm) the areas that require attention might differ from the immediate physical location.

The areas of change/cues/sensation reported are often individual to the practitioner.[12] Several practitioners might report a variety of cues for the same patient or patient condition. For kidney infection, different practitioners might observe the problem in the same position (lower back, for example) although they might describe their sensations as cool, hot, prickly, feeling a pulling or feeling an absence of energy in the field.[13] Through experience, practitioners learn to correlate the sensation they feel with the physical or emotional ailment present. One aspect most healers have in common is the ability to determine the level of intensity of an ailment; usually different healers with similar amounts of experience will pick up the severity of an illness.

During the Therapeutic Touch interaction the patient subjectively experiences a variety of things, most of them sensations such as profound relaxation, heat in the affected area and peripheral flushing (vasodilation).[14] Often patients request to rest since the relaxation is so pleasant a state. Research is in progress to document the physiology of the intense relaxation.

Usually treatment sessions do not last longer than 20 minutes, and there may or may not, depending on the people involved, be a verbal exchange during the treatment stage.

As with all human potentials, each practitioner begins at a different level and develops at a different speed. In addition, there will be variances in the difficulty practitioners experience as they learn this technique. Just as some people learn to swim immediately and others prefer not to develop that skill, so too with Therapeutic Touch. The more one tries to force the development of Therapeutic Touch, the more frustrating the experience can become. For this reason, persons who feel uncomfortable or anxious are asked not to push their learning process until they find the skill occurring. To push it would only be self-defeating and possibly uncomfortable for their patients.

After about six months of experience, practitioners can begin to relax patients, ease pain, decrease elevated temperature and increase blood circulation to the wounded area. Practitioners with two to five years of experience are able to differentiate the primarily physical from emotional symptoms, decrease high blood pressure, and help balance thyroid and diabetic disorders.

Combining Therapeutic Touch and Medical Modalities

Obviously, with conditions necessitating pharmacological treatment, practitioners must be acutely aware that medication levels may have to be scaled down as the body reestablishes its own regulatory system. Since Therapeutic Touch is not a "magical cure" any more than other treatments are, it must be applied in conjunction with the other health modalities appropriate for the disease being treated. One certainly would not deter surgical intervention if a patient had acutely inflamed appendicitis. On the other hand, if one were able to catch the early stages of the imbalance and preventively treat it through Therapeutic Touch, a radical intervention such as surgery might have been avoided. Therapeutic Touch might

In order to support their own recuperative mechanisms, therapeutic touch practitioners should not treat patients when they themselves are ill, angry, anxious or pregnant.

be used to decrease the pain and accelerate the healing in any event.

Since one must be critically conservative when developing therapeutic modalities, Therapeutic Touch practitioners are acutely aware that more research is needed to define the parameters of its effective use. Up to this point Therapeutic Touch has had no ill effects beyond a very rare occurrence of dizziness.[15] Until further research suggests otherwise, Therapeutic Touch practitioners have taken precautions commonly used by practitioners of other developing therapeutic modalities. Beginning practitioners should not work intensely around the head. This is especially pertinent in patients with a history of epilepsy or recent reparative surgery for retinal detachment. In addition, to support their own recuperative mechanisms, practitioners should not treat patients when they themselves are ill, angry, anxious or pregnant. When finishing a treatment session, practitioners should always return (in their own manner) to the meditative centering process, breathing deeply, relaxing and visualizing filling themselves with energy and health.

Developing necessary skills for the Therapeutic Touch modality involves meditation and experiential knowledge of energy fields.

220 BIOFEEDBACK

Biofeedback is yet another noninvasive—yin—modality used to support clients' natural recuperative processes. Through biofeedback training, individuals become active participants in their own health maintenance and recovery.

In nursing education, interpersonal and communication skills, anxiety reduction, family dynamics, crisis intervention, illness care and health education are stressed. Therefore, nurses have the background to learn and apply biofeedback principles and training as another dimension for patient care. The difficult aspect of biofeedback training is counseling clients to help themselves integrate biofeedback into their life. Such skills are taught in the nursing curriculum. Although the instruments used in biofeedback may appear complex, in reality biofeedback is understandable and easily applied.

Alarm Stress Reaction

Until as recently as ten years ago, the body's autonomic nervous system was considered to be independent of personal volition.[15] When an individual experiences a stressful event, the body responds with a cluster of physiological changes designed to prepare for the threat to the human system. This response has been termed the alarm reaction, or stress syndrome,[16] and is commonly experienced as an increase in heart rate, sweat and stomach secretions, a tensing of skeletal muscles and a shunting of blood away from the extremities. When this response is prolonged, the body eventually loses its state of resistance and the person becomes ill.

Biofeedback can be an effective modality for ameliorating conditions that have high components of stress.[17] Biofeedback training enables individuals to interrupt their alarm responses and remain calm in the face of stressful events. Clients learn this control by the combined use of three aspects of training: the instruments, mental/physical exercises and interaction with the nurse.

Biofeedback Instruments

The first element of biofeedback training is the use of electronic instruments that give information about physiological responses that the individual is not normally aware of. The variety of biofeedback instruments is rapidly increasing, but in clinical settings the most frequently used are the electromyograph and the skin temperature monitor.

The physiological information collected by the equipment is translated into several forms of feedback. Trainees have the options of: listening to a tone change pitch, or watching a meter signal, a digital display or a light change intensity or color. The audio mode is often selected, since it involves less mental concentration, allowing clients to focus on their internal awareness.

ELECTROMYOGRAPH

In biofeedback terminology, the muscle activity is measured by electromyography (EMG). The electromyograph records the tension level through electrodes placed on the skin over the desired muscle. These electrodes channel electrical signals from the underlying muscle to the biofeedback equipment, which then converts the raw signal into a meter display or an easily displayed light or sound.

Conditions responsive to EMG biofeedback are anxiety, phobias, tension headache, insomnia, asthma, essential hypertension, bruxism, colitis, ulcer, menstrual distress, childbirth, muscle spasms with pain and torticollis.[18]

SKIN TEMPERATURE MONITOR

The other most widely used modality is skin temperature feedback measured by the thermistor. Peripheral skin temperature biofeedback reflects the circulation resulting from constriction and dilation of the vessels. Increased skin temperature is associated with relaxation.

A thermistor is placed on a finger to measure changes in skin temperature. Feedback temperature changes of 0.1 degree are reported in the form of a meter signal, sound or light. This feedback mode can be used in patients with the circulatory disorders of migraine, Raynaud's disease and a variety of conditions where sympathetic activation (alarm reaction) is implicated.[19]

OTHER INDICES

Other physiological indices currently being used in clinical training are galvanic skin response (GSR), electroencephalographic response, blood pressure and heart rate.[20]

Initially, working with an instrument verifies to clients that they self-regulate the process. Since the goal of biofeedback training is to elicit a relaxed state in clients which they can summon later without the use of instruments, the later stages of training deemphasize the use of the instrument.

Since the goal of biofeedback training is to elicit a relaxed state in clients which they can summon without the use of instruments, the later stages of training deemphasize the use of an instrument.

Daily Exercise

Connecting clients to a biofeedback instrument is not sufficient to obtain lasting success. Biofeedback research substantiates that the most effective changes come from combining complementary relaxation techniques.[21] Adjunctive exercises commonly used are guided imagery exercises,[22] self-hypnosis,[23] breathing exercises,[24] meditation,[25] autogenic training,[26] and yoga.[27]

By doing daily exercises, clients learn to trigger a deep level of relaxation, or the relaxation response.[28]

Precautions

There are some precautions to using biofeedback. When patients use medication, and as the tension levels abate, their bodies become more sensitive and responsive. Physicians prescribing medication should be kept informed about the progress of the biofeedback training, since it directly affects dosage levels. This procedure is particularly imperative with diabetic clients since relaxation reduces the body's need for insulin and insulin coma can occur. Elderly persons and those taking medication for hypo- or hypertension must be carefully observed, for proneness to hypotension would not suggest blood pressure feedback.

222　　Patients with a history of epilepsy should avoid low-frequency EEG training, since it may potentiate epileptic seizure activity.[29] For other precautions and contraindications regarding bruxism, torticollis, cardiac arrhythmias and psychosis, see *Biofeedback* by George Fuller.[30]

Why Biofeedback?

The instruction, "relax . . . take it easy," usually increases a person's tension because the instructor gives no guidance about *how* to relax. Now there are numerous relaxation techniques, including various meditations, yoga and progressive relaxation. What is the advantage of coupling biofeedback with these other techniques?

Through the use of instruments clients receive immediate information about the subtle shifts in their physiological reactions, which they might otherwise not be aware of. Such data can accelerate the process of desired change by providing specific guidance for learning.

Another important quality of the yin modality is its appeal, its "technological mystique." Rather than promoting dependency and passivity, which is often the case in our health care system, in relatively few sessions the biofeedback instrument is no longer needed. Clients learn a control that reduces stress and that enhances their sense of mastery, strength and capability. "Biofeedback is not 1984 with man controlled by machine, but just the opposite, it represents man controlling machine in an effort to control himself."[31]

GETTING BACK TO THE ESSENCE OF NURSING

Nurses, including the author, are increasingly using Therapeutic Touch and biofeedback as yin modalities in dealing with stress-related illness. Yin modalities, of course, will not replace yang interventions, such as surgery or drugs. There will always be clients/patients who choose or who need such interventions. Yin interventions, however, represent another option to offer clients/patients who want to explore the differences and effects of treatments and regimens before making a commitment to more acute intervention.

Yin modalities, increasingly being researched, explored and practiced by nurses, may represent the "getting back to the essence of nursing" that nurses have discussed for decades.

REFERENCES

1. Capra. F. *The Tao of Physics* (Boulder, Colo.: Shambhala Publications 1975).

2. Ibid.

3. Ehrenreich, B. *Witches, Midwives and Nurses, A History of Women Healers* (Old Westbury, N.Y.: Feminist Press 1973) p. 18–19.

4. Ibid. p. 16.

5. Ibid. p. 35.

6. Pelletier, K. *Mind as Healer, Mind as Slayer* (New York: Dell Publishing Co. 1976) p. 244–264.

7. Krieger, D. "Therapeutic Touch the Imprimatur of Nursing." *American Journal of Nursing* 75:5 (May 1975) p. 787.

8. Krieger, D. "The Relationship of Touch, with Intent to Help or Heal, to Subjects' in-vivo Hemoglobin Values: A Study in Personalized Interaction." Paper presented at Ninth American Nurses' Association Research Conference, San Antonio, Texas, March 1973.

9. Krieger. "Therapeutic Touch the Imprimatur of Nursing."

10. Krieger, D. and Peper, E. "Physiological Indices of Therapeutic Touch." *American Journal of Nursing* (in press).

11. Rogers, M. *The Theoretical Basis of Nursing* (Philadelphia: F.A. Davis Co. 1970).

12. Randolph, G. "Developmental Study of Therapeutic Touch Practitioners 1976" (unpublished data).

13. Krieger, D. "The Relationship of Touch, with Intent to Help or Heal."

14. Personal communication with Dolores Krieger, Professor, New York University, March 1977.

15. Pelletier. *Mind as Healer, Mind as Slayer.*

16. Selye, H. *Stress without Distress* (New York: J.B. Lippincott Co. 1974).

17. Aldine-Atherton, Publishers. *Biofeedback and Self Control* (Annuals) (Chicago: Aldine-Atherton, Publishers 1970–1975/76).

18. Brown, B. *Stress and the Art of Biofeedback* (New York: Harper & Row 1977) p. 54–116.

19. Fuller, G. *Methods and Procedures in Clinical Practice* (San Francisco; Biofeedback Institute of San Francisco 1977).

20. Sterman, L. T. "Clinical Biofeedback." *American Journal of Nursing* 75:11 (November 1975) p. 2006–2009.

21. Peper, E. "Biofeedback as a Core Technique in Clinical Therapies." Paper presented at the 81st Annual Convention of the American Psychological Association, Montreal, 1973.

22. Pelletier. *Mind as Healer, Mind as Slayer.* p. 244–264.

23. Sparks, L. *Self-Hypnosis, A Conditioned-Response Technique* (New York: Grune and Stratton 1962).

24. Schwartz, J. *Voluntary Controls* (New York: E.P. Dutton & Co. 1978).

25. Carrington, P. *Freedom in Meditation* (Garden City, N.Y.: Anchor Press 1977) p. 92.

26. Rosa, K. R. *You and A T* (New York: E.P. Dutton & Co. 1973).

27. Patel, C. H. "Yoga and Biofeedback in the Management of Hypertension." *Lancet* ii (November 10, 1973) p. 1053.

28. Benson, H. *The Relaxation Response* (New York: Morrow and Co. 1975).

29. Fuller. *Methods and Procedures in Clinical Practice.* p. 100.

30. Ibid.

31. Ibid.

Stress Management through Hypnosis

Thomas James Daley, R.N., M.S.N.,
*   Hypnotherapist*
School Nurse
Division of Health Services
School District of Philadelphia
Board of Education
Philadelphia, Pennsylvania

Eric L. Greenspun
Hypnotherapist and Certified Instructor
AFL-CIO OPEIU
Philadelphia, Pennsylvania

Not only will men of science have to grapple with the sciences that deal with man, but—and this is a far more difficult matter—they will have to persuade the world to listen to what they have discovered. If they cannot succeed in this difficult enterprise, man will destroy himself by his halfway cleverness.

—Bertrand Russell

THE NURSE IS often considered the front-line health care practitioner whose role includes stress management. One of the less conventional but certainly most innovative techniques for stress management is hypnosis. Symptomatic treatment through drugs, and therapeutic communication and touch have proven and will continue to prove effective in reducing client stress. Once hypnosis is demystified it too, becomes a useful tool to use with clients who have made a commitment to be healthier individuals. The nurse using hypnosis and teaching the client self-hypnosis can assist clients to

226

manage pain and other stress created by illness. Through hypnosis the nurse can also assist clients to relinquish habits that the clients consider detrimental to their health, such as smoking and overeating

White, a pioneer in the field of hypnosis, defines hypnosis as a "meaningful goal-directed striving, its most general goal being to behave like a hypnotized person as this is continuously defined by the operator and understood by the subject. . . . Goal-directed striving (does not) necessarily imply either (conscious) awareness or intention."[1]

This definition implies that there is an agreement between the individual and the hypnotherapist as to what the hypnotic state is, and that that state is unique to each individual. Caprio and Berger have described hypnosis as a sleep-like state in which the subject is self-absorbed as if in fantasy, or is partially withdrawn from reality.[2] The subject does not lose consciousness and might describe the hypnotic state as one of absent-mindedness, or a state of dissociation of consciousness from reality.

Currently scientists are conducting systematic research on how the hypnotic trance is induced. Bandler and Grinder[3] have analyzed the work of Milton Erickson, the father of medical hypnosis, using linguistic analysis techniques to decipher the language of hypnotherapists. They have also studied the nonverbal cues used by hypnotherapists and the models used by human beings to organize their perceptions of the world. Bandler and Grinder emphasize that hypnotherapists use their understanding of how people represent the world in general to induce a trance-like state. Hypnosis may thus be considered

role taking in which clients, in their unique way, sink below "the level of purely conscious compliance and volition and . . . become(s) nonconsciously directive."[4]

There are also physiological theories of hypnosis which postulate that a real physical change occurs in the nervous system during hypnosis.[5] Although these changes have not been demonstrated, research with split-brain patients may reveal the involvement of such mechanisms.[6]

Hypnotherapists sometimes discuss the techniques of hypnosis in the theoretical sense as misdirection of attention.[7] Some subscribe to the theory that hypnosis is the control of thought and action through suggestion.[8] Others consider it to be the temporary inactivation of conscious reason.[9] Precisely put, the client is disassociating the critical and analytical components of thought, thereby allowing the acceptance of suggestion.

BACKGROUND

The use of hypnosis to heal the sick and injured actually dates back to ancient times. Some ancient tribes incorporated dancing, chanting and other consciousness-altering agents into their rituals to heal the sick.[10] Evidence indicates that these hypnotic rituals had some positive effects.[11]

Hypnosis as a subject of scientific inquiry began with the work of Franz Anton Mesmer, a Viennese physician born in 1734.[12] Mesmer learned his craft from Father Gassner, a Catholic priest who used hypnosis to exorcise demons from the bodies of ill persons, thus effecting a "cure." Mesmer and his theories were eventually the object of attack by his contemporaries. Hypnosis as a treatment modality, although kept alive by Charcot and Freud, remained suspect.[13] Until recently the practitioners of hypnosis were viewed, like Mesmer, as charismatic quacks.

Hypnosis eventually became an accepted alternative to pain and death as health care demanded alternatives to conventional medical treatment in situations such as the battlefield where drugs were unavailable and shock was prevalent. Today through the work of such pioneers as Erickson hypnosis is recognized not only as a means of reducing or eliminating pain, but as a means of managing everyday stress.[14,15]

BASIC HYPNOTIC TECHNIQUE

A typical hypnotic induction in which the client learns relaxation is described below. It is only an introduction to the phases of hypnotic technique. NURSES WHO WISH TO USE SUCH TECHNIQUES MUST ETHICALLY AVAIL THEMSELVES OF TRAINING AND EDUCATION IN THE THEORY AND PRACTICE OF HYPNOTHERAPY.

Many people believe hypnosis is time consuming. This is not the case. The basic techniques for hypnosis may take no more than ten to fifteen minutes. This amount of time is based on an unconditioned

---

Today hypnosis is recognized not only as a means of reducing or eliminating pain, but as a means of managing everyday stress.

---

client, one who has not been previously hypnotized. Posthypnotic suggestion for later inductions reduces this time to a matter of seconds.

There are six basic components to hypnosis: pretalk, induction, utilization, awakening, post-talk and assessment.

Pretalk

During the first relaxation period, clients are not told they will be hypnotized. In pretalk, the operator (hypnotherapist) simply explains to the clients what they are going to do that will allow them to relax. The operator explains that the clients will enjoy some remarkable sensations and benefits as a result of the relaxation experience, but to do so they must cooperate. The clients need to understand that they will be entering a state of relaxation in which they will not be unconscious, but will be subconscious, that the experience is much the same as the state that occurs between being totally awake and falling fast asleep.

The subjects are informed that they are undergoing hypnosis after the first relaxation experience. It is therefore necessary to make sure the subject has had a positive first experience. In using any hypnotic technique, the pretalk between the operator and clients must take place in order for the clients to accept the difference in perception smoothly.

Induction

Most hypnotherapists use the standard method of hypnosis induction, procedural or progressive relaxation, which requires ten to fifteen minutes. The procedure is as follows.

228   The operator instructs clients to sit or lie in a comfortable position with the feet uncrossed and teeth unclenched. The clients loosen all tight garments so as not to restrict blood flow, and remove any substances such as chewing gum from the mouth. At this point, the operator may test the suggestibility level of the client, or simply start the induction. Testing the suggestibility level takes time and often becomes a crutch for the operator. Induction can usually be achieved successfully without it.

While clients are getting comfortable, the operator often closes doors and windows to eliminate unwanted stimuli. If this is impossible, the operator instructs the clients to disregard these stimuli using a phrase such as, "You will hear and feel things around you, but they are unimportant now."

Next clients are directed to close their eyes lightly, breathe deeply three times and concentrate on relaxing the crown of the skull. They are then instructed to relax their entire skull down the nape of the neck and to relax progressively the muscles in the face. When this has been completed, the amount of remaining tension is determined. In particular, the operator checks the area between the eyebrows for tension. If it is wrinkled, the operator tells the client to relax the area.

As clients enter hypnosis, they develop a flaccid look on the face. The mouth may droop open. Next, clients are told to relax the neck and large shoulder muscles and to allow the shoulders to droop. They are told that their arms feel very heavy and limp. Their eyelids may be fluttering at this point. This is perfectly normal and a good indication that clients are accepting the technique well. The operator than suggests to the clients that they will inhale relaxation and exhale tension, raising the tone of the voice on relaxation and lowering the tone on tension.

They suggest to the clients that their chest and the small of the back will relax. At this point, the clients should have achieved upper body relaxation. In order to test for upper body relaxation, the operator tells clients that he may touch them anytime but that they should have no fear for he will not harm them, only help them. Then the operator picks up one of the client's hands to test for "limp response." If stiffness is present, he places a hand on the same shoulder and presses down; the hand and arm should become limp. If the limp response is not present, the operator tests the other arm in the same manner, continuing to alternate until he receives a positive response.

The operator continues directing clients to relax until suggestions have been given that include the lower extremities. Now he is ready for the next step.

Utilization

When clients are totally relaxed, they are ready to receive positive reinforcement. The operator should always suggest that clients be peaceful, tranquil, calm and comfortable. Following these suggestions, the operator tells clients that at a specified signal, which could be given at any time in the future, they will return immediately to their present level of relaxation. Such a signal, given while clients are under hypnosis, might be, "At any time, when I point to your forehead and say the words 'deep sleep' you will immediately return to this level of relaxation." This is called a posthypnotic suggestion. Posthypnotic suggestion eliminates the need for lengthy second and subsequent inductions.

At this time, any other beneficial suggestions to reduce discomfort or cope more easily with external situations may be given. The operator should relax clients further with each suggestion given.

Awakening

In most cases, awakening the client is a very simple procedure. Once the beneficial suggestions are given, the operator tells the clients that at the count of five they will feel very good upon awakening, they will feel very calm and at peace with themselves, and they will be in a very healthy, positive state of mind. The operator should start counting in a low tone of voice, increasing the volume as well as the tone until the number five is reached. The operator should also indicate that the clients, on the count of five, will open their eyes and be wide awake.

This entire procedure should be done very slowly. If it is done too quickly, clients may experience a headache, nausea or even vomiting. In the event of a hypnotic hangover, or "hypnotic bends," the recommended procedure is to tell clients to close their eyes and relax. The operator brings clients up again very slowly. Allowing clients enough time to reorient properly may mean the difference between a positive and a negative hypnotic session. This reorienting process is much like the one a patient experiences when first awakening from anesthesia.

If clients have difficulty awakening, the operator should ask them if they understood the suggestion and, if so, why they did not awaken. Sometimes clients enjoy the sensation so much that they do not want to reorient. The operator may tell these clients that if they do not awaken on the count of five they will not be allowed to return to the hypnotic state. The operator may also suggest that the experience of hypnosis, at this time, is very unpleasant and in order to feel more comfortable, the client must awaken. When all else fails and it is absolutely necessary that clients come around, they may be slapped very lightly on the cheek to help orient them.

Post-Talk

When orienting themselves, clients often rub their eyes, straighten their clothes or simply touch their bodies. They should always be allowed sufficient time to physically readjust to the awakened perception. The operator should check for complete reorientation and should verbally emphasize the difference between the two states, the more tangible the relaxed state becomes and the easier it is achieved in subsequent attempts.

Immediately following reorientation, clients experience a heightened suggestibility, and they are especially receptive to

Immediately following reorientation, clients experience a heightened suggestibility. This is the time when goals should be discussed and agreed upon. Goals should be both short and long range.

230 the operator. This period can last as long as four to six hours, but the *most effective* time is within the first hour. This is the time when goals should be discussed and agreed upon. Goals should be both short and long range. They may include experiencing no ill effects after surgery, such as nausea or vomiting, or being able to work easily with other types of surgery. As much positive reinforcement as possible should be given to the client, thereby making it easier to work with a client in future sessions.

Assessment

The last step of this six-step process is the assessment of the client's needs for subsequent lessons in relaxation. The best method for this is observation, which is best accomplished three or four days after hypnosis. The operator should plan a second session for the evaluation and follow-up. During this session the operator observes for the level of relaxation in the client to determine whether subsequent inductions are necessary.

SELF-MANAGEMENT

Once the operator has proven to the clients that they can relax, a program of self-management should be discussed. Here clients are taught how to reinduce themselves in order to reduce their stress levels before attempting to work through a problem. There are many techniques by which clients may reinduce themselves. One very effective procedure is the counting back method. Here the operator instructs clients to sit or lie in a comfortable position with the feet uncrossed and

the teeth unclenched. The eyes should be closed lightly. Clients should then start silently counting backwards from 20, slowly relaxing with each count. The operator explains to the clients that if for any reason they skip a number or lose track of the numbering, they should simply stop and suggest to themselves that they will relax more with each breath they inhale.

Posthypnotic suggestions for continued stress management should also be given at this time. Even if these suggestions are given, the client should feel considerably calmer and more relaxed.

FINGER GRASP METHOD

The previous method of procedural relaxation is very effective for moderate to severe stress. Also very effective for this type and more pronounced stress is the "finger grasp method."

In this technique, the body positions of both operator and client are important. The operator stands facing the seated client and extends two fingers of both hands so that they point directly at the other hand; the elbow and forearm of the operator should be parallel to the floor. The seated client then grasps each of the set of fingers with the back of the hand facing the ceiling, similar to the grasping reflex of an infant.

The operator instructs the client to shut the eyes lightly and squeeze the fingers as tightly as possible and then to relax. This procedure is repeated until the client is incapable of squeezing tightly. All the while, the operator suggests the impending incapability of the client to squeeze hard.

Suggestions of fatigue are also given. As the client's ability to squeeze decreases the hands should be lowered, thus increasing the difficulty in squeezing due to the position of the wrists.

The operator then starts deepening the client's relaxation state with the inhalation method described previously. Once the client is totally relaxed, each of the other steps should be followed just as in the basic technique.

Certainly there is potential for nurses to use hypnosis in many areas of health care. However, for clients to benefit from hypnosis, operators need to spend time refining and reinforcing their skills. Several of us who have completed an approved course of study in hypnosis meet periodically to do just that. Nurses must begin to think of themselves as tour guides who can open doors into areas that clients never dreamed possible. It is the client who must want to pass through those doors.

REFERENCES

1. White, R. "A Preface to a Theory of Hypnotism." *Journal of Abnormal Social Psychology* 36:4 (October 1941) p. 477–506.
2. Caprio, L. and Berger, J. R. *Helping Yourself with Self Hypnosis* (Englewood Cliffs, N. J.: Prentice-Hall, Inc. 1963.
3. Bandler, R. and Grinder, J. *Patterns of the Techniques of Milton Erickson, M.D.* vol. 1 (Cupertino, Calif.: Meta Publications 1975).
4. Ibid. p. 7.
5. Shor, R. E. "Three Dimensions of Hypnotic Depth." *International Journal of Clinical and Experimental Hypnosis* 10 (1962) p. 23–38.
6. Diamond, S. and Beaumont, K. *Hemisphere Function in the Human Brain* (New York: John Wiley & Sons, Inc. 1974).
7. Kroger, W. S. and Fezler, W. D. *Hypnosis and Behavior Modification: Imagery Conditioning* (Philadelphia: J. B. Lippincott Co. 1976).
8. LeCron, L. M. and Bordeaux, J. *Hypnotism Today* (N. Hollywood, Calif.: Wilshire Book Co. 1976).
9. Gindes, B. S. *New Concepts of Hypnosis* (N. Hollywood, Calif.: Wilshire Book Co. 1976).
10. LeCron and Bordeaux. *Hypnotism Today.*
11. Ibid. p. 17.
12. Ibid. p. 17.
13. Ibid. p. 25–27.
14. Kroger and Fezler. *Hypnosis and Behavior Modification.*
15. Erickson, M. H. *Advanced Techniques of Hypnosis and Therapy* (New York: Grune and Stratton 1967).

Anxiety/Stress and the Effects on Disclosure between Nurses and Patients

Margie N. Johnson, R.N., Ph.D.
Associate Professor
Psychiatric Mental Health Nursing
Texas Woman's University
Dallas Center
Dallas, Texas

INDIVIDUALS who encounter the health care system today are largely dissatisfied with the care they receive. This observation is quite perplexing, particularly since methods designed to deal with consumer dissatisfaction have been an increasing concern of nurses, practitioners, educators and researchers for well over two decades. Literature addressing the unrest among patients as well as discontent among those responsible for providing quality care is abundant. Explanations for this state of affairs are varied, and any attempt to isolate a single reason would be futile. Most appropriately, questions about methods used to cope with the problem of patient dissatisfaction might be raised.

Dissatisfaction related to various stresses perceived by the hospitalized individual is the focus of this investigation. What might nurses do to assist clients/patients in coping with stresses? How might nurses deal with their own stress and dissatisfac-

234 tion with their current functions in relation to patient care?

Recently a study was done to determine if a relationship could be found between self-disclosure and anxiety (stress response) in selected nurses and patients in a clinical setting. The study stemmed from a basic belief that investigation of how nurses and patients cope with stressful events in a clinical setting can play a large part in building a useful knowledge base for improving nursing practice.

CONCEPTUAL FRAMEWORK

The conceptual framework for the study was based on literature and research which suggested that self-disclosing individuals tend to be healthier, mentally and physically, than individuals who do not self-disclose.[1-3] Self-disclosure is defined as a voluntary process of revealing one's personal data, such as beliefs, values, feelings and perceptions, to another person; it involves being known to another in a specific way that one wants to be known.[1] The literature further speculates that anxiety adversely affects one's level of self-disclosure; that is, persons experiencing significant levels of anxiety will not disclose information about themselves.[4] The study addressed the question of whether or not a relationship between these two phenomena (anxiety and self-disclosure) in selected groups of nurses and hospitalized patients can be established.

According to Volicer, hospitalization is an event which increases anxiety in nearly all individuals who are hospitalized.[5] Increased anxiety is often precipitated by stresses such as separation from family and familiar surroundings, fear of the unknown and inability to fully understand the complex nature and consequences of illness. In addition, certain cultural and/or ethnic beliefs may have an effect on patients' attitudes toward their illness and hospitalization. Furthermore, and perhaps most importantly, there is the factor of communication between patients and health care professionals, especially nurses, which may contribute in varying degrees to patients' anxiety levels. Tagliacozzo interviewed samples of patients in a large urban hospital and found that 68% of them reported they had refrained from expressing their feelings, desires, fears, or criticisms to either nurses or physicians. Also, some of the patients cited instances in which being a "good patient," self-controlled and minimally dependent, was reinforced by positive reactions from the personnel.[6] Skipper observed 86 patients between the ages of 40 and 60 years, and found that they refrained from communicating with the nurses due to a fear of negative reactions from them, a fear of receiving unsatisfactory answers to their questions and a perception that nurses were always too busy and overworked.[7]

Wooldridge et al. discussed the importance of communication and psychological support of the patient by the nurse. They contend that a basic sociopsychological principle is that individuals' definition of their current situation is strongly affected by their reaction to the "significant others" in the immediate social environment.[8] This implies that what nurses communicate or do not communicate when they are with patients will have important implications for patients and their perception of their hospitalization and illness. It follows that all interactions between nurses and patients have real and/or symbolic meaning for the patients. Therapeutic communication theory that deals with factors contributing to increase or decrease in quality communication between persons could serve as a useful adjunct to this framework.

Finally, Robinson proposed that an individual admitted to a hospital brings not only an illness but a definitive mental set. This mental set will influence the manner in which the individual assumes the patient's role during the course of hospitalization. The manner in which ill persons respond to hospitalization will be influenced by their fantasies about the institution and the professional people in it. The protective mechanisms patients use to buffer against anxiety will assist in fending off the uncomfortable feelings that beset them as they face confinement.[9] Use of various protective behaviors by the patient may produce the reverse effect.

Rather than bringing about a comforting response, there may be an increase in discomfort, fear and withdrawal.

Figure 1 demonstrates the framework synthesized from the literature. From the patients' viewpoint, stress is brought on by the complexities of illness and hospitalization. The onset of stress leads to an increase in anxiety responses and a decrease in the amount of meaningful self-disclosures. Nursing intervention which includes self-disclosure brings about an increase in patients' self-disclosure and an accompanying decrease in patients' levels of anxiety. As a result, patients are more able to cope with stress factors encountered during hospitalization.

Presumably, nurses also experience anxiety as a result of stress experienced in the work situation which may be influential in deterring meaningful interactions with patients. Aasterud observed that nurses exhibit anxiety in the work setting and use a variety of maladaptive defenses to cope with these experiences. She stated that

FIGURE 1. INFLUENCE OF STRESS ON LEVELS OF ANXIETY AND SELF-DISCLOSURE WITH PROPOSED CHANGES FOLLOWING EFFECTIVE NURSING INTERVENTION

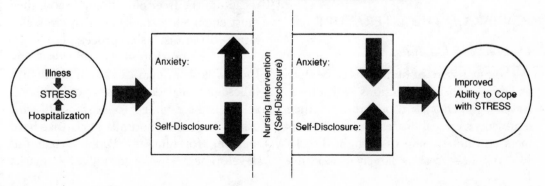

236 many hospital procedures and nursing care practices are viewed as intrusive and victimizing to the patient. Nurses are often unaware of their anxiety about such practices, since historically they have perceived themselves as being supportive, caring and helpful to patients. Aasterud further observed that nurses tend to establish a social defense system which includes the performance of ritualistic tasks in order to avoid change, thus restricting meaningful contact with patients.[10] Finally, Skipper hypothesized that when nurses limit communication with their patients, they avoid the anxiety-producing situation of having patients question or evaluate nurses' knowledge, performance or authority.[7]

There seems to be sufficient support for the contention that both nurses and patients resist the urge to express their real feelings and problems. Patients may conceal information about themselves because nurses and other health care personnel do not share information about themselves with patients. Proposed in the present investigation is that the interpersonal patterns of communication, specifically that of self-disclosure, that exist between nurses and patients are related to stress and anxiety.

REVIEW OF THE LITERATURE

Construct of Self-Disclosure

The true nature of humans is to be open and free in their interactions with others. Revealing personal thoughts to others represents a critical process in the development and functioning of thought. Disclosure of one's ideas is largely responsible

Children have little "verbal continence" and seem unaware of what it means to keep thoughts and feelings to themselves. This period of free self-disclosure ends when the child is negatively reinforced by adults as a result of disclosures.

for the reduction of egocentric thought and the augmentation of socialized thought that is observed concomitantly with development. Piaget maintains that children have little "verbal continence" as they learn to speak, and seem unaware of what it means to keep thoughts and feelings to themselves. This period of free self-disclosure ends when the child is negatively reinforced by adults as a result of disclosures. In other words, the early relationship developed between children and significant others is influential in later development of adult propensities to self-disclose.[11]

Within the life span of the average individual, more factors function to inhibit rather than encourage their natural disclosing tendency. Authentic self-disclosure as viewed by Jourard is rare among today's people. Thus, if people are to recapture the free spirit of childhood, they must engage in experiences that are facilitative to the disclosing process.

One central hypothesis advanced by Jourard is that "man can attain health and fullest personal development only insofar as he gains courage to be himself with others and when he finds goals that have meaning for him."[1(p ix)] People attain full development by shedding the masks which alienate them from themselves and from significant others. The courage to know oneself and to be known by others implies the existence of an interpersonal relationship, that begins with self-disclosure on the part of one individual to another. Such disclosure is risky and may necessitate a recall of those forces described earlier by Piaget which operated during childhood to prevent disclosure. The opportunity for establishing a climate for free and open exchange must be a goal of nursing activities.

Cozby summarized a group of studies related to self-disclosure and mental health. He observed that the self-disclosure/mental health relationship is curvilinear, suggesting that individuals who seldom disclose anything about themselves may be unable to establish close relationships with others. In contrast, individuals who freely disclose a great deal about themselves may be perceived by others as being maladjusted. The medium level self-disclosers may impart considerable information about themselves to someone who is very close and hence maintain a moderately close relationship—not too close to be offensive, but close enough to establish meaningful social bonds.[12]

ANTECEDENT CHARACTERISTICS

Personality, age, sex, race, ethnic group and social class, culture and religion are some of the antecedent factors influencing self-disclosure.

The amount of mutual disclosure in a dyad reflects personality characteristics of the two individuals. When low-disclosing subjects were paired with high disclosers, the low-disclosing subjects increased their disclosure output to match the level of the high-disclosers.[13]

As individuals age, the amount they disclose to others, especially parents and same-sex friends, gradually diminishes. However, disclosures to opposite-sex friends or spouses increase from the age of 17 up to about the mid-40s and then drop off.[14] With increased age, the communicative intimacy of relationships with others diminishes, possibly as a function of the disengagement phenomenon espoused by Henry and Cumming.[15]

Jourard and Lasakow reported that females have higher self-disclosure scores than males. The low disclosure of males was felt to be directly associated with less empathy, less insight and a shorter life span than females.[16]

When the variables of race and social class are considered, blacks disclose less than whites and Mexican-Americans disclose less than blacks.[17-19] Some data suggest that racial differences in self-disclosure may be due to social class factors. Jaffee and Polansky obtained no differences in disclosure scores between lower-class blacks and lower-class whites.[20] Mayer reported that middle-class women disclosed more about their marital difficulties than did working-class women.[21]

Cross-culturally, Lewin found that Americans disclose a great deal about themselves and make friends easily, but do not develop highly intimate relationships. In contrast, Germans do not disclose as much about themselves, but develop very close relationships with a few others.[22]

Jewish males disclose at significantly higher levels than Baptist, Methodists and

238 Catholics, with the latter three not differing significantly from one another.[23] Cooke obtained a significant correlation between disclosure to parents and religious behavior (e.g., frequency of church attendance) of sample subjects.[24]

SELF-DISCLOSURE AND SELECTED PARAMETERS

Certain parameters of self-disclosure that have been studied include amount of disclosure, depth of disclosure, intimacy level, duration, disclosures over time and target group selected as disclosure recipients.

In a study using eight subjects, Jourard reported that revealing too little or too much about oneself seemed to be equally unacceptable. As friendship is developing, too great or too small an acceleration in the rate and amount revealed may retard or sever a developing relationship.[25]

Intimacy and duration of disclosure appear to be partially related, with a correlation coefficient of 0.42 between the two variables.[26] There is, however, an inverse relationship between amount and intimacy of disclosure such that individuals disclose less about more intimate topics.[27,28] Individuals generally are more willing to disclose "public" (attitudes, tastes and work) information than "private" (money, personality and body) information.

Individuals are generally more willing to disclose "public" (attitudes, tastes and work) information than "private" (money, personality and body) information.

Taylor found that over periods of one, three, six, nine and 13 weeks, pairs of high-disclosers reported more mutual self-disclosures than did pairs of low-disclosers, although the rate of the increase over time was similar for both groups. There was a rapid increase in nonintimate disclosures, and a slow, gradual increase in intimate disclosures over time for both groups.[29]

Target groups selected for disclosure vary in the amount of disclosure made to them. Both college and high school students indicate more disclosures made to mothers than to fathers.[30,31] Persons and Marks reported that their subjects disclosed most to interviewers who were most similar to themselves in personality profile.[32] These findings are consistent with the assumption that self-disclosure is dependent on the closeness of the relationship between the subject and target. There were no studies found on disclosures made to nurses as a target group.

INTERPERSONAL RELATIONSHIPS

Social approval, dependency and power, liking, reciprocity and therapeutic outcome are factors that influence self-disclosure in interpersonal relationships. Colson found that subjects' disclosures were greatest in positive evaluation conditions and lowest in negative evaluation conditions.[33] Investigation of dependency and self-disclosure by Altman and Haythorn indicated that high-dependency dyads were more intimate and showed a more active pattern of social interaction than did the low-dependency dyads.[27] Thibaut and

Kelly demonstrated that the constraints of first encounters may prevent forming meaningful relationships. In the case of strangers however, when the time limit of the encounter is brief, significant disclosure may occur. The longer the interacting period between strangers is expected to be, the more constrained the relationship will be.[34]

Individuals generally resist entering into relationships in which the other person holds a great deal of power. For example, a study by Kounin et al. revealed that individuals feel more at ease and reveal more negative things about themselves with a nonpowerful counselor.[35]

Worth et al. concluded that more disclosures are made to liked individuals (on initial impressions) and individuals liked most those who disclosed most to them.[36]

A number of studies have supported the idea that reciprocity in self-disclosure between individuals is important for a stable relationship. Wiegel et al. asked their subjects how much they had actually disclosed in the past, how much they would initiate, and how much they would disclose in response to initiation by the other person. The subjects indicated they would disclose most in response to initiation of self-disclosure by the other person.[37] In a related study by Chittick and Himelstein, the authors manipulated subjects' disclosures directly by asking confederates to vary the amount they disclosed when introducing themselves to the subjects. Subsequent disclosure from the subjects varied proportionately to the confederate's disclosure.[38]

The importance of full client disclosure for therapeutic outcome has been documented. Truax and Carkhuff found significant correlations between therapist and client disclosures reporting that the level of client disclosure appeared to be a predictor of final outcome.[39] Powell found that subjects disclosed more when the interviewer responded to subjects' self-references with open self-disclosure than when approval-supportive or reflected-restatement techniques were used.[40] Further, Drag concluded that the interviewer who discloses, in addition to eliciting greater disclosure from subjects, is rated more trustworthy and more positive than the interviewer who does not self-disclose.[41]

An obvious limitation of the data on patterns and practices of self-disclosing behavior is an almost complete lack of validation of the process in a clinical setting. The present study differs from most of the work reported above in that a clinical setting is used.

A Construct of Anxiety

Anxiety is perhaps one of the most frequently appearing phenomena in psychological literature. Its theoretical and operational definitions are laden with semantic confusion. This has led to vague and interchangeable use of the term in the research literature. Also, considerable lack of agreement regarding the nature of anxiety, conditions that arouse it and specific past and/or current experiences that make an individual vulnerable to it are prevalent.

Freud regarded anxiety as "something felt," an unpleasant affective state or

240   condition. Freud modified his original conception concerning the origin of anxiety, initially defining anxiety as being repressed libidinal excitation. He later defined anxiety as being a signal that indicated the presence of a dangerous situation. He then differentiated between objective anxiety and neurotic anxiety largely on the basis of whether the source of the danger originated from the external world or from internal impulses.[42]

Mowrer proposed a "guilt theory" to explain anxiety, stating that anxiety comes not from acts which the individual would commit but dares not, but from acts which he has committed but wished that he had not. If an individual behaves irresponsibly, with too much self-indulgence and too little self-restraint, then anxiety is experienced.[43]

An "interpersonal theory" posited by Sullivan characterized anxiety as an intensely unpleasant state or tension arising from experiencing disapproval in interpersonal relations. Once aroused, anxiety distorts the individual's perception of reality, narrows the range of stimuli perceived and causes those aspects of the personality that are not acceptable to be dissociated.[44]

May described a "learning theory" approach to anxiety. The anxiety phenomenon is viewed as apprehension cued off by a threat to some value which the individual holds essential to existence. While the capacity to experience anxiety is innate, the particular events or stimulus conditions evoking it are largely learned. May proposes that an anxiety reaction is normal if it is proportionate to the objective danger and does not involve repres-

sion. Anxiety is abnormal if reactions are disproportionate to the objective danger, but not the subjective danger, and repression is involved.[45]

Tillich described anxiety from an existentialist point of view by defining it as a type of fear resulting from the threat of nothingness or nonbeing. He noted that a

---

Tillich described anxiety from an existentialist point of view as a type of fear resulting from the threat of nothingness or nonbeing.

---

common feature of most theories of anxiety is an emphasis on unresolved conflicts between structural elements of the personality.[46]

Lazarus and Averill described anxiety as an emotion that is based on the appraisal of a threat which entails symbolic, anticipatory, and uncertain elements that result when cognitive systems no longer enable an individual to relate meaningfully to the external world.[47]

Anxiety at low levels is useful and is associated with mastery over oneself and the environment. Anxiety serves to expand one's awareness of an existing or potential threat. Extreme anxiety, however, can be so severe as to disrupt ongoing behavior. In acute panic states the individual may flee blindly in any direction, disregarding his usual responsibilities. At this point, anxiety becomes so severe that no response is capable of lessening it.

Spielberger et al. have expanded definitions for two specific types of anxiety, state anxiety and trait anxiety:

State anxiety is conceptualized as a transitory emotional state or condition of the human organism that is characterized by subjective, consciously perceived feelings of tension and apprehension and heightened autonomic nervous system activity. A-state may vary in intensity and fluctuate over time.

Trait anxiety refers to relatively stable individual differences in anxiety proneness, that is, to differences between people in the tendency to respond to situations perceived as threatening with elevation in A-state intensity.[48]

For the present study, the conceptualization of anxiety factors by Spielberger et al. has been selected.

The relevance of the anxiety study for nursing is couched within the framework formulated by Jourard, who proposed that there is a relationship between one's ability to self-disclose and one's level of anxiety; and that self-disclosing behavior in one person encourages the other to self-disclose, thereby reducing anxiety in both persons.[1] If nurses can be taught the skills of appropriate self-disclosure communication, patients may find it easier to cope with stresses of illness and hospitalization.

THE STUDY

Study Questions

The study addressed two major research questions. First, is there a relationship between nurses' levels of state/trait anxiety and their levels of self-disclosure to patients? Second, is there a relationship between patients' levels of state/trait anxiety and their levels of self-disclosure to nurses?

Methodology

SUBJECTS, VARIABLES AND INSTRUMENTS

Nurse and patient subjects in the study were from four types of hospital units: (1) medical, (2) surgical, (3) psychiatric and (4) critical care. The 70 nurses who took part were RNs and LVNs currently engaged in full-time practice. Patients (N = 68) were individuals between the ages of 21 and 60 years who had been hospitalized in one of the specialty units at least five and no more than eight days. The independent variables of the study for nurses were: their nursing specialties (hospital unit), age, race, education program (RN or LVN) and years of nursing experience. For patients, the independent variables were their hospital unit, age, sex, race and level of education. The dependent variables for both nurses and patients were their scores on the instruments.

The two instruments used in this study were the Jourard Self-Disclosure Questionnaire (JSDQ) and the State-Trait Anxiety Inventory (STAI). The JSDQ, developed by Jourard in 1958,[1] was designed to measure verbalized aspects of self-disclosure defined as a voluntary act of revealing personal data about oneself including beliefs, values, feelings and perceptions to another person. The JSDQ instrument is divided into six areas: work, money, personality, body, attitudes and opinions and taste and interest. The nurses were asked to indicate to what extent they had discussed content in each of the 30 statements with patients; and the patients were asked to indicate to what extent they had disclosed the content in each of the 30 statements with a nurse. Since each ques-

242   tion could receive a score of 0 = no disclosure, 1 = some disclosure or 2 = full disclosure, the total range of disclosure scores could be from zero to 60.

The STAI was developed by Spielberger et al.[48] This instrument consists of two self-report scales for measuring the two anxiety concepts, state anxiety and trait anxiety, as previously defined. The locus of the stressful events for patients' state anxiety was their hospitalization, and for nurses' state anxiety it was their present work situation. The frame of reference of trait anxiety for patients was when they were not ill, or hospitalized, and for nurses it was when they were not in their work situation. Although originally developed as a research instrument for investigating anxiety responses in normal (nonpsychiatrically disturbed) adults, the STAI has also been found to be useful in the measurement of anxiety in normal subjects as well as neuropsychiatric, medical and surgical patients. Each subscale of the STAI, state anxiety and trait anxiety, is composed of 20 items. The range of possible scores for each scale varies from a minimum of 20 (low anxiety) to a maximum of 80 (high anxiety).

SETTING

The setting for this study was a 775-bed public general hospital that provided extensive inpatient, outpatient and emergency services to a large urban indigent population in the southwestern United States. The hospital provided all major health services and a variety of special medical and surgical therapies, as well as psychiatric services. The four specialty units were chosen due to the nature and diversity of patients' illnesses and a diversity in the type of nursing care given.

DATA COLLECTION

Nurses and patients who volunteered to participate and met the above criteria were included in the study sample. Subjects were requested to answer both questionnaires and to provide the necessary demographic data (e.g., age, sex, race, level of education or nursing experience and hospital unit). The questionnaires were enclosed in large envelopes that included instructions, a letter explaining the potential risks and benefits of subjects' participation and a form for subjects to sign indicating that participation was voluntary. Data-collection procedure for nurses went according to the established protocol. However, for patients it was necessary to use the interview schedule technique due to difficulties encountered by some patients in reading the items and in recording their responses. The average length of each interview was approximately 20 minutes. The data-collection period for nurses required two weeks and for patients about eight weeks.

ANALYSIS OF DATA

The data were analyzed descriptively and inferentially on all respondents across all variables. Means and standard deviations were computed on all data. One-way analyses of variance were used to determine if any significant differences existed among nurses, among patients and between nurses and patients on self-disclosure and anxiety. Scheffe F-tests were computed in those cases of significant F ratio in which more than two variables were involved. The Spearman-Brown correlation coefficient was obtained to determine the relationship between the levels of self-disclosure and anxiety in both groups of subjects. A $p < 0.05$ level of statistical significance was used as the criterion for rejection of hypotheses.

BASIC ASSUMPTIONS

Before and during the course of this study three basic assumptions were made: (1) that nurses and patients would respond to the data-gathering instruments candidly; (2) that the method of selecting nurses and patients would equalize among and within all units any effects due to different diagnoses, and number of hospitalizations on patients would equalize any effects due to different areas of specialty for nurses; and (3) that the method of data collection on patients would not vary significantly from one interviewer to another since they received their training and instructions from the researcher.

LIMITATIONS

The generalizability of this study is limited by the fact that all data were collected in one hospital; therefore, any conclusions and generalizations that are reached may be applicable only to this particular population and sample.

PILOT STUDY

A pilot study was conducted using the instruments, the research design and the methodology previously described. The pilot study provided support that the design and methodology employed in the study were sound.

As a result of the pilot study, two changes were made in conducting the larger study. One of the changes was to shorten the 60-item self-disclosure instrument to a 30-item measure by using only the odd items, due to the inordinate amount of time required by subjects to complete it and the seemingly fatiguing effect on the respondents, especially patients. The other major change was the decision to use research assistants as interviewers to assist those patients who would have difficulty recording their responses due to physical limitation.

DISCUSSION OF FINDINGS
RELATED TO NURSES

Measures of State/Trait Anxiety among Nurses

Tables 1 and 2 contain a compilation of data relative to the mean values of state anxiety and trait anxiety among nurses.

When nurse subjects were grouped according to area of nursing specialty (hospital unit), it was shown that nurses on the psychiatric unit reported significantly lower levels of state anxiety than nurses on the medical unit and the surgical unit. On measures of trait anxiety, nurses on the psychiatric unit also reported significantly

When nurse subjects were grouped according to area of nursing specialty, it was shown that nurses on the psychiatric unit reported significantly lower levels of state anxiety than nurses on the medical unit and the surgical unit.

TABLE 1

Mean Levels of State Anxiety among Nurses across All Variables

Hospital Unit	N	$\overline{X}$	S.D.	Age	N	$\overline{X}$	S.D.	Race	N	$\overline{X}$	S.D.	Educational Program	N	$\overline{X}$	S.D.	Years of Nursing Experience	N	$\overline{X}$	S.D.
Med.	18	37.83	9.62	18-34	44	35.87	10.78	White	39	35.72	10.54	LVN	23	30.87	7.11	1-5	37	35.27	10.11
Surg.	19	37.32	12.16	35-44	19	29.63	7.26	Nonwhite	31	32.32	8.99	RN	47	35.85	10.79	6-10	11	35.00	13.63
Psych.	17	28.94	5.19	45+	7	36.14	7.71									11+	22	32.05	7.41
CC	16	32.06	8.51																

TABLE 2

Mean Levels of Trait Anxiety among Nurses across All Variables

Hospital Unit	N	$\overline{X}$	S.D.	Age	N	$\overline{X}$	S.D.	Race	N	$\overline{X}$	S.D.	Educational Program	N	$\overline{X}$	S.D.	Years of Nursing Experience	N	$\overline{X}$	S.D.
Med.	18	35.83	9.48	18-34	44	36.68	8.60	White	39	35.21	8.68	LVN	23	33.61	9.23	1-5	37	37.11	9.14
Surg.	19	39.47	8.82	35-44	19	32.68	7.31	Nonwhite	31	34.87	8.13	RN	47	35.77	7.94	6-10	11	29.64	6.95
Psych.	17	30.35	5.11	45+	7	31.28	7.95									11+	22	34.32	6.41
CC	16	33.94	6.93																

lower levels than nurses on the surgical unit. These findings indicate that psychiatric-mental health nurses perceive fewer anxiety-producing events in their current work situation. They also have a lower tendency or disposition toward anxiety, which may be due to their specific training and experience in working with psychiatric patients. In addition, psychiatric-mental health nurses could be already sensitized to the psychological implications of the research instruments, and thus deliberately guard against reporting their own anxiety tendencies.

When the subjects were grouped according to type of education program they completed, it was shown that LVNs reported significantly lower levels of state anxiety than RNs; however there were no significant differences in their mean trait anxiety scores. This finding may reflect the possibility that RNs have more responsibility and are exposed to more anxiety-producing events in the job situation than LVNs.

When the nurses were grouped according to their years of nursing experience, it was shown that nurses with one to five years of nursing experience reported significantly more trait anxiety than nurses with six to ten years of experience. This finding may be indicative of the possibility that nurses with more experience have acquired relative security in their work situation and thus their disposition to respond to anxiety-producing events is lessened.

Age and race did not seem to be factors influencing differences in nurses' self-reported levels of state or trait anxiety.

Measures of Self-Disclosure of Nurses to Patients

Table 3 contains mean levels of self-disclosure of nurses to patients. The variables analyzed were hospital unit, age, race, educational program and years of nursing experience. When the subjects were grouped according to type of educational program they had completed, LVNs reported disclosing significantly more to patients than RNs. It may be that LVNs disclose more to patients than RNs because, as mentioned before, they are less anxious than RNs. Or it may be that LVNs have more opportunity to disclose to patients because they spend more time in direct contact with them. It should be noted that as a single group (LVNs and RNs combined) the disclosures made by nurses to patients were very low in number compared to disclosures made to other target groups. Mean-level disclosures shown in Table 3 are compared with the highest possible value of 60 obtainable in this category.

When the subjects were grouped according to hospital unit, age, race and years of nursing experience, there were no significant differences in the nurses' reported levels of self-disclosure to patients.

Relationship between State/Trait Anxiety and Self-Disclosure of Nurses to Patients

In studying the correlations of state/trait anxiety and self-disclosure of nurses to patients (see Table 4), significant relationships were found when the data were analyzed for nurses according to age. In

TABLE 3

Nurses' Mean Levels of Self-Disclosure to Patients across All Variables

Hospital Unit	N	X̄	S.D.	Age	N	X̄	S.D.	Race	N	X̄	S.D.	Educational Program	N	X̄	S.D.	Years of Nursing Experience	N	X̄	S.D.
Med.	18	3.50	4.42	18-34	44	7.34	8.88	White	39	6.72	7.46	LVN	23	9.74	10.29	1-5	37	6.57	7.83
Surg.	19	8.89	10.98	35-44	19	6.32	7.17	Nonwhite	31	7.23	9.01	RN	47	5.97	6.53	6-10	11	7.55	7.87
Psych.	17	7.59	6.93	45+	7	6.14	6.15									11+	22	7.27	9.05
CC	16	7.81	8.09																

TABLE 4

Spearman-Brown Rank Order Correlations between Levels of State Anxiety/Trait Anxiety and Self-Disclosure of Nurses to Patients[a]

Hospital Unit	N	SA/SD	TA/SD	Age	N	SA/SD	TA/SD	Race	N	SA/SD	TA/SD	Educational Program	N	SA/SD	TA/SD	Years of Nursing Experience	N	SA/SD	TA/SD
Med.	18	-0.24	-0.09	18-34	44	-0.15	0.01	White	39	-0.46[c]	-0.33[b]	LVN	23	-0.02	0.04	1-5	37	-0.03	0.01
Surg.	19	-0.11	0.07	35-44	19	-0.39	-0.43	Non-white	31	-0.04	0.11	RN	47	-0.28[b]	0.21	6-10	11	-0.45	-0.18
Psych.	17	-0.39	-0.04	45+	7	-0.76[c]	-0.28									11+	22	-0.30	-0.39
CC	17	-0.11	-0.36																

[a] SA = State anxiety, TA = Trait anxiety, SD = Self-disclosure
[b] = p .05.
[c] = ±p .01.

nurses who were 45 years of age and older, there was a significant negative correlation between state anxiety and their level of self-disclosure to patients.

In white nurses, there was a significant negative correlation between state anxiety and self-disclosure; and between trait anxiety and self-disclosure to patients.

When the data were analyzed according to education program, RNs reported a significant negative correlation between state anxiety and self-disclosure to patients.

From a total of 28 correlations computed across the 14 variables, 23 were negative and four of these (mentioned above) showed a significant negative correlation. This implies a strong tendency for support of the research proposition, that as anxiety levels tend to increase, levels of self-disclosure tend to decrease.

DISCUSSION OF FINDINGS RELATED TO PATIENTS

Measures of State/Trait Anxiety among Patients

Tables 5 and 6 show a compilation of data relative to the mean values of state anxiety and trait anxiety among patients. When the patients were grouped according to hospital unit, those on the psychiatric unit reported significantly higher levels of state anxiety than patients on the medical, surgical or critical care units. This finding does not seem unusual since many of the patients on the psychiatric unit in this study had anxiety reactions as a diagnosis. On measures of trait anxiety there were no significant differences among patients grouped by hospital unit.

This result may indicate that when not in the hospital, psychiatric patients may be similar to other patients; but when hospitalized, they experience or report higher levels of anxiety than patients on other units. It is also possible that specific characteristics of the psychiatric unit may contribute to the reported high anxiety levels. This speculation seems credible since no significant differences were discovered between these patients on any of the other independent variables.

Measures of Self-Disclosure of Patients to Nurses

Table 7 contains mean levels of self-disclosure of patients to nurses. The variables analyzed were hospital unit, age, sex, race and level of education.

For patient subjects, none of the independent variables seem to have a significant influence on the differential levels of patients' self-disclosure to nurses. Furthermore, when compared with other target groups, patients' self-disclosures to nurses were lowest. Mean-level disclosures shown in Table 7 are compared with the highest possible value of 60. Although none of the values reported were significant, the low tendency across all variables suggested that patients disclose very little to nurses. The patients' low levels of self-disclosure to nurses possibly is a consequence of their reaction to the low levels of disclosures by nurses to patients.

Relationships between State/Trait Anxiety and Self-Disclosure of Nurses to Patients

Correlations demonstrating the relationship of state/trait anxiety and self-disclo-

TABLE 5

Mean Levels of State Anxiety among Patients across All Variables

Hospital Unit	N	X̄	S.D.	Age	N	X̄	S.D.	Sex	N	X̄	S.D.	Race	N	X̄	S.D.	Level of Education[a]	N	X̄	S.D.
Med.	17	41.12	5.60	18-34	21	45.76	14.80	M	27	42.81	13.40	White	33	48.53	14.65	N/HS	32	44.22	13.65
Surg.	17	44.61	15.65	35-44	13	49.38	14.81	F	41	47.22	13.92	Nonwhite	35	42.29	12.16	S/HS	25	45.24	13.14
Psych.	17	57.18	13.36	45+	34	43.79	12.81									S/Col	9	48.89	17.38
CC	17	38.59	10.58													F/Col	2	53.00	11.31

[a] N/HS = No high school; S/HS = Some high school; S/Col = Some college; F/Col = Finished college

TABLE 6

Mean Levels of Trait Anxiety among Patients across All Variables

Hospital Unit	N	X̄	S.D.	Age	N	X̄	S.D.	Race	N	X̄	S.D.	Sex	N	X̄	S.D.	Level of Education[a]	N	X̄	S.D.
Med.	17	45.18	10.23	18-34	21	44.24	15.68	White	33	45.97	15.70	M	27	46.59	13.03	N/HS	32	46.75	14.69
Surg.	17	40.83	10.96	35-44	13	46.69	13.41	Nonwhite	35	47.43	13.22	F	41	46.68	15.62	S/HS	25	47.16	14.69
Psych.	17	53.06	17.84	45+	34	48.12	14.47									S/Col	9	48.67	14.34
CC	17	48.12	15.83													F/Col	2	29.50	6.36

[a] N/HS = No high school; S/HS = Some high school; S/Col = Some college; F/Col = Finished college

TABLE 7
Patients' Mean Levels of Self-Disclosure to Nurses across All Variables

Hospital Unit	N	X̄	S.D.	Age	N	X̄	S.D.	Race	N	X̄	S.D.	Sex	N	X̄	S.D.	Level of Education[a]	N	X̄	S.D.
Med.	17	11.65	8.15	18-34	21	10.19	10.22	White	34	8.74	9.08	M	27	6.85	6.80	N/HS	32	9.28	9.79
Surg.	17	8.18	8.15	35-44	13	11.08	10.51	Nonwhite	34	10.46	10.26	F	41	10.88	10.46	S/HS	25	10.12	8.96
Psych.	17	9.12	11.85	45+	34	8.03	8.37									S/Col	9	5.44	5.61
CC	17	8.18	7.79													F/Col	2	16.00	21.21

[a]N/HS = No high school; S/HS = Some high school; S/Col = Some college; F/Col = Finished college

TABLE 8
Spearman-Brown Rank Order Correlations between Levels of State Anxiety/Trait Anxiety and Self-Disclosure of Nurses to Patients[a]

Hospital Unit	N	SA/SD	TA/SD	Age	N	SA/SD	TA/SD	Race	N	SA/SD	TA/SD	Sex	N	SA/SD	TA/SD	Level of Education[d]	N	SA/SD	TA/SD
Med.	17	0.04	-0.33	18-34	22	-0.25	-0.27	White	34	-0.29	-0.16	M	27	-0.09	-0.23	N/HS	32	0.08	-0.24
Surg.	17	-0.50[b]	-0.13	35-44	22	0.35	-0.76[c]	Non-white	34	0.08	-0.46[c]	F	41	-0.14	-0.33[b]	S/HS	25	-0.40	-0.45[c]
Psych.	17	0.15	-0.36	45+	34	-0.04	-0.08									S/Col	9	-0.50	0.03
CC	17	0.23	-0.21													F/Col	2	Insufficient Sample	

[a]SA = State anxiety; TA = Trait anxiety; SD = Self-Disclosure
[b] = p .05.
[c] = p .01.
[d]N/HS = No high school; S/HS = Some high school; S/Col = Some college; F/Col = Finished college

250 sure of patients to nurses are shown in Table 8.

Several significant correlations were found. Patients on the surgical unit reported a significant negative correlation between their state anxiety and self-disclosure to nurses. Patients aged 35 to 44 reported a significant negative correlation between their trait anxiety and self-disclosure to nurses.

When data were analyzed by race, non-white patients reported a significant negative correlation between trait anxiety and self-disclosure to nurses.

Finally, a significant negative correlation was discovered when the patients were grouped according to levels of education. Patients with some high school education reported a significant negative correlation between their trait anxiety and self-disclosure to nurses.

From a total of 28 possible correlations between state/trait anxiety and self-disclosure to nurses computed across the 14 variables, 22 were negative and five of these (mentioned above) were statistically significant. This finding, which is similar to the finding with nurse subjects, implies a strong tendency for support of the research proposition, that as anxiety levels tend to increase, levels of self-disclosure tend to decrease.

IMPLICATIONS FOR NURSING

The findings in this study indicate two important implications for nursing: (1) there is slight but preliminary evidence that anxiety responses to stress have a negative effect on individuals' (nurses and patients) levels of self-disclosure; (2) low reciprocal self-disclosure occurs between nurses and patients.

The positive and therapeutic outcomes that can be anticipated from moderate levels of self-disclosure necessitate a close examination of this communication pattern. For nurses in a clinical setting, the stress encountered in intensive care units, emergency departments and other areas where there are high mortality rates can be

---

The stress encountered in intensive care units can be detrimental to the effective functioning of the nurse. In effect, nurses tend to decrease their communications with each other as well as with patients.

---

detrimental to the effective functioning of the nurse. In effect, nurses tend to decrease their communications with each other as well as with patients. Some high-stress areas have instituted stress-release discussion groups for their staff in an effort to keep to a minimum the untoward reactions from long exposure to unrelenting stress situations.

Nurse theorists have proclaimed that nursing is a practice discipline and that the practice begins with and continuously involves clients and patients. To improve practice, research must be designed to explore those variables and relationships that influence the interaction between nurses and patients. Development of nursing theories would then be useful to the extent that they addressed and directed the practice of nursing.

The findings of this study point to

critical deficiencies in our data base about nurses and patients in regard to the phenomena (anxiety and self-disclosure) examined. Therefore, the following studies could be undertaken: (1) an investigation into the factors which facilitate or inhibit self-disclosure between nurses and patients in the clinical setting; (2) an experimental

study to examine the therapeutic and/or social effects of reciprocal self-disclosure between nurses and patients to determine whether or not patients value this intervention; (3) additional research into the factors contributing to the development of stress and anxiety in nurses and hospitalized patients.

REFERENCES

1. Jourard, S. M. *The Transparent Self* (New York: Van Nostrand Reinhold Company 1971).
2. Johnson, D. *Reaching Out* (New Jersey: Prentice-Hall, Inc. 1972).
3. Prophit, Sr P. "The Relationship of the Psychological Construct of Self-Disclosure to Post Coronary Adjustment." Ph.D. Dissertation, The Catholic University of America 1974.
4. Jourard, S. M. *Self-Disclosure: An Experimental Analysis of the Transparent Self* (New York: John Wiley & Sons, Inc. 1971).
5. Volicer, B. J. "Patients' Perception of Stressful Events Associated with Hospitalization." *Nurs Res* 23:3 (May-June 1974) p. 235-238.
6. Tagliacozzo, D. L. "The Nurse from the Patient's Point of View" in Skipper, J. K. and Leonard, R. C., eds. *Social Interaction and Patient Care* (Philadelphia: J. B. Lippincott Co. 1965).
7. Skipper, J. K. "Communication and the Hospitalized Patient" in Skipper, J. K. and Leonard, R. C., eds. *Social Interaction and Patient Care* (Philadelphia: J. B. Lippincott Co. 1965).
8. Wooldridge, P. J., Skipper, J. K. and Leonard, R. C. *Behavior Science Social Practice and the Nursing Profession* (Cleveland: The Press of Case Western Reserve University 1968).
9. Robinson, L. *Psychological Aspects of the Care of Hospitalized Patients* (Philadelphia: F. A. Davis Co. 1972).
10. Aasterud, M. "Defenses Against Anxiety in the Nurse-Patient Relationship" in Lawrence, H. and Schwartz, J., eds. *The Psychodynamics of Patient Care* (Englewood Cliffs, N. J.: Prentice-Hall, Inc. 1972).
11. Piaget, J. *The Language and Thought of the Child* (New York: World Press 1962).
12. Cozby, C. P. "Self-Disclosure, Reciprocity and Liking." *Sociometry* 35:1 (March 1972) p. 151-160.
13. Jourard, S. M. and Resnick, J. L. "The Effect of

High-Revealing Subjects on the Self-Disclosure of Low-Revealing Subjects." *J Humanist Psychol* 10:1 (Spring 1970) p. 84-93.
14. Jourard, S. M. "Age Trends in Self-Disclosure." *Merrill-Palmer Quarterly* 7:3 (July 1961) p. 191-197.
15. Henry, W. E. and Cumming, E. "Personality Development in Adulthood and Old Age." *J Project Techn* 23:4 (December 1959) p. 383-390.
16. Jourard, S. M. and Lasakow, P. "Some Factors in Self-Disclosure." *J Abnorm Soc Psychol* 56:1 (January 1958) p. 91-98.
17. Jourard, S. M. "Self-Disclosure in Britain, Puerto Rico, and the United States." *J Soc Psychol* 54:1 (August 1961) p. 315-320.
18. Dimond, R. E. and Hellkamp, D. R. "Race, Sex, Ordinal Position of Birth and Self-Disclosure in High School Students." *Psychol Rep* 25:1 (August 1969) p. 235-238.
19. Littlefield, R. M. "An Analysis of Self-Disclosure Patterns of Ninth Grade Public School Children in Three Selected Sub-Cultural Groups." Ph.D. Dissertation, Florida State University 1968.
20. Jaffee, P. E. and Polansky, N. A. "Verbal Inaccessibility in Young Adolescents Showing Delinquent Trends." *J Health Human Behav* 3:2 (Summer 1962) p. 105-111.
21. Mayer, J. E. "Disclosing Marital Problems." *Social Casework* 48:1 (May 1967) p. 342-351.
22. Lewin, K. "Some Social Psychological Differences Between the United States and Germany" in Lewin G., ed. *Resolving Social Conflicts: Selected Papers on Group Dynamics 1934-1946* (New York: Harper & Row 1948).
23. Jourard, S. M. "Religious Denominations and Self-Disclosure." *Psychol Rep* 8:1 (January-June 1961) p. 446-448.
24. Cooke, T. F. "Interpersonal Correlates of Religious

252

Behavior." Ph.D. Dissertation, University of Florida 1962.

25. Jourard, S. M. "Self-Disclosure and Other Cathexis." *J Abnorm Soc Psychol* 59:3 (November 1959) p. 428-431.

26. Vondracek, S. I. and Vondracek, F. W. "The Manipulation and Measurement of Self-Disclosure in Pre-Adolescents." *Merrill-Palmer Quarterly* 17:1 (1971) p. 51-58.

27. Altman, I. and Haythorn, W. W. "Interpersonal Exchange in Isolation." *Sociometry* 28:4 (December 1965) p. 411-426.

28. Fitzgerald, M. P. "Self-Disclosure and Expressed Self-Esteem, Social Distance and Areas of the Self Revealed." *J Psychol* 56:2 (October 1963) p. 405-412.

29. Taylor, D. A. "The Development of Interpersonal Relationships: Social Penetration Process." *J Soc Psychol* 75:1 (June 1968) p. 79-90.

30. Himelstein, P. and Lubin, B. "Attempted Validation of the Self-Disclosure Inventory by the Peer Nomination Technique." *J Psychol* 61:1 (September 1965) p. 13-16.

31. Dimond, R. E. and Munz, D. C. "Ordinal Position of Birth and Self-Disclosure in High School Students." *Psychol Rep* 21:3 (December 1967) p. 829-833.

32. Persons, R. W. and Marks, P. A. "Self-Disclosure with Recidivists: Optimum Interviewer-Interviewee Matching." *J Abnorm Psychol* 76:3 (Part 1) (December 1970) p. 387-391.

33. Colson, W. N. "Self-Disclosure as a Function of Social Approval." (Unpublished Manuscript, University of Florida 1965).

34. Thibaut, J. N. and Kelly, H. H. *The Social Psychology of Groups* (New York: Wiley, 1959).

35. Kounin, J., et al. "Extent of Clients' Reactions to Initial Interviews." *Human Relations* 9:3 (August 1956) p. 265-293.

36. Worthy, M., Gray, A. L. and Kahn, G. M. "Self-Disclosure as an Exchange Process." *J Personality Soc Psychol* 13:1 (September 1969) p. 59-63.

37. Wiegel, R. G., Wiegel, V. M., and Chadwick, P. C. "Reported and Projected Self-Disclosure." *Psychol Rep* 24:1 (February 1969) p. 283-287.

38. Chittick, E. V. and Himelstein, P. "The Manipulation of Self-Disclosure." *J Psychol* 65:1 (January 1967) p. 117-121.

39. Truax, C. B. and Carkhuff, R. R. "Client and Therapist Transparency in the Psychotherapeutic Encounter." *J Counsel Psychol* 12:1 (Spring 1965) p. 3-9.

40. Powell, W. J. "Differential Effectiveness of Interviewer Interventions in Experimenter Interview." *J Consult Clin Psychol* 32:2 (April 1968) p. 210-215.

41. Drag, L. R. "Experimenter-Subject Interaction: A Situational Determinant of Differential Levels of Self-Disclosure." Master's Thesis, University of Florida 1968.

42. Freud, S. *An Outline of Psychoanalysis* (New York: W. W. Norton & Co. 1949).

43. Mowrer, O. H. *Learning Theory and Personality Dynamics* (New York: Ronald Press 1950).

44. Sullivan, H. S. *The Interpersonal Theory of Psychiatry* Perry, H. S. and Gauiel, M. L., eds. (New York: W. W. Norton & Co. 1953).

45. May, R. *The Meaning of Anxiety* (New York: Ronald Press 1950).

46. Tillich, P. *The Courage to Be* (New Haven, Connecticut: Yale University Press 1952).

47. Lazarus, R. S. and Averill, J. R. "Emotion and Cognition" in Spielberger, C. D., ed. *Anxiety: Current Trends in Theory and Research* (New York: Academic Press 1966).

48. Spielberger, C. D., Gorsch, R. L. and Lushene, R. E. *Manual for the State-Trait Anxiety Inventory* (Palo Alto, Calif.: Consulting Psychologists Press 1970.)

Part V
Stress and the Caregiver

Stress Management and the Nurse

David E. Hartl, Ed.D.
*Assistant Professor of Public
   Administration
University of Southern California
National Consultant in Management and
   Organization Development and Adult
   Education
Los Angeles, California*

STRESS AS A PERSONAL EXPERIENCE

BEFORE STRESS can be discussed as an abstract notion it is critical to understand that stress is a *personal* experience. It is a condition that is best understood when thought of not as a phenomenon that goes on "out there" in the environment but as a phenomenon that takes place within one's own body. From that personal experience it is possible to both better understand what causes stress and to deal with its symptoms in a deliberate and effective manner.

WHAT IS STRESS?

Stress has as many definitions as there are authors who write about it. However, there is a general tendency to define stress as *that physical and emotional experience which results from a requirement to change from the condition of the moment to any other condition.* Everyone experiences some

255

256 degree of stress virtually all the time. To be alive is to be experiencing some stress; absence of stress would indicate death.

Problems relating to stress become apparent when there is *too much stress*, or too much for *too long*. How much stress we can endure and for how long depends upon individual capacity. What does seem clear is that too much for too long can be destructive. Lazarus writes:

> It has become increasingly apparent that stress is important as a factor in illness in general and in chronic illness in particular. Many present day illnesses cannot be explained in terms of a single "cause". Research suggests that a significant portion of the population seeking medical care is suffering from stress-based illness.[1(p57)]

Stress is a physical and emotional phenomenon. Some symptoms of prolonged stress include hypertension or high blood pressure, cardiovascular diseases and general relative ill health, as well as emotional outbursts and unexplained lapses in performance and memory.

The human system's capacity for sustaining relatively high degrees of stress for short periods is rooted in our early evolutionary needs for a "fight or flight" response to danger. Under conditions requiring an intense focus of energy, the human system has the ability to release hormones into the blood stream, increase blood supply to the skeletal muscles and slow down the gastrointestinal process—efforts that ready the body for activities and performances that are often truly extraordinary. During periods of perceived danger, the system is out of balance in a fashion approximating an out-of-balance environment. After the danger passes, the system will seek to revert naturally to a balanced condition or homeostasis. This condition is not stress free; it is only without the excess stress that was present for a brief time during the period of danger. Today's dangers come not from saber-toothed tigers as was the case for our evolutionary ancestors, but from more subtle sources. Nonetheless our systems still react as they did ages ago.

NURSES AND PERCEIVED DANGER

Nurses often experience danger (or stress) as a continuing condition in their lives by virtue of their choice of profession. There is danger from sickness or injury among patients for whom they are responsible, or danger from the effects of inaccurate doses of medication, and inaccurate or insufficient information about a patient's condition. There is danger for the nurse at other levels of experience—insufficient resources to meet the needs and wants of patients; not enough time to provide needed patient care and attention; pressure from having to decide which patient gets what attention.

There is perceived danger inherent in the nature of the medical profession. As a professional hierarchy, it is often made more confusing or confounding by the complexity of accountability lines—requirements to meet new administrative procedures and changing technical demands; having to deal with new legislation and regulations calling for more paper work; changes in supervisors, subordinates or physicians; novel medical or administrative circumstances for which there are no clear guidelines; having to deal with ethical issues involving one's own performance or the performance of a nursing colleague or physician.

The nurse's life away from the job is also filled with ongoing conditions and specific events that induce feelings of danger. The works of Holmes and Rahe and subsequently Cochrane and Robertson have produced a list of life events and changes that often are perceived as a danger to the individual's well-being and produce stress.[2,3] Sample events on the lists include changes in social life, place of residence, marriage, divorce, death of a family member, major accident, serious illness, etc. Examples of ongoing conditions that frequently induce stress are long drives to work each day, subway commuting, a seemingly endless upward spiral of living costs, etc.

Figure 1 illustrates some of the sources of stress for the nurse. The four quadrant matrix used is based on a summary framework of sources of stress developed by Adams.[4]

Developing an Early Warning System

In the face of perceived danger the human system automatically seeks to take care of itself by going into "red alert."

Certain physiological actions are called into being to enable the system to deal with the danger. This creation of a particularly alert state often develops below a level of awareness. When the need for acute energy has passed, a person becomes aware of the previous state of "red alert" or stress. It is during the build-up to the stressed state that it becomes critical for a person to notice what is going on within the self.

Developing a capacity to observe one's self at all times is a necessary function of the body's early warning system. It is this process that enables us to assess whether or not such a state is appropriate to the real situation. For example—a call comes from the emergency ward with the information that an accident victim is arriving and needs transfusions and preparation for immediate surgery. The nurses' systems go into "red alert" and they begin to function with a heightened sense of purpose and clarity. Fast movements seem easy; all the right things get done at the right time; tested procedures and medical practices are set in motion. A veneer of outward calm settles over systems strung tight with acute perception. It takes only the briefest moment of self-observation to know that

FIGURE 1. SOURCES OF STRESS

	On the job	Away from work
Recent events	New physician, new policies, more work, reorganization, etc.	Death in the family, marriage, accident, new residence, etc.
Ongoing conditions	Medical hierarchy, patient care, too few resources, etc.	Unusual hours at home, spiraling costs, problems with children, etc.

258 this condition of stress is entirely appropriate to the real circumstance. And so a body system continues to perform inwardly and outwardly under stress to meet the real emergency.

However, there are times when the same internal response may not be so appropriate. Suppose a supervising nurse attempts to enforce a hospital policy with one of the staff nurses and the staff nurse refuses to cooperate. The nurse has threatened the supervisor's authority in public. Rather than confront the nurse on the spot, the supervisor allows the situation to drift and everyone returns to work. It could be that it was a bad day anyway and it just did not seem like a good idea to reprimand the nurse at the time, but it is very likely that what the supervisor takes back to work will be a lot of stress. The supervisor's system reacts to the perceived danger of authority that is questioned or challenged—muscles tense, the mouth goes dry, the mind races with fantasized arguments and reasonable excuses and plots how to respond or act at the next encounter with the staff nurse.

Stress that is not noticed or dealt with at the time of its initial occurrence can create a particularly fertile place for similar stress-producing situations to grow—*often magnified by the original unresolved stress.*

The most critical step in reducing inappropriate stress is developing an "observer." Create a piece of the self that is always watching *in here* while the rest is watching or doing something *out there.* That observer is the early warning system that provides one with choice. With an observer a person can choose whether to stay with a stress response to danger or not. Without the observer, there is no reality testing device and one can become captive of uncontrolled stress response.

Testing for Reality

There are two realities that require testing to keep stress within appropriate bounds—subjective reality and objective reality. *Subjective* reality is that which exists within one's own experience. *Objective* reality is that which exists outside the self in the environment. Both realities are germane to the effort to maintain a balanced equilibrium because the two can—and often do—impact on each other. Whether they impact, and how, is often more a matter of choice than is thought.

One's degree of choice is a function of how well self-response can be perceived and separated from environmental response. Two questions seem appropriate at all times: "Does what I am perceiving in the environment have anything to do with me?" and, "Is my response to what I am perceiving the experience that I want (i.e., will it get me what I want)?"

For example, when there is an emergency accident case and a need for immediate preparation for surgery, etc., that situation could have something to do with the individual as a nurse, and the response (activation of the stress mechanisms) could be just the response needed and wanted to provide the special energy and acuity necessary to deal with the emergency.

However, when an unfortunate confrontation with a staff nurse might spoil the whole day, the supervisor may decide that the experience was clearly objective and relevant only to the *role* of supervisor. It could be decided that there was no immediate danger to one as a person or to anyone else—only an authority problem to be dealt with at an appropriate time.

The first level of issue is to be sure that what one sees is really what is there. Maybe that staff nurse had to challenge authority for private reasons, but nothing personal was intended. The second level is to notice what is going on within one's self in response to what was seen. Once the nurse takes notice of the self with the "observer," there is an opportunity to choose the reality of a personal experience. The nurse may choose not to have a stress response when that will not serve one or further one's purposes as a nurse.

Memories and feelings that sometimes distort objective realities and evoke internal responses of stress are experiences that often go deep into the past. Many of those memories and feelings have long since been lost to awareness through habitual use of accustomed presence. They are no longer perceived as separate from that which is objectively in the environment *right now*. They are like sun glasses through which the world is viewed that give color and shading to what is seen. It is difficult even to notice the sun glasses until, one day, they are taken off (made separate) and the world looks different.

As nurses are able to separate the self in their own minds, from what is seen in the environment and from the response to what is seen, they can use rational processes to make judgments about actions that may be taken to assure that their own best interests, as well as the best interests of others, are served. Much of the stress that is experienced is perpetuated by an unwillingness to look after one's own best interests. Instead, people often respond from habit or from values that were learned long ago that are no longer relevant to their present circumstances.

A value prevalent among nurses is unselfish service to others. If living out this value means nurses ignore their own wants and needs they virtually guarantee themselves an inappropriately high level of stress as an ongoing condition in life. Being willing to get what is wanted or needed, and to regard getting those things as important, is what Selye calls "altruistic egoism" or a healthy concern for one's self.[5(p69)] A healthy person in the self has much more to offer to the world.

Much of what we see and experience as "reality" is a function of our attitudes. According to Selye, a person can "convert a negative stress into a positive one [or] 'eustress'" by reforming attitudes toward either specific events or ongoing conditions.[5] Eustress, a word Selye coined, uses the Greek prefix "eu" meaning good or positive as in "euphoric." By shifting attitudes from negative to positive, especially toward ourselves, it is suggested that the experience of distress can be converted to an experience of eustress. In this way we can reduce the ongoing level of inappropriate stress carried through life.

DEALING WITH FEELINGS

Dealing with feelings involves a four-step process:

1. Notice the feeling or sensation; acknowledge that something is going on at a level of emotional experience right now.

260

2. Give the feeling a label such as anger, hurt, sadness, fear, resentment, etc., or humor, delight, enthusiasm, joy.
3. Make a decision as to whether or not the feeling or cluster of feelings is appropriate to the present situation being perceived in the environment.
4. Give expression to the feelings in a way that is safe, will get what is wanted or needed and will do no harm to another.

Noticing the Feelings

Noticing feelings requires developing an awareness of physical sensations and emotional responses in addition to an awareness of thoughts and actions. Schooling and training equip people for sensitivity to thoughts and actions but very little deliberate attention is generally given to developing sensitivity to feelings and physical sensations. In fact some children are plainly encouraged to deny feelings and bodily sensations.

It is more likely that feelings and physical sensations will be noticed if they are conceived as something a person *has* rather than as something a person *is*. It is often easier to evaluate and discard an idea than to do the same for a feeling.

A person's body is the best information source about feelings being experienced. Anger, for example, is identifiable not only from the sensing of emotion but also from noticing that the muscles across the shoulders and back of the neck are tight. Anxiety is often reflected through clumsiness of the hands and feet; embarrassment shows as a flushed face; fear can be reflected by stomach muscles that are in a knot; etc. Learning to read physical body sensations can help identify emotional experience.

Labeling the Feelings

The next step in dealing with feelings is giving an emotional experience a conceptual frame of reference. As people think about feelings they apply what they know to the experience of the feeling and then manage the feeling as they would an idea. The process of labeling the feeling begins the thinking process. People experiencing anger, for example, recognize the feeling from prior experience and label it accordingly. As they think about the anger they have, they consider the fact that every time they have acted from anger in the past it has brought them trouble, so they do not allow their energy to be used to act on the anger. They are now in a better position to think about what they will do and make deliberate decisions.

Deciding the Appropriateness of Feelings

Knowing how appropriate a feeling is to the present situation in the environment puts people back in control of their rational processes. Feelings carried from previous situations can be left out of present considerations. This does not mean those previous feelings have been dealt with; they have simply been deliberately left out of considering the present circumstances.

Expressing Feelings

There are many safe ways in which feelings can be expressed. Frustration, anger and other feelings that get in the way of clear decision making can be dealt with in any of a variety of ways from intensive therapy sessions to daily jogging. Whatever method of safe expression a person uses, it is important for there to be regular opportunity for expressing feelings. Cleaning up feelings through expression is something like housework—no matter how much one does it, there is always more to do.

METHODS OF REDUCING STRESS

In this country the most common method of seeking immediate stress reduction is the use of medicines, alcohol and other drugs. While these methods provide some relief from the acute awareness of symptoms of stress, they only serve as a temporary support until the basic problems can be dealt with. There are obvious dangers inherent in the use of substances to secure relief from stress symptoms. The risk of developing a dependency on a drug is genuine and the cost of sustaining the use of drugs or medicines can be quite high. Having stress symptoms masked by a substance can give the illusion of well-being so that basic problems are neglected. Substances can have effects on performance other than just to reduce the awareness of stress symptoms. Nonetheless, in emergency situations of acute dysfunctional stress, some medication may be a measure of resort.

Methods other than the use of substances can be effective in stress reduction. Environmental changes, attitude changes, diet control, physical activities, relaxation techniques, therapeutic involve-

ment and emotional need fulfillment are but a few.

Environmental changes can include anything from changing place of work or residence to investing money in a new rug or painting. For a nurse, bringing about changes inside the work place may be more difficult. Immediate or surrounding work areas, hallways and meeting areas are often dull, boring, institution like and otherwise not a pleasure to be near. Somewhere in the dim dark past somebody who must have been very wise decided that the only colors of paint that could be kept clean enough for a medical facility were white, beige or medium green.

A factor that influences both the effectiveness and efficiency of changes in the work environment is the level of stress such concerns induce in staff members. Making changes that have the effect of short-term inconvenience for long-term stress reduction among staff may be a beneficial trade-off. Changing job placement or duties for brief periods, or changing the methods used to get a certain job done can add variety and relief from some environmental sources of stress.

Health care institutions are filled with environmental circumstances that can contribute to stress among nurses. Some degree of stress can be expected, therefore, whenever one chooses to work in such an institution. Developing coping processes to deal with environmental stressors is especially important and it is appropriate to expect individuals to adapt to these organizational circumstances to a certain degree.

Some health care institutions, however, have such intense and extensive environ-

262 mental stressors that even well-developed individual coping processes are inadequate to deal with them. Under these conditions it is important to remember that organizations and institutions are invented to *enhance* self-esteem and effectively provide products and services. When these basic purposes are abridged due to excessive environmental stressors, it becomes necessary for the organization to monitor and adapt its requirements so these stressors do not exceed the coping processes of its members.

Attitude changes deal with creating a positive set of attitudes toward self, others and things that will bring about required results. Creating new personal and professional goals is an exercise that can help examine what one thinks to be really important.

Rogers contends that developing a posture of "unconditional positive regard" toward self and others provides an opening in a person through which positive and enhancing data can be communicated in both directions—outward to others and inward from others.[6(p34)] This circumstance of unconditional positive regard accepts the premise that each person has an intrinsic value—unconditionally worthy no matter what situation, behavior or feelings are represented.

The ability to forgive, to totally cancel whatever blocks one from holding self or others as anything less than totally worthy human beings, is a reformation of attitude that can release stress. Following closely to this is developing the ability to understand the needs and circumstances of others as they see them.

Self-honesty alleviates the stress that goes with self-punishment for lying or misrepresenting. Acceptance of the truth, even when it includes behaviors, thoughts and feelings that could be viewed with alarm, is easier to live with than a lie that seems to keep growing in complexity.

Diet control provides virtually direct influence over many bodily functions associated with stress. Intake of caffeine and sugar throughout the day tends to exacerbate other stress responses. A diet deficient in any of the major food groups, minerals and vitamins that is sustained over time will contribute to stress symptoms. Eating a balanced diet, taking vitamin supplements, drinking enough water, using natural instead of processed sugar, and avoiding, when possible, unnecessary chemical additives to food, help maintain the body for full functioning.

Physical activities aid in stress reduction. Regular exercise develops new and greater capacities in several areas of function especially when the exercise pushes the system to about double the resting heart rate for brief sustained periods of time. A physical exercise program done with proper guidance does not push the system too far or too fast. An important key to achieving the stress reduction benefits from exercise is that the activity be regular and sustained.

Physical activity—washing the car, cleaning the yard, washing windows, painting walls—can have the effect of expressing stress from the person into the work, if the work is done with attention and purpose. It does not help as a stress reduction method if the labor itself adds to or causes frustration. It helps only if the physical labor is given full attention, and pleasure is taken in the result.

A hobby or avocation that allows for

creativity and fun is another major stress reduction outlet. No matter what the activity, it must be given full attention and provide enjoyment while doing it even if it is only for a few minutes a day. Having safe times and places in which one can physically express feelings that would otherwise go unexpressed is also important.

Relaxation techniques can be mastered relatively quickly and can provide an immediate or planned occasion to quiet down the physical system as well as the mind. There is an easy five-step technique that can be used when things have been particularly hectic and stress is high:

1. Find a comfortable place to sit.
2. Place feet flat on the floor.
3. Close eyes.
4. Breathe steadily and with purpose for about five minutes.
5. Take particular notice of the parts of the body that feel tense and will them to relax.

This technique relaxes the body and leaves the mind free to identify what is really wanted or needed from the present situation and then have the calm energy to get it.

There are a variety of ways of relaxing and slowing down the physical and mental processes that involve more elaborate and disciplined practices. Activities such as transcendental meditation, bioenergetics, autogenics, biofeedback, etc. are all methods that can be used regularly to provide a time during the day to quiet down, relax and experience more energy within one's self for the tasks at hand.

Change of pace or scenery can bring about immediate stress relief. Taking a brief walk outside, carefully washing hands and face, listening to music for a few minutes, massaging the face and forearms briefly, looking out a window at a tree or clouds in the sky, are all examples of brief moments of interruption that can help reduce stress of the moment if they are done with intent and attention.

Therapeutic involvement, for many in the health care professions, is a natural extension of their own clinical work and serves to help work through issues in their personal and professional lives that come from experiences in the past—sometimes as far back as childhood. Nurses may find that many of the values and attitudes they formed as children are of great benefit in the present and may have even been determining factors in the choice of becoming a nurse in the first place. However, there may be other values and attitudes, beliefs and feelings learned as children that still trigger stress responses which are no longer appropriate to the present or serve one's best interests. Engaging in a therapeutic experience can help uncover some of those old and dysfunctional experiences and leave them behind.

Emotional need fulfillment assures that needs for positive attention, recognition and appreciation are being met on a consistent basis. People can give themselves positive strokes by acknowledging their own uniqueness, talents and worth as persons who are good and do good things. Positive strokes should be given to others whenever occasion permits and if there is no convenient occasion, create one. A nurse feeling the need for acknowledgement or appreciation should ask for a stroke and accept it when offered. Be careful about giving too much credence to

264 others' behavior that may evoke feelings of being ignored or having attention distracted. Nurses can feel free to reject negative strokes from themselves and others that are not appropriate or deserved.

In sum, stress is a profoundly personal experience and to do anything about it one must deal with the self and environment. Stress cannot be reduced for long without coming to terms with the self and the environment. The mind cannot reduce stress; it can only direct attention to feelings and the body where stress is experienced. When nurses can give attention to their total selves—ideas, feelings and physical sensations—then they are in control of their place in the world.

Nurses clearly have the intelligence, training and judgment to make sound decisions for action when the decision-making processes are uncontaminated by emotion. One should not act *from* feeling; one should act from judgment and perhaps, *with* feeling. Once the feeling content is separated from the process of rational consideration and included as but one factor among many, the making of a good decision—unfettered by stress—will virtually take care of itself.

Above all a sense of humor, and the perspective that goes with it, is perhaps the greatest stress reducer there is.

REFERENCES

1. Lazarus, R. S. "Proceedings of the National Heart and Lung Institute Working Conference on Health Behavior." DHEW (NIH, 77-868) Washington, D.C., 1977.
2. Holmes, T. H. and Rahe, R. H. "The Social Readjustment Rating Scale." *J Psychosomatic Res* 11:2 (August 1967) p. 213-218.
3. Cochrane, R. and Robertson, A., "The Life Events Inventory." *J Psychosomatic Res* 17:2 (1973) p. 135-139.
4. Adams, J. D. "Improving Stress Management." *Social Change* 8:4 (1978) p. 2.
5. Selye, H., interviewed by Laurence Cherry. "On the Real Benefits of Eustress." *Psychology Today* 11:10 (March 1978) p. 69.
6. Rogers, C. R. *On Becoming A Person* (Boston: Houghton Mifflin Co. 1961) p. 34-35.

Assertiveness: Freeing the Nurse to Practice

Gloria Ferraro Donnelly, R.N., M.S.N.
Mental Health—Psychiatric Nursing
Specialist
Assertiveness Facilitator
Episcopal Hospital
La Salle College
Philadelphia, Pennsylvania

NURSES WANT CHANGE! Listen to the rhetoric! Look at the nursing literature—the nurse as a change agent. Look at the nurse's role—expanded, extended to nurse practitioner, nurse midwife, clinical specialist, independent practitioner. Look at the health care system—changing laws, rapidly changing organization, computerized technology. Nursing is indeed preoccupied with change—how to plan it, how to initiate it, how to predict it and how to control it.

Change is constant in today's complex health care delivery system. It occurs at different rates in different settings and even more puzzling at different rates in the same setting. It is quite common to find nursing departments readily adjusting to the complexities of technological advances in patient care while simultaneously agonizing over whether or not to change the traditional hospital dress codes. Even though today's nurse functions at a higher technical level, the decision-making pro-

266 cess in direct patient care can be dramatically altered by changing the traditional handmaiden image that society, physicians and even nurses hold of nursing. Can nurses free themselves from the dilemma that the technical nature of practice has changed, but the image of "nurse" has not?

Assertiveness training is a self-care, self-responsibility tool increasingly used by practicing nurses to free themselves from the inhibiting effects of working in the health care system. Assertiveness training is a behavior modification technique that began concurrently with the flourishing women's rights movement in the sixties. Since its inception, assertiveness training has become much more than a technique to manipulate small pieces of behavior. Today assertiveness training can be coupled with other holistic approaches to healing, such as nutritional counseling, physical therapy, exercise and meditation.[1] Problems related to being assertive are usually only part of a total presenting complaint picture that varies from person to person. Nonassertive and/or aggressive behavior are often accompanied by stress or tension related symptoms such as headache, pains across shoulders, muscle tension and fatigue. One nurse who completed a five-week assertiveness course no longer needed to rely on the "6 or 7 aspirins" previously taken during the course of an eight-hour shift. Practicing assertive behavior had relieved a somatic manifestation of stress.

ASSERTIVENESS: STATE OR TRAIT?

Assertiveness is not a personality trait that can be precisely labeled and quantified although there are behavioral assessment scales that reveal one's tendency to be assertive. Assertiveness is rather, a relative behavioral characteristic that is situation dependent. Assertive behavior renders a person free "to act in his (her) own best interests, to stand up for himself (herself) without undue anxiety, to express his (her) honest feelings comfortably, or exercise his (her) own rights without denying the rights of others."[2]

Assertiveness is a part of everyone's behavior repertoire. Although one's tendency in certain situations may be toward

---

Assertiveness might be conceptualized as the integration of aggressive and nonassertive tendencies that free the individual to act.

---

nonassertive behavior or aggression, everyone is appropriately assertive in certain situations that require the behavior. Assertiveness might be conceptualized as the integration of aggressive and nonassertive tendencies that free the individual to act. (See Figure 1.) However, operationally defining assertive behavior and assertive training is an endeavor that is still in its early stages.[3]

Assertive-Nonassertive: The Difference

Nonassertive behavior is a passive, hesitant or submissive response toward an individual or group. Nurses behaving nonassertively deny themselves expression for fear of incurring the wrath of someone in the clinical setting hierarchy, or to avoid hurting someone else's feelings. Assertiveness training, as developed by Wolpe, was

FIGURE 1. ASSERTIVENESS AS INTEGRATED BEHAVIOR

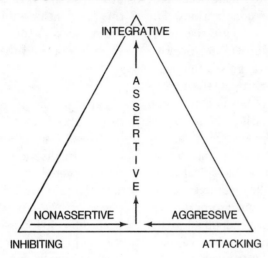

originally used to treat individuals with passive or inhibited life style.[4] Through the use of behavioral rehearsal with the assertiveness facilitator, the client learns to integrate assertive responses into behavior patterns by modeling the assertive responses of the facilitator.

Nurses who chose to participate in assertiveness training often describe situations that appear, on the surface, to be quite benign. One nurse described a situation in which the unit coordinator had assigned the nurse's primary patient to another staff member. "In the past, I would have gritted my teeth and accepted the situation. This time I approached the unit coordinator and said, 'I prefer to keep Mr. Smith as my patient.' The coordinator changed the assignment immediately. There were no repercussions."

Persons who behave nonassertively in any arena of life often allow others to choose for them, and often they do not achieve their goals. Wolpe's theory links nonassertive behavior to anxiety. He postulates that assertiveness training is indicated for persons who in interpersonal situations experience "unadaptive anxiety responses that prevent them from saying or doing what is reasonable and right ... suppression of feeling may lead to a continuing inner turmoil which may produce somatic symptoms and even pathologic changes in predisposed organs ..."[5] For many nurses the anxiety that blocks responses in clinical situations is often related to low self-esteem as a nurse. As one participant in an assertiveness course said, "I could never speak out! I'm only a nurse!"

Assertive-Aggressive: The Differences

Assertiveness training is also utilized to assist persons in recognizing and revising aggressive behavior in interpersonal situations. Aggression is attacking behavior with the goal of demeaning, blaming, accusing or humiliating the other person. The terms assertive and aggressive are

268 often confused since for males the term aggressive has positive connotations. For example the description "aggressive salesman" may conjure up more positive images than the term "aggressive nurse."

A nurse who resorts to aggressive behavior may have difficulty deciding to revise the behavior. Aggressive behavior is common in traditional, hierarchial, bureaucratic settings. Occasionally, as nurses move up the ladder of a traditional practice-setting hierarchy, they feel freer to use aggressive behavior. Nurse-to-nurse aggression may accomplish individual goals; however, it may become divisive to a work group of a unit or a department.

Assertiveness training is also used to help persons (1) recognize their expressions of aggressive behavior and (2) utilize the assertive skills to revise the behavior. One simple assessment technique is to increase awareness concerning the use of "I" versus "you" messages. Persons behaving aggressively have a tendency to begin many of their responses to others with the word "you." Persons behaving assertively are instructed to formulate "I" messages. "I" messages facilitate a freer expression of feeling, opinion or belief from the perspective of self. "I" messages also safeguard the person from slipping into aggressive behavior.

For example, an IV therapy team nurse walked into a patient's room and the family began to scream at the nurse because their mother had been left in the chair. The nurse might have responded aggressively by saying to the family, "You're overreacting! The staff will put your mother back in bed." Instead, the nurse replied assertively, "I understand how upsetting this can be. I don't work on this unit, but I do think you should talk to the nurse who took care of your mother. I'll help you find that nurse!"

"I" Messages

Participants in assertiveness training often express hesitation about freely using "I" messages. Are not "I" messages too egocentric? Is there a danger that they will be interpreted as bragging or boasting? In assertiveness training, focus on self-perspective is crucial. This, however, has been difficult for women operating within the cultural stereotypes of traditional feminine behavior. Even many professional mental health workers consider the emotionally healthy woman to be passive and emotional, easily influenced, less objective, less competitive, less independent and less adventurous than the well-adjusted man.[6] Therefore "I" messages may at first seem alien to a nurse who has been socialized into a traditional female role.

With practice, "I" messages become easier and finally automatic. Integrating the "I" message into one's response pattern is an important element of becoming assertive. One difficulty that assertiveness training participants initially have is prefacing aggressive statements with phrases such as "I think" or "I feel." For example. "I think you have a problem with your anger!" is an aggressive message even though it technically begins with "I." "I am becoming very angry" might be a more appropriate response. Instead of evaluating the behavior of another, the response focuses entirely on the speaker. Concentrating on how one phrases responses is an important part of the self-assessment process.

Self-Assessment

The popular assertiveness literature contains many questionnaires and scales used to raise one's level of self-awareness concerning assertive, nonassertive and aggressive behavior.[7-11] Some assertive facilitators suggest that participants keep logs or diaries for a week or two. Table 1 is an example of such a log. Self-awareness includes a focus not only on the verbal component of the message but also on the nonverbal component. During an interpersonal encounter, the person is instructed to be aware of posture, voice tone and quality, eye contact, hand gestures, facial expressions and muscle tone. Videotaping is often used in assertiveness sessions so

that participants can retrospectively assess their response behavior. In group assertiveness training, group members use each other for feedback. Assessment is an ongoing process throughout the period of training and beyond.

PROCESS OF ASSERTIVENESS TRAINING

Participants in an assertiveness training course learn that simple imitation of another's assertive responses does not always work. Learning to be assertive can be compared to learning a complex motor skill, such as riding a bicycle or practicing aseptic technique. An experienced operating room nurse practices aseptic technique with ease, but a novice may violate several rules and make errors before the behavior

TABLE 1

Sample Assertiveness Log

Setting, situation and date	Behavior, body cues, effect, physical reactions, feelings	Behavioral response (What I did or said and in what manner)	What I would like to have done or said	What hindered me from doing what I wanted to do

Learning to be assertive can be compared to learning a complex motor skill, such as riding a bicycle or practicing aseptic technique.

becomes automatic. Similarly, with experience participants automatically respond assertively.

During assertiveness training, individual rights are emphasized and explained. Behavioral rehearsal, relaxation training, role playing and modeling the trainer's behavior may occur. Group discussion takes place and participants share experiences using assertive behavior. Assertiveness training is not a highly systematized clinical procedure. It is a "combination of many therapeutic procedures, rather than a relatively well-defined therapy logically derived from psychological theory."[12] Participants are also instructed to use verbal response techniques that facilitate assertive behavior. (See Table 2.)

Assertiveness training programs are presented in various formats from one-day workshops to 10 or 12 weekly sessions. It is best to investigate the philosophy and approach of the facilitator before investing in assertiveness training. Finding an assertiveness facilitator compatible with one's value system may be an important factor in influencing positive outcomes.

OUTCOMES TO ASSERTIVE BEHAVIOR

Assertiveness training workshops help not only the individual nurse but also the health care institution. Self-reports on success with assertive behavior reveal that nurses feel freer to speak out, to question and to offer suggestions and opinions in clinical situations. This pattern directly affects the quality of patient care. Nurses may feel freer for instance to question clinical routines that have not respected the individual needs of clients, as in the following situation.

In a coronary step-down unit the established routine was for all patients to be readied for morning care and for breakfast at 7:30 AM. A nurse, who was taking an assertiveness course, was caring for a patient who was sleeping soundly at 7 AM. The nurse decided not to awaken the patient who had been having difficulty sleeping. While the nurse was bathing another patient, the head nurse came into the room and asked, "Can I get your sleeping patient ready for breakfast? Don't you think you should wake him?" The nurse replied, "Thanks, but no. I want him to sleep as long as he needs to. I'll call dietary and order a special tray. I think it is most important for this patient to get some rest." The head nurse shrugged and left the room.

The assertive nurse in this situation attributed success to practicing the principles of assertiveness training. The nurse chose not to be intimidated by the routine or by the authority figure attempting to enforce the routine. Instead, the nurse decided what was best in this situation, and acted calmly using "I" messages to convey a position. There were no after-effects reported in this situation, except that the patient got his needed rest, and the nurse was free to practice.

After assertiveness training some nurses

TABLE 2

Assertive Communication Techniques

---

1. Broken Record

A systematic assertive communication skill in which you are persistent and keep saying what you want over and over again without getting angry, irritated or loud.

By practicing to speak like a broken record you learn to be persistent and to stick to the point of discussion and to continue to say what you want. This technique helps you to ignore all side issues brought up by the other party.

2. Workable compromise

A technique to use with an equally assertive person to work out a compromise. A workable compromise is one in which your self-respect is not in question.

3. Free Information

A listening skill in which you evaluate and then use the free information that people offer about themselves. It accomplishes two things; it facilitates conversation and it prompts others to respond easily and freely.

4. Self-disclosure

Assertively disclosing information about yourself—how you think, feel and react to the other person's free information—permits social communication to flow both ways. This technique should be used with free information, because to elicit more free information you must be willing to self-disclose.

5. Fogging

A technique to assertively cope with manipulative criticism. You neither deny any of the criticism, nor get defensive nor attack with criticism of your own. Instead you send up a fogbank. It is persistent. It cannot be clearly seen through. And it offers no resistance to penetration. By fogging you offer no resistance or hard psychological striking surfaces to critical statements thrown at you.

6. Negative assertion

A technique to cope with criticism or with your own errors and faults by openly acknowledging them. This technique is to be used only in social conflicts, not in physical or legal ones.

7. Negative inquiry

An assertive, nondefensive response that is noncritical of the other person and prompts that person to examine his/her own structure of right and wrong. For example, "I don't understand. What makes you think nurses are stupid?"

Sources:
1. Alberti, R. E. and Emmons, M. *Stand Up, Speak Out, Talk Back.* (New York: Pocket Books 1975).
2. Bloom, L. Z., Coburn, K. and Pearlman, J. *The New Assertive Woman.* (New York: Dell Publishing Co., Inc. 1975).
3. Smith, M. *When I Say No I Feel Guilty!* (New York: Bantam Books 1975).
4. Fensterheim, H. and Baer, J. *Don't Say Yes When You Want to Say No!* (New York: Dell Publishing Co., Inc. 1975).

---

report fewer stress-related somatic complaints, such as headaches, generalized fatigue, neck stiffness and muscle tension. These results may be attributed to the self-care, self-responsibility orientation that is stressed during the training sessions or to the freeing of responses that were previously blocked. An increased level of self-awareness may result in "taking better care" of self as a psychophysiological being. With a holistic-eclectic framework, assertiveness training can be coupled with

272

After assertiveness training some nurses report fewer stress-related somatic complaints, such as headaches, generalized fatigue, neck stiffness and muscle tension.

other modalities to help clients maximize their health potential.[13]

After nurses have mastered techniques for assertive behavior, they have reported teaching the principles to their clients. An occupational health nurse offers assertiveness sessions to clients working in a large publishing firm. A school nurse is conducting sessions with adolescent girls. Nurses have also reported sharing the assertiveness literature with their colleagues and students. Several nurses have formed assertiveness self-help groups for staff in their own clinical settings.

Increasing the number of assertive nurses in the health care system may have other far reaching effects. The power of the nurses in policy making may increase considerably. Individuals who behave assertively, freely offer their input instead of waiting to be asked. Unfortunately, social tradition in nursing has been so strong that many female nurses "who find

themselves in a position of direct power for the first time go to some extremely awkward means to keep this power hidden, to keep themselves from being seen in a position so contrary to the feminine role."[14] Assertiveness training made available on a wide scale may revitalize and reshape the health care system since nurses numerically dominate the system.

ASSERTIVENESS AS INTEGRATED BEHAVIOR

Within a holistic framework, assertiveness might be considered an integrated form of behavior. (See Figure 2.) Assertive behavior transcends the traditional male and female role models that are so pervasive in the health care system today. Assertiveness with its focus on self provokes the realization that a person is free to be fully human, without being limited to outmoded sexual stereotypes. Such persons take charge of their actions and evaluate their environments. They operate from a self-perspective rather than on the basis of external directives. They convey a confidence in their actions that does not invite opposition. If opposition

FIGURE 2. A HOLISTIC VIEW OF BEHAVIOR

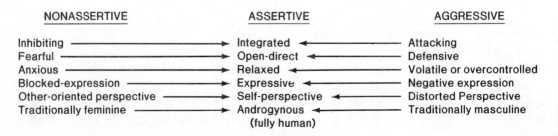

NONASSERTIVE	ASSERTIVE	AGGRESSIVE
Inhibiting ⟶	Integrated ⟵	Attacking
Fearful ⟶	Open-direct ⟵	Defensive
Anxious ⟶	Relaxed ⟵	Volatile or overcontrolled
Blocked-expression ⟶	Expressive ⟵	Negative expression
Other-oriented perspective ⟶	Self-perspective ⟵	Distorted Perspective
Traditionally feminine ⟶	Androgynous ⟵	Traditionally masculine
	(fully human)	

surfaces, an assertive person is self-confident enough to reevaluate the situation.

Assertiveness training is not a controlling technique; it is a freeing process that encourages the individual to take care of self. And caring for self frees the nurse to care for others.

REFERENCES

1. Emmons, M. "Assertion Training within a Holistic-Eclectic Framework" in Alberti, R.E., ed. *Assertiveness: Innovations, Applications, Issues* (San Luis Obispo, Calif.: Impact Publishers 1977) p. 337–347.

2. Alberti, R. E. "Assertive Behavior Training, Definitions, Overview, Contributions" in *Assertiveness: Innovations, Applications, Issues* p. 22.

3. Frazier, J. R. and Carver, E. J. "Some Comments on the Problem of Defining Assertive Training." *Comprehensive Psychiatry* 16:4 (July/August 1975) p. 369–373.

4. Wolpe, J. *The Practice of Behavior Therapy* (New York: Pergamon Press 1969).

5. Ibid. p. 61.

6. Broverman, I. K. et al. "Sex Role Stereotypes and Clinical Judgements of Mental Health Workers." *Journal of Consulting and Clinical Psychology* 34:1 (1970) p. 1–7.

7. Alberti, R. E. and Emmons, M. L. *Your Perfect Right* (San Luis Obispo, Calif.: Impact Publishers 1970).

8. Bloom, L. Z., Coburn, K. and Pearlman, J. *The New Assertive Woman* (New York: Dell Publishing Co. 1975).

9. Butler, P. *Self-Assertion for Women* (San Francisco: Harper & Row, Publishers 1976).

10. Smith, M. J. *When I Say No, I Feel Guilty!* (New York: Bantam Books 1975).

11. Fensterheim, H. and Baer, J. *Don't Say Yes When You Want to Say No!* (New York: Dell Publishing Co. 1975).

12. Frazier and Carver. "Some Comments on the Problem of Defining Assertive Training." p. 69–70.

13. Emmons. "Assertion Training within a Holistic-Eclectic Framework." p. 339.

14. Butler. *Self-Assertion for Women* p. 289.

Effecting Time Management

Charold L. Baer R.N., Ph.D.
Professor and Chairperson
Department of Medical-Surgical Nursing
University of Oregon Health Sciences Center
  School of Nursing
Portland, Oregon

Charge nurse Paul Smith approaches staff nurse Sara Jones and asks, "Sara, are you ready to give the change of shift report?" Flustered, Sara replies, "Heavens no! It can't be that time already!" Paul responds, "It certainly is! Doesn't time fly when you're having fun? Oh, by the way, what kind of response did Mrs. Shaeffer have to the tube feedings you started this afternoon, and does Mr. Williams know his dietary restrictions well enough to be discharged today?"

Now more harried than ever, Sara says, "Mrs. Shaeffer hasn't had any tube feedings yet, Mr. Williams hasn't had any diet teaching evaluation, Mr. Simpson hasn't had his dressing changed and Mr. Ransom and Mr. Johnson have not been ambulated. In addition...."

Paul quickly interrups, "Good grief, what have you been doing all afternoon? Why didn't you say you were having problems getting things done?"

Sara replies, "Well, I thought I could get everything done, so I started with some easy thing first, like washing Mr. Ransom's hair. Then Dr. Everett asked me to help him with

276

his research study by drawing a couple of tubes of blood from four of my patients. It sounded easy enough, but those patients have really bad veins and it took forever to get the blood samples. I was just getting ready to start working with my patients again when you came, but I've run out of time. There never is enough time to do everything I need to do."

INCIDENTS LIKE THIS occur repeatedly every day in almost every hospital in the country. Nurses seem to continually encounter stressful situations because they never have enough time to complete their patient assignments. The lack of proper time management results in a decreased level of satisfaction for the nurse, which in turn adds to the internal stress level.

Figure 1 depicts a schematic representation of this stress-producing formula. A brief analysis of the formula indicates that if nurses could deal with their time problems, they could then increase their performance levels, therefore increasing their satisfaction and decreasing their stress.

The problem is to find how nurses can better manage their time in order to decrease their stress. The following aspects are important: (a) the concept of time; (b) general perspectives on time; (c) myths of time management that affect the practicing nurse; and (d) how and why time is wasted.

THE CONCEPT OF TIME

Time is one of the most important, most discussed and most often misused resources available to human beings. As Lakein suggests, time is life.[1] We cannot have one without the other. Our lives seem to revolve around time. For example, we plan our lives according to specific times for getting up in the morning, arriving at work, carrying out procedures, administering medications, going to lunch, leaving work, participating in evening activities and going to bed. We also use time as a common excuse, for example: I can't stay, I haven't time; I can't help, I haven't time; I can't go, I haven't time; I can't write, I haven't time. In addition, we frequently misuse time because we tend to waste it.

Time is one of the most important, most discussed and most often misused resources available to human beings.

FIGURE 1. SCHEMATIC REPRESENTATION OF THE STRESS-PRODUCING FORMULA

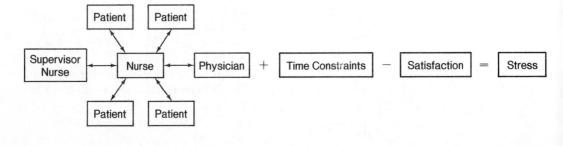

Time is also a unique and inconsistent resource. It is unique in that it cannot be accumulated or saved. Mackenzie clearly emphasizes this point when he refers to time as being something that we are forced to spend, whether we choose to or not, at a fixed rate of 60 seconds every minute. He adds that it is an irretrievable commodity that cannot be turned on and off like a machine or replaced like a man.[2] Time appears to be inconsistent because no one seems to have enough of it, yet everyone has all there is that is available.[3] Time is one resource that is distributed equally to all individuals regardless of need, wealth or academic achievement.

These facts provide some insight into why we often do not have enough time. Since all the time that exists is equally available to each of us, we are incorrect in referring to deficient amounts of time. So, if the problem is not the amount of time, then what is it?

The problem is us. It is not how much time we have, but rather how we use that time that helps us decrease our stress levels. That is why understanding time and its mismanagement will help us learn how to better manage ourselves in relation to time.

PERSPECTIVES ON TIME

Each individual has a specific perspective on time. That perspective has been influenced by our personality, education, and culture, as well as socioeconomic factors. The specific way in which we view time will influence the degree of stress that we encounter when we mismanage our lives in relation to time. Therefore it is logical that we should try to understand how we view time.

How do you see time? Do you see it as a fleeting, active, tense, acute concept, or as quiet, static, soothing and blunt? When you must remember a date in history, do you underestimate or overestimate the time that has elapsed since the event occurred? If you were to check the time indicated by your watch right now, would it be faster, slower or the same as the exact time? If your answers to the above questions were: (1) fleeting, active, tense and acute; (2) an underestimation; and (3) faster, you have a perspective on time that belongs to a high achiever.[4]

In that respect, you are similar to most nurses in their concept of time, since most nurses tend to be high achievers. Because they are high achievers, nurses are more likely to encounter stress if they mismanage their time. The reason for this becomes clear if we analyze some of the common characteristics of high achievers.

Webber has identified the high achiever as someone who gains satisfaction through the process of achieving a goal and not just in the goal itself. He also adds that the high achiever needs the intrinsic satisfaction that results from: (1) performing a task well and meeting high standards; (2) trying to overcome difficult but not impossible obstacles; and (3) trying different, novel and creative ways to solve problems.[5] Thus, as high achievers, nurses need to perform challenging tasks at a high level in order to gain internal satisfaction. When they cannot do this due to mismanagement of their time, they feel stress. How

278 should nurses manage their time more effectively? To answer that question, we first need to examine the common myths that are associated with the management of time that might affect the clinically practicing nurse.

COMMON MYTHS OF TIME MANAGEMENT

Some of the common myths of time management that might affect nurses are those related to activity, decision level, delayed decisions, delegation, omnipotence, overworking, efficiency, hard work, open door, problem identification, time saving, time shortage, time flies and time is against us.[6]

The *activity* myth says that those who are the most active get the most done. This is a myth because activity cannot be confused with results. For example, nurses can become involved in a flurry of activity in running from room to room trying to organize their working environment, checking linen, thermometers, etc, without ever getting anything done.

The *decision level* myth says that the higher the level at which a decision is made, the better the decision. This is a myth because decisions should be made at the lowest possible level because those individuals have the most pertinent facts. Nurses often allow their supervisors or charge nurses to make out their daily patient assignments without providing input. The results are that many times the nurse is assigned a patient care load that is in conflict with his or her performance capabilities.

The *delayed decision* myth says that by delaying the making of a decision, the quality of the decision will be improved. This is a myth because the longer it takes to make a decision, the more crucial and difficult the decision becomes. For example, the nurse who assesses a patient's level of consciousness and notices a slight deviation from normal, but cannot decide whether to notify the physician because the deviation is slight, is merely setting the stage for a stressful event.

The assumption that *delegation* of activities to others will save time, worry and responsibility is another myth. In actuality, it takes more time to delegate a task than it does to do it, and the delegator still retains the responsibility. Thus nurses who try to save time by delegating a difficult dressing change to someone else without adequate

---

Nurses who try to save time by delegating a difficult dressing change to someone else without adequate explanation may only be making more work for themselves because they are still responsible for the patient's dressing.

---

explanation may only be making more work for themselves because they are still responsible for the patient's dressing when it becomes saturated due to improper placement.

Another common myth is that of *omnipotence*, or the "if I do it myself it will be done faster and better than if anyone else does it" complex. This is a myth because you will have to continue to perform all those tasks because you are not teaching anyone else to do them. An example is the nurse who has attended special classes to learn a specific technique or procedure, such as peritoneal dialysis. The nurse then hoards the information rather than sharing with others, and as a result must be called in on all shifts when the need for that specific technique arises.

Overworking is a common myth that thrives on the feeling that an individual is indispensable. Obviously this is a myth because no one is indispensable. This myth is best demonstrated by the nurses who constantly work double shifts, postpone vacations and assume double patient-care assignments because they are certain that the patients and hospital could not survive without them.

The myth of *efficiency* assumes that the most efficient worker is also the most effective worker. This is a myth because one can be very efficient while doing the wrong task. Efficiency is doing things right, while effectiveness is doing the right things right.[7] In caring for an individual with one leg in a cast, a nurse may be very efficient in providing medications to decrease pain, but might not be very effective if the pain were due to edema resulting from a too tight cast.

Hard work is another myth that implies that the harder individuals work the more they get done. This is a myth because hard work does not ensure that things will get done, instead being well organized in working toward the goal will. For example, a nurse can work very hard with a patient getting him mentally ready to ambulate, but unless a plan exists for when he should walk and how far, the goal may never be attained.

The *open door* approach to helping other team members is another myth because nurses can become so involved in helping other team members with their tasks and patient assignments that the nurses' own patients suffer. Sara, the staff nurse in the beginning, is a perfect example of this myth. Sara was so busy helping Dr. Everett that she did not have time to meet the needs of her patients.

The myth that *identifying the problem* is the easiest part of the problem-solving process is very common in time management. Problem identification is a myth because identifying the right problem is a difficult task. As a result, individuals often waste energy trying to solve the wrong problem. A prime example is the nurse who works very creatively at trying to increase a patient's appetite and does not see that the real reason he is not eating well is because his dentures do not fit properly.

Time saving is probably the biggest myth of all. Time cannot be saved, it can only be better utilized. A nurse who takes short cuts in delivering care may not be saving time but instead be creating problems for the future. One example is the nurse who teaches a patient the mechanics of how to care for his open wound, but not the underlying principles. After discharge the patient tries to adapt the procedure at home and grossly contaminates the wound. The patient is then readmitted with a more serious problem.

Another common myth is that of *time shortage*. We complain of not having enough time, but that is a myth because we all have the same amount of time. The key to this myth is in the mismanagement

280 of the time. An appropriate example is Sara: if she had not decided to wash Mr. Ransom's hair and to assist Dr. Everett, she would have had sufficient time to complete her assignments.

The assertion that *time flies* is also a myth. The illusion that time is flying is usually attributable to inadequate planning. The nurses who try to do everything for every patient in an eight-hour period of time are only setting up stressful situations because they cannot get everything done.

The last common myth related to time management is that *time is against us*. This is a myth because time is inanimate and cannot fight us. Instead we fight ourselves by mismanaging our time. Sara's example of mismanagement is a significant demonstration of how nurses can and do mismanage time.

HOW AND WHY NURSES WASTE TIME

Mackenzie identified 35 time wasters related to the functions of management.[8] Some of those time wasters are used by nurses. They include:

1. not having objectives, priorities or daily plans;
2. shifting priorities without a sound rationale;
3. leaving tasks unfinished;
4. not setting time limits;
5. daydreaming;
6. attempting too much at once;
7. experiencing personal disorganization;
8. duplicating efforts;
9. confusing lines of responsibility, communication and authority;
10. understaffing;
11. over involvement in routine details;
12. delegating ineffectively;
13. making numerous mistakes;
14. being unable to say no; and
15. not listening.

It does not take much imagination to see how these time wasters add to the nurse's stress level. How nurses can better manage their time to decrease this stress is the next question.

MANAGING TIME

Segmentation

The first part of successfully managing time is to separate those things that you have control over from those that you do not. Webber refers to this process as *segmentation*.[9] For example, nurses may not be able to control the time they need to

---

The first part of successfully managing time is segmentation , separating those things that you have control over from those that you do not.

---

report for work, but they can control what they do while they are there. Nurses may not be able to control the therapies that a patient needs, but they can control the order and time at which the therapies are done. Nurses may not be able to control the number of patients that they are assigned to care for, but they can control how they will proceed in providing that care.

Concentration

The second part of Webber's process for managing time is *concentration*, or systematically controlling those things that can be controlled.[10] This part of the process involves planning, organizing and implementing activities to control the use of one's time.

PLANNING

Planning is the most important step in managing one's time. It includes: (1) setting priorities, (2) scheduling, and (3) establishing the "to do " list.

Many different approaches can be used in setting priorities. Among the various approaches are the ABC Approach, the Pareto Principle and continuums. The ABC Approach, as devised and explained by Lakein, consists of performing the following activities: (a) listing everything that needs to be done; (b) assigning an A to high-value items; (c) assigning a B to medium-value items; (d) assigning a C to low-value items; and (e) doing all A items first, all B items second and all C items third.[11]

The Pareto Principle, often called the 80-20 rule, states that 80 percent of the time expended produces 20 percent of the desired results and 20 percent of the time expended produces 80 percent of the desired results.[12] The idea in employing this principle is to set priorities to select the most productive activities by deciding what not to do and learning to say no.

Still another method of setting priorities is to place things that need to be done on two separate continuums; one continuum is related to importance and the other to urgency.[13]

No matter which method of priority setting is used, it is imperative that the nurse know which things are the most

important to be accomplished during the work day.

Once the nurse has identified the priorities for the day, it is then important to devise a *time schedule* for dealing with the priorities. A written plan appears to be best for high achievers perhaps because high achievers cannot bear to deviate from what challenges them in black and white. A schedule is important to nurses because it focuses their attention on using blocks of time to accomplish the priorities and tasks at hand. It is important also that the schedule be flexible so that it can be altered as the patient's needs change.

Many times making a list of what needs to be done is the first step in accomplishing the tasks. Nurses should formulate daily "to do" lists in order to make the best use of their time. Being able to cross an item or two off a list each day helps minimize stress.

ORGANIZING

Organizing oneself and the environment is an important part of managing or controlling time. It includes practicing (1) no detourism and (2) mental wastebasketry.

Practicing *no detourism* essentially means organizing the working environment so that there are no distractions from the priorities. Part of no detourism is removing clutter from the environment. If nurses have an organized environment within which to work, they are more likely to adhere to the task at hand and to experience less stress.

Practicing *mental wastebasketry* means organizing one's mind in order to deal with the established priorities. This involves employing selective perception so

282 that one attends only to those things at hand and allows useless information to be discarded. For nurses this means concentrating only on those things that have high priority for their patients and tuning out the other irrelevant data.

IMPLEMENTING

Implementing refers to carrying out those activities that help individuals control their time. Such activities include: (1) attacking the priorities; (2) avoiding procrastination and escape: (3) rewarding yourself; and (4) continuing to succeed.

In controlling one's time, the first activities to be implemented should *attack the priorities*. When the priorities are completed, move on to other tasks. Nurses need to begin early to deal with the priorities they have identified for the patient. This initial activity will do much to decrease their stress levels.

It is important that individuals be able to identify when they are *procrastinating* or trying to *escape* from working on a priority. Once they have admitted to themselves that they are procrastinating, they can set

---

Nurses can motivate themselves to do the tasks they are procrastinating about by thinking about what can be accomplished next once they finish the present task.

---

time limits on the priorities, stress the benefits of getting the task done, eliminate some of the things that promote procrastination and learn how to say no. Nurses tend to procrastinate in doing routine, involved procedures. They prefer more challenging, short-term procedures. Nurses can motivate themselves to do the tasks they are procrastinating about by thinking about what can be accomplished next once they finish the present task.

It is important that individuals *reward themselves* when they adhere to their plans and effectively control their time. For nurses, such rewards might include taking a coffee break when one does not usually do so, or attending an inservice conference when normally there is not sufficient time.

Once individuals master the art of managing and controlling their time, it is important that they strive to *continue to succeed*. Lakein suggests programming to succeed by: (a) planning whenever harried or overwhelmed; (b) keeping involved in priorities; (c) avoiding favorite escapes; (d) maintaining a positive attitude; (e) doing something for themselves every day; and (f) resisting doing easy but unimportant tasks.[14] Needless to say, this programming also applies to nurses.

If we go back now and analyze Sara and her time problem, we can easily see that if she had: (1) planned for managing her time by setting priorities, making a time schedule and establishing a "to do " list; (2) organized her mind and working environment by practicing no detourism and mental wastebasketry; and (3) implemented activities to control her time such as attacking the priorities, avoiding procrastination and escape and learning to say no, she would not have been involved in the stressful situation that occurred. Thus, it seems that Sara and other nurses can decrease their stress levels by learning how to manage and control their time more effectively.

REFERENCES

1. Lakein, A. *How to Get Control of Your Time and Your Life* (New York: The New American Library 1974) p. 11.

2. Mackenzie, R. A. *The Time Trap* (New York: McGraw-Hill Book Co. 1972) p. 2.

3. Mackenzie, *The Time Trap.* p. 1.

4. Webber, R. A. *Time and Management* (New York: Van Nostrand Reinhold Co. 1972) p. 11–16.

5. Webber, *Time and Management.* p. 13–14.

6. Mackenzie, R. A. "Myths of Time Management," *The Business Quarterly* (Spring 1974) as excerpted in *Notes and Quotes* 410 (September-October 1974) p. 2.

7. Mackenzie, "Myths of Time Management." p. 2.

8. Mackenzie, *The Time Trap.* p. 86.

9. Webber, *Time and Management.* p. 60.

10. Webber, *Time and Management.* p. 73.

11. Lakein, *How to Get Control of Your Time and Your Life.* p. 28–29.

12. Mackenzie, *The Time Trap.* p. 52.

13. Webber, *Time and Management.* p. 84

14. Lakein, *How to Get Control of Your Time and Your Life.* p. 149.

Coping with Stress through Peer Support

Susan P. Epting, RN, MSN
Instructor of Nursing
Gwynedd-Mercy College
Gwynedd Valley, Pennsylvania
Formerly Staff Development Instructor
American Oncologic Hospital/
Fox Chase Cancer Center
Philadelphia, Pennsylvania

BURNOUT—physical and emotional exhaustion resulting from stress—has recently become a much discussed topic among professionals as well as nonprofessionals. Although found in many groups of people, this syndrome is particularly prevalent among health care providers. One especially vulnerable group are nurses working in chronic illness settings such as oncology units.

It is known that this stress-induced syndrome occurs, and several hypotheses have been made regarding its causes. But what can be done to cope with this problem? At American Oncologic Hospital/ Fox Chase Cancer Center the administration's view is that the best way to deal with burnout is to prevent it in the first place. For this reason, two innovative approaches to handle high levels of stress have been implemented: recovery days and psychosocial support groups.

286 DEFINING STRESS

The concept of stress is not new. Authors have been describing and attempting to define it for decades. Hartl identified a general tendency to define stress as "that physical and emotional experience which results from a requirement to change from the condition of the moment to any other condition."[1]

This definition stipulates that the presence of stress implies a change. Any change, whether it be positive or negative, carries with it some additional stress. Holmes and Rahe developed a "social readjustment rating scale" in which they assign numerical values to the amount of impact that certain life events have on the individual.[2] These specific life changes range from minor violations of the law to the death of a spouse. Also included in their list are seemingly positive events such as outstanding personal achievements and vacations. By looking at these events, which are both positive and negative, one can see that any change results in some stress to the person. How stress is experienced depends on the capacity of the individual to adapt. It is a personal experience and is therefore different for everyone. For example, public speaking may be very easy for one person and exceedingly stressful for another.

Not all stress is bad. Everyone experiences some degree of stress almost all the time. To be under no stress would be equivalent to death. The body must be prepared to deal with unexpected or unavoidable events so that it is not destroyed. It is necessary to have some pressure so that motivation continues. Some individuals find stress, such as work deadlines, to be beneficial. It is common to hear the statement, "I work better when the work must be finished by tomorrow." This person is saying that increased amounts of stress produce more motivation resulting in a higher level of productivity.

Problems related to stress arise when the degree of stress remains too high for a prolonged period of time. Again, what is too much stress or what length of time is too long depends on the individual and his or her capacity to cope. One person may be able to deal with large amounts of stress for a long time before developing problems, whereas another individual may manifest symptoms of high levels of stress after only a short time.

HOW STRESS IS MANIFESTED

Stressors elicit a response from a person's entire body—from the psyche as well as the physiology. Hans Selye defined stress as "a nonspecific response of the body to any demand, whether it is caused by, or results in, pleasant or unpleasant conditions."[3] On the basis of this definition, Selye coined the phrase *general adaptation syndrome* (GAS) to refer to this response. The GAS consists of three stages: (1) alarm reaction, (2) stage of

When a stressor is present, the body prepares to either fight or flee the stress-producing event. The human system mobilizes its energies, causing several physiological processes to go into action.

resistance, and (3) stage of exhaustion. These three phases describe how the body reacts in the presence of stressors.[4]

The first stage, that of the alarm reaction, is better known as the "fight or flight" response. When a stressor is present, the body prepares to either fight or flee the stress-producing event. The human system mobilizes its energies, causing several physiological processes to go into action. Hormones are released into the blood stream, the blood supply to the skeletal muscles is increased, and the gastrointestinal processes are slowed down. All these processes allow the body to defend itself against the stressor.

The alarm reaction can be portrayed by the following example. A new graduate nurse, Ms. R., walks onto the oncology unit for her first day of orientation. She is assigned to Mr. H. who has just undergone a thoracotomy for carcinoma of the lung. He has chest tubes connected to a pleur-evac, a nasogastric tube to straight drainage, a Foley catheter, oxygen by nasal cannula, and a peripheral intravenous line for the administration of antibiotics. Mr. H. also has a subclavian line through which he is receiving total parenteral nutrition. The amount of hyperalimentation fluid flowing through the subclavian line is monitored by an infusion pump. As the nurse prepares to assist Mr. H. with his morning care, the alarm on the pump sounds. Not accustomed to working with this equipment, the nurse panics at the sound of the alarm. Ms. R. begins to feel her heart rate and her respiratory rate increase. If her blood pressure was monitored, it would be found to be elevated. Studies have shown that blood glucose and serum sodium increase while the level

of serum potassium decreases. Gastric secretions increase, pupils dilate, muscles tense, and digestion slows. The body is preparing itself for extraordinary activities requiring an intense focus of energy. It is ready to either fight or flee the stressful event.

No one can continually exist in such a state of alarm. So after a few weeks of working with patients such as Mr. H., Ms. R. will become accustomed to the infusion pump alarm. She will react with deliberate actions when the alarm sounds. Her body will overcome the stressor and adapt to it. Selye referred to this phase as the stage of resistance.

As the body's resistance to the stressor increases, it begins to adapt. The body's processes repair any damage done during the alarm reaction phase and normal functioning returns. However, if the source of the stress is not removed or if the amount becomes overwhelming and the person cannot effectively deal with it, the ability to adapt is lost. A state of exhaustion occurs and the organism can no longer fight back. The result may be susceptibility to diseases such as gastrointestinal ulcers, hypertension, or myocardial infarction. Eventually the organism may die from the effects of prolonged stress. This phase, called by Selye the stage of exhaustion, corresponds to the syndrome called *burnout*.

BURNOUT

McConnell defines burnout as the "syndrome exhibited by nurses who have either depleted or exhausted their emotional and physical energies in dealing with the stressors of the work environment."[5] The nurse

288 who reaches this point has passed through the alarm reaction and resistance stages.

The nurse who is "burned out" can no longer cope with stress and demonstrates this fact through numerous signs and symptoms. It is important to keep in mind that the presence of one or two signs or symptoms does not necessarily indicate burnout. However, when several manifestations are present together and for extended periods of time, burnout may be imminent. Signs and symptoms indicating burnout can be divided into two categories: physical and psychosocial or behavioral.[6]

Physical symptoms

One of the initial symptoms a person experiences when becoming burned out is fatigue. The nurse who works day shift feels tired on awakening in the morning and finds it hard to get up for work. Many times this fatigue appears to be justified since these individuals often feel that only they can provide adequate care for their patients. They are tired because they tend to stay at work several hours later than required and perhaps work double shifts or on their days off.

There are other physical signs that reflect the influence of too much stress. These include: gastrointestinal problems such as diarrhea, nausea, and vomiting; persistent colds; back pain; weight loss or perhaps weight gain; loss of appetite; and increased susceptibility to infections. The individual may also experience headaches, insomnia, dyspnea, and angina.[7,8]

Behavioral symptoms

Persons nearing burnout can be identified by their behavior. Some individuals become increasingly irritable, rigid in their thinking, resistant to change, and tend to find fault more quickly. They may experience behavior changes.[9] People who were once withdrawn may suddenly become outgoing and vice versa. They may develop negative, cynical attitudes about coworkers, thereby contributing to difficulties in working with others. The individuals reach a point where they are no longer able to cope and become indifferent to their jobs and other health care personnel. They are no longer enthusiastic about their work and find it hard to concentrate.

The nurse may also experience more frequent periods of moodiness and depression, which may be reflected in increased periods of crying for no apparent reason. Mrs. T., a staff nurse at American Oncologic Hospital/Fox Chase Cancer Center, identified another typical sign of burnout—taking problems home after work. "I know I've had it when I take my problems home to my husband and children." In this case, Mrs. T. was unable to emotionally detach herself from the job. She was overinvolved with the patients and could not stop thinking about them during time off from work. This fact further contributed to dreams she had at night. Mrs. T. complained of frequent dreams about patients, their family members, and cancer in general. Conflict-laden dreams and subsequent depression can both contribute to the nurse's feelings of fatigue and reluctance to get out of bed for work.

Other signs of approaching burnout are especially important from an administrative point of view. Increased periods of absenteeism and tardiness, greater numbers of incident reports completed for accidents on the job, and an increase in the turnover rate of personnel are just a few of these signs. In addition, the work output decreases.

All these signs and symptoms may be indicative of too much stress. Health professionals, as stated previously, are prone to the development of burnout. For several reasons, oncology nurses are particularly susceptible to developing this syndrome.

CAUSES OF BURNOUT IN ONCOLOGY NURSES

Although many factors can be cited as possible causes of burnout, there is no single cause that is always present. Some contributors apply to any nurse whereas others are specific to those working for extended periods of time in chronic illness settings such as oncology. Stressors in the health care environment can be divided into three main areas: (1) the health care environment; (2) other health care personnel; and (3) patients and their family members.[10]

Environmental causes

Within the work environment itself there are various factors that are potential stressors. Insufficient amounts of supplies or continuous problems in obtaining supplies for the floor are definitely stressful for the nurse. The physical layout of the facility can also produce a great deal of stress. A nurse who must continuously walk from the patient's room to the utility room at the opposite end of the hall may become tired and distressed. Sometimes the unit is too small to accommodate the number of patients, or the area around the nurses' station does not have enough room

to accommodate several nurses, physicians, and other personnel at the same time. Tempers flare, and needless frustrations result.

A major contributor to burnout is a constant shortage of staff. Associated with this may be an increase in the number of critically ill patients. When the staffing is short and the number of patients who require complete care increases, the result is an increased workload on a staff that is probably overworked already. These nurses will cope as best they can, but they become frustrated because they know that much more could be done if there were more staff present.[11]

Professional relationships

Another area of potential stress is that of relationships with other health care personnel. Ineffective communication results in difficulties for all concerned. Huckabay and Jagla found that the communication problems between staff members and the nursing office, and between staff members and physicians were more pronounced than among staff members and between staff members and other departments. They believed that this occurred because physicians and nursing administrators are seen as superiors who have authority over the nurse.[12] Wherever poor communication exists, it is very stressful for all personnel.

Personality conflicts between staff members, lack of a strong, positive leader, misunderstandings about roles, unhappiness with the job, and lack of support from peers or superiors all have been identified as stressors.[13,14] These factors always exist when there are several people working together. However, it is necessary

290 to try to minimize such situations so that too much stress can be prevented.

Relationships with patients and their families

Perhaps the biggest source of stress to the nurse working in a chronic illness setting is relationships with the patients and their families. Oncology nurses are vulnerable to a high degree of stress because of the type of patient they care for. The nature of the disease, in itself, evokes anxiety. Despite the fact that the treatment of malignancies has vastly improved over the past decade, cancer is still a threatening illness in our society. Those health professionals working on a unit or in an institution where all the patients are hospitalized for cancer may find it particularly stressful, since all they see are oncology patients. Therefore, oncology in itself is a stressor.

In some respects, the oncology nurse's emotions are more at risk than those of the physician who works in oncology.[15] There are two reasons for this fact: (1) nurses, collectively speaking, are with the patient 24 hours per day; and (2) the presentation that the patient makes to the physician differs from that made to the nurse.

The physician is usually with the patient for only a few minutes a day, so the nurse must handle many situations without the help of a physician. Nurses are constantly in the presence of the patients and their families. Further, when the physician makes rounds, the patient will usually try to appear emotionally composed. The oncologist sees the patient as emotionally well controlled, but the patient is unable to keep up this cheerfulness during the entire shift. The nurse must then deal with the feelings that the patient does not share with the physician.

Robinson identified two major psychological issues with which nurses must struggle.[16] These two issues are common among nurses working with chronically ill patients and their families. The first deals with identification with patients, particularly those who are dying. These nurses are forced to recognize the existence of their own mortality. The degree of identification is directly proportional to the amount of contact with the patient.[17] Nurses frequently identify with patients whose age approximates their own, with patients who remind them of themselves, or with those patients who are friends or family members of people they know.

Secondly, all health care personnel experience guilt resulting from a sense of having failed their patients. Health professionals are educated in how to treat patients so their health improves. But cancer patients often die—a constant reminder of failure. At the subconscious level, care givers are angry at the patient for not responding to care. Consciously, this anger is experienced as guilt because being angry at the patient is intolerable.[18]

A final factor that can contribute to burnout is communication problems. In

All health care personnel experience guilt resulting from a sense of having failed their patients. Health professionals are all educated in how to treat patients so their health improves. But cancer patients often die—a constant reminder of failure.

addition to the problems resulting from communication difficulties between staff members, these problems also exist at times between patients, their families, and staff. At times family members or the physician do not want the patient to know the diagnosis. This situation puts nurses in a stressful position because they are not able to relate honestly to the patient. One task of nurses is to help the patient and family to go through the stages of the grieving process in preparation for death. It is not possible to do this when the truth is being withheld. The stress of having to deal with this problem day after day can sometimes become too great.

All these factors are potential sources of stress for nurses working with chronically ill patients such as those with malignancies. How can nurses protect themselves from experiencing emotional breakdowns in the face of these stressors? The answer must lie somewhere within the health care system.

COPING WITH STRESS

The best way to deal with stress is to eliminate or minimize the stressors. This is not always realistic, however, so one must search for alternatives. Besides removing the causative factors, an attempt can be made to prevent burnout by strengthening the coping mechanisms of those under stress. Prevention can be accomplished by: (1) being cognizant of the signs and symptoms of burnout; (2) psychologically "unplugging" from the work environment; and (3) developing supportive family or peer networks.

Nurses can all become aware of the signs and symptoms of burnout through continuing education. Attendance at workshops on the subject of stress or reading about the topic is helpful. Once nurses are knowledgeable about stress and its sometimes deleterious effects, they can identify these effects in their coworkers as well as themselves.

Nurses need to "unplug" from their jobs when they go home. All nurses take thoughts about patients home at times, but each needs to be able to develop methods of relaxing and forgetting. Physical activities such as jogging, swimming, or bicycling are helpful to some people, whereas others prefer hobbies such as needlecraft or ceramics. Practicing relaxation techniques can also be helpful. It is important to choose an activity one enjoys. An outlet that is not enjoyable will itself become a source of stress. When vacation days are available, it is often good to take a few days off from work. It is not always necessary to go on a trip; sometimes just a break from the job will be helpful.

A PROGRAM TO PREVENT BURNOUT

At the American Oncologic Hospital/ Fox Chase Cancer Center, a program was set up to aid in the prevention of burnout. Each fulltime staff nurse is eligible for five paid recovery days per year. When things get rough and the nurse can no longer cope, that individual requests a recovery day. If staffing is limited, the recovery day may not be granted for the following day. But knowing that he or she will shortly have an extra day off helps the nurse to cope better. If all five recovery days are not used during the year, the time is

292 converted into paid sick time to be used as necessary.

No one can exist and function without the support of family and peers. Family members and friends can allow the nurse to ventilate about work experiences but can also limit such discussions if appropriate.[19] Peers are very helpful in discussing issues related to patients, families, and staff. It is sometimes supportive to know that a colleague has the same feelings and frustrations as oneself. For these reasons, the author established psychosocial support groups for nursing personnel at the American Oncologic Hospital/Fox Chase Cancer Center.

PEER SUPPORT GROUPS

The literature dealing with the use of support groups for staff members is fairly limited. Newlin and Wellisch discuss the need for such groups on their oncology unit. They follow a program consisting of two forms of support networks, one formal and one informal. The formal support mechanism consists of weekly meetings where the nurses are able to discuss any issue important to them at the time.[20]

Stillman and Strasser set up a similar program in their critical care unit. Their approach focuses on allowing the nurses to openly discuss their anxieties, in addition to assisting them to develop effective communication skills. Evaluation of the groups has shown that the nurses have developed increased competence and confidence in relating to patients, coworkers, and physicians. There has also been a request for additional group seminars.[21]

Maslach, in her research on burnout, found support groups to be of significant benefit to health professionals. Her findings show that burnout rates are lower for those individuals who are able to share their feelings with colleagues. They are not only able to ventilate their frustrations but are able to get constructive feedback from their peers.[22]

Using the literature as a basis, the administration at American Oncologic Hospital/Fox Chase Cancer Center conducted an assessment to determine the need for psychosocial support groups for nursing staff. The assessment was conducted in both an informal and a formal manner. Questionnaires eliciting interest were formally sent to all nursing personnel. In addition, the author conducted informal discussions with the members of the nursing staff.

On the basis of this assessment, several support groups were set up starting in January 1979. The author currently conducts one group for each of the three shifts. The intention was that since the nursing staff works permanent shifts at this institution, all individuals would be available to attend the same group each week.

Several weeks before the first meeting of each group, each member of the nursing staff received a memorandum explaining the rationale behind the institution of support groups as well as specifics such as dates and times for meetings.

Characteristics of facilitators

It was decided that group facilitators should possess three characteristics: (1) they should be nurses with experience in oncology; (2) they should have some education in psychiatric nursing; and (3) they should be in a staff rather than a line position.

These three factors were identified for several reasons. During the needs assessment it was requested that a nurse facilitate the groups because staff members felt they would be more comfortable with a person who had worked in situations similar to their own. In essence, they felt they could better identify with another nurse. It is also important that the group facilitator have some training in psychiatry. At times emotional topics arise and there must be someone present who can help the participants handle these emotions. Finally, many nurses find that they are not able to honestly relate their frustrations and feelings if the group leader is in a position of authority over them. This fact was substantiated when a member of the nursing administration attempted to facilitate a group, only to find that the members were not able to ventilate comfortably.

Based on these three requirements, the author was chosen as the facilitator for the groups. The author is a nurse with oncology experience as well as graduate education and experience in psychiatric nursing. In addition, she works in a staff position in the staff development department. Despite these facts, the author had to prove herself to the members of the group. Since she had only worked at the hospital for four months, she was not known to everyone. Also, her office is located within the nursing administration suite, raising some doubts in the minds of the nursing staff as to whether she could be trusted to keep confidential the information revealed in the group meetings. After about six weeks, this leadership issue was mostly resolved.

Membership

When the project began, 15 members of the nursing staff were assigned to each group. Head nurses were included, but supervisors were not. The membership was limited, and only designated members could attend so that the group process could develop. This approach was later modified, because attendance at the group sessions varied depending on the time schedules on the floor. The groups are now open to all the people who work on each shift, with the average attendance being 15.

Meetings

The initial meeting of each group was important. Besides orienting the members to the purposes and structure of the peer support network, several issues had to be addressed. Confidentiality was the most important of these issues. Matters discussed in the sessions must never leave the room. This is the responsibility of the leader as well as the members of the group. It was also stressed that attendance would not be mandatory, and people would be free to leave the room whenever they desired.

The group members were asked to think about what they hoped to achieve through meeting and discussing mutual feelings and issues. It is important that the goals be those of all of the members and not merely those of the leader. Unless the group strives toward objectives they are interested in, little effort will be put into meetings and little will be achieved. Some goals identified were: (1) to be able to verbalize job frustrations; (2) to develop better rapport among the staffs of the

294 different units; (3) to improve patient care by learning to meet patients' psychosocial needs; (4) to establish increased cohesion among coworkers; and (5) to improve communication with the nursing administration.

Each group meets weekly for one hour and follows a similar format. At the end of each meeting a topic is chosen for discussion at the next session. Topics have included: reasons for working in a hospital that is entirely oncology, stress and burnout, death and dying, overinvolvement with patients, difficulties with families, pain control, and working with young adult patients. When used, these previously chosen topics usually stimulate further discussions. If there is an issue on the minds of the members when the meeting begins, that will be discussed instead of the previously chosen topic. For example, one week a terminally ill woman receiving high doses of intravenous narcotics was admitted to the hospital. Nurses were upset about the legalities of the situation as well as euthanasia. Clearly, this presented a crisis that had to be resolved immediately. The topic for discussion identified the previous week was set aside and discussed the following week.

Initial obstacles to successful groups

When the groups first began, several trends arose in each. These trends are not surprising; they are common to most groups in the early stages of their formation. One of the early issues was leadership. As stated previously, group members did not know whether they could trust the author as their leader. Not only did they question her sincerity, but also her qualifications since she does not give direct patient care. These concerns were not always voiced directly but they came up in other ways such as discussions about administration, differences in the roles of the RN and LPN and physicians—all of which focused on authority issues. Questions about leadership are frequently found in groups as members struggle to establish their place in the leadership hierarchy.[23] The issue of authority later lost significance as group cohesiveness began to develop.

Initially the groups focused on superficial rather than emotionally sensitive issues. Topics such as lack of adequate floor space, requirements to work week-

Questions about leadership frequently arise in groups as members struggle to establish their place in the hierarchy. The issue of authority loses significance as group cohesiveness begins to develop.

ends, and lack of refrigerators on some floors were addressed. The establishment of a working group is a long process. Individuals cannot be expected to reveal their deepest feelings immediately. Once trust is established among all participants in the group, more feelings are shared.

In addition, several norms could be identified when examining the process occurring in the early groups. These included a desire not to say anything that was not "nice" about other members, and a general rule that members would not disagree with each other. These issues are common to beginning groups; after about six weeks they began to diminish in frequency as the members began to discuss more important issues.

Difficulties encountered in setting up groups

When setting up the support group system the author encountered some difficulties. The initial group meetings were held from 2:30 P.M. to 3:30 P.M. From an administrative viewpoint, this time was ideal because only a minimal amount of overtime had to be paid. However, since it covered the time period during change of shift, many nursing personnel were not able to attend the meetings. No matter what time is scheduled for the group, the patients are the priority, and the floors are sometimes busy.

Turnover in the nursing staff plays another important role in the development of group process. The result of turnover is that group membership is unstable. It is therefore difficult for the group process to develop since attendance at the meetings differs each week.

Several members of the nursing staff did not have a clear understanding of the purpose of developing peer support groups. And some individuals were just not interested in such activities but attended in order to get off the floor. As a result, it was sometimes difficult to encourage the group to identify goals they hoped to accomplish.

Other problems have been identified elsewhere in the article. When setting up support groups, it is necessary to have patience, enthusiasm, and perseverance.

There are many frustrations, but the mechanism of peer support will work if the facilitator and the group members are committed to the group. Without such a commitment, the difficulties may be insurmountable.

A group leader must be flexible, willing to take some extra responsibility, and ready to restructure the groups as necessary. Each set of people is different, so the same format will not function well for all groups. Plans must be modified again and again until the best solution is reached. It is hard work requiring dedication on the part of group members as well as the facilitator. But evaluation shows the results are worth all the efforts put into such a project.

Evaluation of the groups

Although the system of peer support groups at American Oncologic Hospital/ Fox Chase Cancer Center has been functioning since January 1979, no formal evaluation has been conducted yet. Several reasons account for this fact, the most important being that the group structure has had to be changed numerous times. The system does appear to be stable now so a formal evaluation is being planned, with the results to be published at a later date.

Informal evaluations have been conducted throughout the course of the past year. The positive and negative aspects of the groups have been discussed at several meetings. These critiques have resulted in modifications such as changes in meeting times, group membership, and the type of format followed (structured versus unstructured).

296 The author plans to conduct a formal evaluation shortly. Several criteria will be examined in terms of changes effected by the use of formal support groups. The author has developed hypotheses about trends she expects to find as a result of the group meetings.

1. Nurses spend increased amounts of time with the patients and families.
2. A decreased amount of sick time is used by nurses.
3. More collaboration occurs between nursing units.
4. Fewer recovery days are used.
5. Nurses are more able to handle patients' psychosocial needs as evidenced by a change in the number and type of social service consults.
6. The rate of turnover among nursing personnel has decreased.

An informal examination has shown some progress toward these results. The amount of sick time used has decreased and there has been a decrease in the turnover rate of nursing personnel. Variables other than the support groups have most likely influenced these changes. However, the changes have occurred since the implementation of the groups and recovery days. A more formal, structured evaluation is expected to substantiate these results.

High levels of stress present for prolonged periods of time have been shown to have damaging effects among health care providers, especially those working in chronic illness settings such as oncology. A system of peer support groups is one manner in which individuals can discuss their mutual feelings and frustrations while learning to deal with the stress found in their professional and personal lives.

REFERENCES

1. Hartl, D.E. "Stress Management and the Nurse." *Advances in Nursing Science* 1:4 (July 1979) p. 91.
2. Holmes, H. and Rahe, R. "The Social Readjustment Rating Scale." *Psychosomatic Research* 2:4 (April 1967) p. 214.
3. Selye, H. *The Stress of Life* 2nd ed. (New York: McGraw-Hill 1978) p. 74.
4. Ibid. p. 36-38.
5. McConnell, E. "Burnout and the Critical Care Nurse." *Critical Care Update* 6:8 (August 1979) p. 5.
6. Ibid. p. 5-14.
7. McConnell, E. "Burnout—How It Affects You." *Ross Laboratories' Public Health Currents* 19:5 (September-October 1979) p. 21-24.
8. Patrick, P.K.S. "Burnout: Job Hazard for Health Workers." *Hospitals* 53:22 (November 16, 1979) p. 87-90.
9. McConnell. "Burnout and the Critical Care Nurse." p. 5-14.
10. Bilodeau, C.B. "The Nurse and Her Reactions to Critical-Care Nursing." *Heart Lung* 2:3 (May-June 1973) p. 358-363.
11. McConnell. "Burnout—How It Effects You."
12. Huckabay, L. and Jagla, B. "Nurses' Stress Factors in the Intensive Care Unit." *Journal of Nursing Administration* 9:2 (February 1979) p. 21-26.
13. Bilodeau, C.B. "The Nurse and Her Reactions to Critical-Care Nursing."
14. Gunderson, K. et al. "How to Control Professional Frustration." *American Journal of Nursing* 77:7 (July 1977) p. 1180-1183.
15. Newlin, N.J. and Wellisch, D.K. "The Oncology Nurse: Life on an Emotional Roller Coaster." *Cancer Nursing* 1:6 (December 1978) p. 447-449.
16. Robinson, L. *Psychological Aspects of the Care of Hospitalized Patients* (Philadelphia: F.A. Davis Co. 1976).

17. Newlin, N.J. and Wellisch, D.K. "The Oncology Nurse."

18. Ibid.

19. Ibid.

20. Ibid.

21. Stillman, S.M. and Strasser, B.L. "Helping Critical Care Nurses with Work-Related Stress." *The Journal of Nursing Administration* 10:1 (January 1980) p. 28–31.

22. Maslach, C. "Burned-Out." *Human Behavior* 5:9 (September 1976) p. 16–22.

23. Thelen, H.A. and Dickerman, W. "Stereotypes and the Growth of Groups" in Bradford, L.P., ed. *Group Development* (LaJolla, California: University Associates 1974) p. 73–80.

Stress Research in Clinical Settings

Margery Garbin, R.N., M.S.N.
Psychiatric Liaison Nurse
Mercy Catholic Medical Center
Darby, Pennsylvania

On a recent busy day, Ms. Scott, a staff nurse on a medical–surgical unit, was assigned to care for six seriously ill patients. She recognized that Mr. Jones, who was recovering from a myocardial infarction, was extremely tense. Ms. Scott talked to him about his tension and learned that he attributed it to inactivity and to worrying about his health and business affairs. Ms. Scott taught Mr. Jones progressive relaxation while visualizing himself in a relaxing environment. After the exercise, Mr. Jones felt much more comfortable.

Ms. Scott, who was behind in her work, then hurried to pour medications. The head nurse asked her, "Did you change Mr. Brown's dressings?" Ms. Scott snapped, "I'll do it as soon as I can. I only have two hands!"

NURSES ARE GENERALLY aware that patients experience stress as they cope with illness, hospitalization and uncertainty about the future. Recognizing a patient's stress, nurses, like Ms. Scott, often suggest relaxation exercises or other

300 stress-reduction activities. Less often, however, do nurses apply their understanding of stress to themselves in the work situation.

Nurses acknowledge that their work is often very stressful, and they can quickly list numerous causes of stress in the work environment. Nevertheless, they do not often analyze their situation and apply stress management strategies to themselves. More often high levels of stress among the nursing staff are manifested as somatic complaints, intra-staff bickering and scapegoating. A high staff turnover rate may also reflect nurses' attempts to escape a stressful environment, yet they often enter other situations that are equally stressful. The pressures faced by nurses, especially in busy, understaffed, inner-city hospitals, will probably not decrease in the near future. What can change is the way that nurses respond to the causes of stress and handle them.

An inservice education project to teach stress management techniques to nurses was recently implemented at Episcopal Hospital in Philadelphia. The aims of the project were: (1) to increase the nursing staff's ability to recognize their own responses to stress, and (2) to acquaint them with a variety of coping strategies to handle stress. These strategies include relaxation techniques, visualization, meditation and assertiveness training. By encouraging the project, nursing administrators hoped to convey support to the nurses under stress. Both administrators and educators shared the hope that the project would lead to a reduction of staff tension and to greater staff retention.

In the process of developing research strategies to measure the effectiveness of the project, several problems became evident. First, there was disagreement and confusion about the concept of stress and, therefore, about stress research. Second, there are limitations to applied research studies done in the field, such as clinical or work settings. Both of these issues have implications not only for research but for any application of stress-management techniques in clinical settings.

ISSUES RELATED TO THE CONCEPT OF STRESS

The concept of stress is a broad one which incorporates a wide range of problems and situations. It has been the concern of investigators in such fields as physiology, sociology, psychology, nursing, medicine and others. The way that

---

The way that stress is conceptualized depends on the special focus of interest of the particular investigator in the particular field.

---

stress is conceptualized depends on the special focus of interest of the particular investigator in the particular field. In a broad sense, however, stress serves as an integrating concept among the biopsychosocial sciences, suggesting fundamental connections among them.

Selye, the endocrinologist who introduced the concept of stress to the sciences, defines stress as a nonspecific physiological response of an organism to evocative agents which he terms *stressors*. He places great importance on stress as a physiological response within an organism, not to be confused with the external events (stressors) which bring about the response.[1]

Selye further emphasizes the concept of physiological nonspecificity: "stress is the nonspecific response of the body to any demand."[2] He named this response the General Adaptation Syndrome (GAS) which proceeds in three phases. The first phase is the alarm reaction, characterized by adrenal enlargement, gastrointestinal ulcers, thymicolymphatic evolution and other clinical, structural and chemical changes. The second phase is the adaptive stage characterized by optimal adaptation of the organism. The third phase is exhaustion, when the acquired adaptation is lost. For Selye, occurrence of the GAS defines the occurrence of stress.

The GAS occurs not only under unpleasant conditions but also under conditions of exercise, surprise or passion, not generally thought of as stressful. Although the same response pattern may be produced through entirely different processes (e.g., a passionate kiss or a game of tennis), the psychological meanings of the two states are completely different. This nonspecificity or generality of response may cause problems to researchers since determining the event or situation which elicits the response in a real-life setting may be difficult.

Also, psychological research has repeatedly shown that responses to a psychosocial stimulus may vary widely from one individual to another, or from one time to another in the same person. The responses depend on a multitude of intervening, interacting variables related to an individual's personality, history, coping style, etc. In fact, future stress research may focus more on idiosyncratic psychobiological patterns than on common response patterns to stressors.[3]

The popular use of the term *stress* often differs from Selye's terminology by denoting an external force (stimulus) acting on a person rather than the physiological response described by Selye. Therefore, Selye's term *stressor* overlaps with such concepts as "life stress," "environmental stress" and "work stress." Confusion results when the broad term *stress* is used to refer both to the sources of stress (stimuli) and to the effects of stress (responses).

Psychological Stress and Stress Response

Problems also arise in defining what kinds of situations or what properties of situations are stressful. For instance, "psychological stress" has been used to describe the impact of a variety of environmental conditions: crowded or isolated, challenging or boring, rapidly changing or repetitious, authoritarian or unstructured, among others. The stress associated with this wide range of situations may represent several, or many, different kinds of stress, rather than a single phenomenon. In addition, it is difficult to estimate, much less measure, stressful properties of a situation to establish quantitatively the degree of stress in different situations.

Often individuals differ in their response to the same stressful situation. Nurses, for instance, differ in the amount of stress they perceive in such settings as an intensive care unit or a psychiatric unit. Olsen found that operating room nurses' perceptions of various stressors varied with length of operating room experience, education and responsibility.[4]

302 Cleland studied the effect of work environment stressors on performance in two nursing tests. She found that nurses who scored high in need for social approval had a sharp decline in performance when the situational stressors increased. Conversely, the performance of nurses with low need for social approval increased when situational stressors increased.[5] Both of the studies indicate that a variety of intervening variables influence the responses of nurses to stressful situations.

In the ongoing study at Episcopal Hospital, nurses were asked to respond to 27 "nursing stressor" items to determine what they perceived as stressful in the work environment. Nurses were asked to indicate on a scale from 1 (no stress) to 5 (extreme stress) how stressful each of the 27 items was to them. A mean score was computed for each item. For this study, a mean score of 3.0 or greater was considered an indication of perceived stress.

The variability of perceived stress was evident in the range of scores for the items. Scores for several items ranged across the scale from "no stress" to "extreme stress," even among nurses working on the same units and the same shifts. The six items shown in Table 1 had mean scores of 3.0 or more and were therefore perceived as stressful by the group as a whole.

Broad Definition of Stress

Stress, in addition to referring to extreme environmental conditions, has also been used by researchers as a substitute for a variety of psychological concepts, such as anxiety, frustration, tension, arousal and emotional distress.[6] In psychological research, the existence of

TABLE 1

Nursing Stressors in the Work Environment

Stressor	Mean Score
1. Heavy workload, making total patient care impossible	3.55
2. Making a mistake	3.37
3. Lack of support from peers or head nurse	3.19
4. Cardiac arrest	3.19
5. Lack of communication with physicians	3.04
6. Inadequate equipment, supplies, or work space	3.00

Note: Data incomplete; based on first 76 questionnaires returned.

stress is often inferred from the presence of emotional states such as anxiety or from physiological indices such as heart rate or galvanic skin response (GSR). Again, however, there are marked individual differences in the indices, with subjects often not responding to environmental conditions as the experimenter intended or predicted. The individual's perception and appraisal of the environmental situation seems to be a crucial mediator of stress.

The difficulty in defining stress is related to the fact that human beings interact with the environment in a complex, holistic manner. Efforts have been made, therefore, to define stress broadly in terms of the interaction of individual and environment. Stress occurs when an individual or larger social system is confronted with an environmental demand that exceeds his or her response capability and the consequences of not adapting are serious.[7] The subjective aspects of stress are of crucial importance. That is, an environmental demand leads to stress only if individuals anticipate that they will not be able to cope with it, and only if the consequences of failure to cope are perceived to be important.[8] In this model, the individual is regarded as an active, adaptive, coping organism, rather than as a passive or reactive organism.

This paradigm regards stress as a central concept with heuristic value, not as a rigorous, scientific concept with hypothetico-deductive power.[9] Stress research, then, is focused on selected, clearly delineated aspects of the person–environment interaction. In fact, Mason suggests that researchers use the term "stress" as sparingly as possible, and "adhere to terms for stimulus and response parameters which are as operationally sound and descriptive as possible," at least until the need for a

---

While the conceptual definition of stress may be broad and nonspecific, the operational definitions in stress research should be worded in terms of specific concepts that can be measured.

---

more generic term becomes evident.[10] Thus, while the conceptual definition of stress may be broad and nonspecific, the operational definitions in stress research should be worded in terms of specific concepts that can be measured.

ISSUES RELATED TO METHODOLOGY

In addition to the conceptual issues, there are also methodological issues in stress research. The investigators' research

strategies will reflect their different aims and their differing uses of the term *stress*. The criteria chosen to define and measure stress may be physiological, psychological or social behaviors.

The criteria selected imply value judgments concerning which behaviors are important and which responses or levels of behavior are better or poorer. For instance, a researcher might hypothesize that nurses with a certain personality pattern, such as internal locus of control, will perform better in a given stressful situation. It is tempting to assign a positive value to this behavior and to conclude that nurses with internal locus of control are better adjusted or healthier.

Although the individual behaves and responds as a whole, there are as yet no holistic measuring tools available. Rather, there are a wide variety of techniques for measuring stress-related variables. These include: (1) indices referring to physiological properties (GSR, EEG, blood pressure, heart rate, etc.), (2) indices related to psychological properties (personality tests, problem-solving performance, psychiatric records, etc.), and (3) indices referring to properties of behavior in various settings (questionnaires measuring task performance, aspects of interpersonal relations, observation of speed and quality of task performance, production records, etc.).[11] Each of these measures has strengths and weaknesses.

For instance, one major problem in physiological measures is the wide range of intra-individual and inter-individual differences unrelated to specific stressor conditions. Because a person's score on a test may differ from one day to the next, serious questions about reliability of

304 measurement are often raised. Even the time of day may make a difference in how a person responds to a stressor.

Another frequently encountered problem is the vulnerability of subjective psychological reports to reactivity effects. That is, the subject who knows that he is being tested may alter his behavior to the psychological demands of the testing situation.

Ethical issues are especially important in stress research. In laboratory settings, stressful conditions are created, and unpleasant, possibly traumatic, effects may be evoked. The investigator is obliged to minimize the unpleasant experiences, to fully inform the subject about the purposes and procedures and to explain after the experiment the exact nature of the procedure, especially if deceit is involved (e.g., asking subjects to solve unsolvable problems).

The ethical necessity of informed consent introduces the possibility that the study may be biased by the subjects' awareness of what the investigator hopes to find. The question of how much information to give to protect the rights of subjects while avoiding bias is, therefore, a serious issue. However, the potential danger of long-term adverse effects, such as lowered self-esteem, must be recognized by every investigator as an unacceptable hazard in stress research.[12]

LIMITATIONS OF APPLIED RESEARCH

Laboratory research and field research can be viewed as opposite ends of a research continuum. Laboratory research tends to involve basic research, aimed at discovering new knowledge and contributing to theory development. Field research tends to involve applied research, aimed at using knowledge to achieve goals relevant to the real world. The differences between most laboratory and field research, however, are not sharp but are matters of degree. Many studies share elements of both laboratory and field research; these would fall midway on the research continuum.

Field research in nursing has the appeal of taking place in actual clinical settings and, therefore, maximizing realism. This appeals to nurses who are eager to see immediate application of knowledge to clinical problems. On the other hand, the realism poses problems of control.

Control of numerous extraneous variables must be a major concern of a field researcher. In field studies, as in real life, a multitude of variables interact in complex ways. A laboratory setting can provide tight control of many variables, but such control is limited in natural settings.

Field studies are, therefore, vulnerable to problems of internal invalidity. That is, the investigator may not be able to say with confidence that the experimental manipulation was responsible for the change in the subjects' behavior, since there were uncontrolled extraneous variables present. The extraneous variables may have contributed significantly to the results of the study.

In contrast, laboratory studies are vulnerable to problems of external invalidity. For instance, results of stress research based on a narrow sample in a tightly controlled laboratory setting often cannot be generalized to a larger population or to a more realistic stress situation. To be meaningful, a study should aim for strength in both internal validity and external validity.[13]

A number of potential practical problems are related to field studies. In real-life situations randomly assigning subjects to experimental and control groups may not be possible. In stress research, this has resulted in many studies done with no control group or one-shot case studies which are methodologically weak. Other potential problems include financial limitations, the need to spend much time and energy collecting data and a possible lack of cooperation by subjects.

Field research requires skill in persuasion and interpersonal relationships. This is especially true in the early stages of the project when administrators of an institution must be convinced that this research is important, safe and necessary. Much time and effort must be spent on these preliminaries in order to elicit the cooperation of key people needed to get the research accomplished. As Kerlinger says, "The field researcher needs to be a salesman, administrator and entrepreneur, as well as an investigator."[14]

RESEARCH IN THE WORK SETTING

The work place has been called an ideal setting for stress-prevention programs since it provides access to large groups of people who encounter stressful situations every day.[15] Certainly a hospital work setting provides numerous individual–environment interactions that potentially

A hospital work setting provides numerous individual-environment interactions that potentially lead to stress. Nurses, therefore, are a group of workers who might benefit from stress-reduction practices.

lead to stress. Nurses, therefore, are a group of workers who might benefit from stress-reduction practices.

In the work setting there are three general stress factors to consider. The first factor is concerned with the characteristics of the individual. People bring their personality patterns to the work setting; some are more predisposed to stress or have more difficulty coping with stressful situations.

Second are the sources of stress in the work environment. These are numerous and varied, including such stressors as poor relationships at work, role conflict in the organization, lack of participation in decision making and factors intrinsic to a particular job (e.g., ICU nurse).[16]

Third are the sources of stress outside the work environment. Outside sources of stress which influence the well-being of a worker include such factors as family problems, financial worries and life crises. All of these factors interact in the stress process.

Figure 1 illustrates the factors influencing the nurse's perception and response to stressors in the work setting. The nurse also influences the environment and can modify stressors and supports at home and at work. The interaction model of work-related stress reflects the complexity of

306 FIGURE 1. STRESS: INDIVIDUAL/ENVIRONMENT INTERACTION

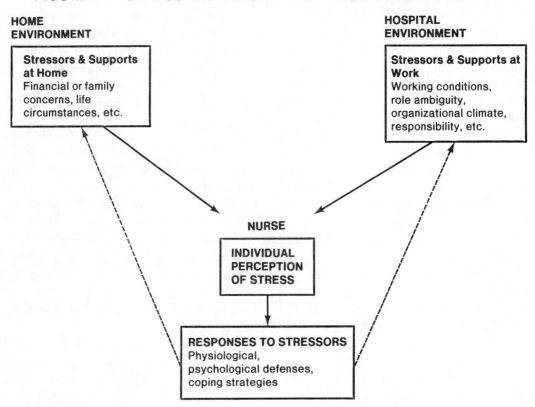

HOME
ENVIRONMENT

**Stressors & Supports
at Home**
Financial or family
concerns, life
circumstances, etc.

HOSPITAL
ENVIRONMENT

**Stressors & Supports at
Work**
Working conditions,
role ambiguity,
organizational climate,
responsibility, etc.

NURSE

**INDIVIDUAL
PERCEPTION
OF STRESS**

RESPONSES TO STRESSORS
Physiological,
psychological defenses,
coping strategies

stress in a real-life setting and the difficulty of controlling so many variables.

Field studies in the work setting present additional problems related to getting the full participation of employees. Both administrators and employees must be oriented to the project to obtain informed consent and support for the project. Otherwise the workers may have little motivation to participate in the study or may regard the project with suspicion. Suspicion is likely to be especially high when the data to be collected are about stress behaviors. The employees' right to privacy must be protected. Even when scrupulous efforts are made to maintain confidentiality, workers may not be willing to give candid responses if they fear that administrators might use the data in some way to evaluate their personality or performance.

Participation in the study may itself create a problem. People respond to any attention paid to them. Almost any change, any experimental treatment or just the knowledge that a study is being done, will bring about changes in people (the Hawthorne effect). This effect can be controlled by having one or more control groups receive different treatments and later comparing the results of all groups for significant differences.

The issues and limitations of studying stress in clinical situations are concerns of both the researcher and the clinician using stress-reduction techniques. Both must avoid the confusion related to the concept of stress by clarifying and defining stress for themselves in a way that reflects their purposes. Both must also be aware of the presence of multiple factors which may influence their experimental or clinical treatment. Important questions to consider include:

1. What is my conceptual definition of stress?

2. What is my operational definition of stress?

3. Are reliable and valid measuring instruments available to measure the variables?

4. Can subjects' rights to informed consent be protected without biasing the project?

5. What are the environmental variables which may influence the project? Can they be controlled?

6. Are resources such as time, money, energy, and expert assistance available to support the project?

Providing answers to these questions may help the investigator or clinician to cope with the stress inherent in the process of planning stress research or stress-reduction projects.

REFERENCES

1. Selye, H. *The Stress of Life* (New York: McGraw-Hill Book Co. 1956) p. 64.

2. Selye, H. "A Code for Coping with Stress." *Association of Operating Room Nurses Journal* 25:1 (January 1977) p. 35.

3. Appley, M. H. and Trumbull, R. *Psychological Stress* (New York: Appleton-Century-Crofts 1967) p. 4.

4. Olsen, M. "OR Nurses' Perception of Stress." *Association of Operating Room Nurses Journal* 25:1 (January 1977) p. 43–47.

5. Cleland, V. S. "The Effect of Stress on Performance. A Study of the Effect of Situational Stressors on the Performance of Nurses—Modified by Need for Social Approval." *Nursing Research* 14:4 (Fall 1965).

6. Appley and Trumbull. *Psychological Stress*. p. 1.

7. House, J. S. "Occupational Stress and Coronary Heart Disease: A Review and Theoretical Integration." *Journal of Health and Social Behavior* 15 (March 1974) p. 13.

8. McGrath, J. E. *Social and Psychological Factors in Stress* (New York: Holt, Rinehart and Winston 1970) p. 15–17.

9. McGrath. *Social and Psychological Factors in Stress*. p. 11.

10. Mason, J. W. "A Historical View of the Stress Field." *Journal of Human Stress* 1:2 (June 1975) p. 35.

11. McGrath. *Social and Psychological Factors in Stress*. p. 41–57.

12. "The Nurse in Research: ANA Guidelines on Ethical Values." *Nursing Research* 17:2 (March–April 1968).

13. Kerlinger, F. N. *Foundations of Behavioral Research* 2nd ed. (New York: Holt, Rinehart and Winston 1973) p. 324–325.

14. Kerlinger. *Foundations of Behavioral Research*. p. 408.

15. Peters, R. K., Benson, H., and Porter, D. "Daily Relaxation Response Breaks in a Working Population: I. Effects on Self-reported Measures of Health, Performance, and Well-being." *American Journal of Public Health* 67:10 (October 1977) p. 946.

16. Cooper, C. L. and Marshall, J. "Occupational Sources of Stress: A Review of the Literature Relating to Coronary Heart Disease and Mental Ill Health." *Journal of Occupational Psychology* 49 (1976). p. 14–21.

Perceived Stressors and Satisfiers of Critical Care Nursing

James W. Grout, MA
Associate Specialist

Susan M. Steffen, RN, MS
Lecturer

June T. Bailey, RN, EdD
Professor
School of Nursing
University of California
San Francisco, California

IN A LARGE health care center, there may be a half dozen or more specialized intensive care units (ICUs). Whether they emphasize the critical care of the medical, surgical, respiratory, cardiopulmonary, neurologic, pediatric, or neonatal patient, they all are designated for seriously ill patients requiring continuous observation by highly skilled nurses. The work environment of such ICUs has limited space, little privacy, constant activity, and a bewildering array of sophisticated and noisy monitoring devices. They are unusual too in the urgency with which critical tasks must be performed and the level of stress that nurses must tolerate.

These situational and psychological stressors have been amply documented in the literature.[1-12] Many studies, however, have been based on experiences with a single unit or with a limited number of

Writing of this article has been supported by DHHS, NIH, Stress Reduction Training Program for Intensive Care Nurses, nursing special project grant D10 NU02072.

310 nurses. One objective of the authors' project was to broaden this data base by surveying a large sample of nurses to learn more about the stressors and satisfiers for nurses working in the ICU.

THE SURVEY SAMPLE

The regional survey, which was conducted in fall 1977, consisted of a sample of 1,238 intensive care nurses working in 74 hospitals in the nine counties of the San Francisco Bay Area. A national survey of nurses who were members of the American Association of Critical Care Nurses also was conducted and has been reported.[13] Site visits were made by members of the project staff to 89 ICUs, which included the following specialized units: regular intensive care, combined intensive care and coronary care (ICU/ CCU), surgical, medical, respiratory, intensive care nursery, pediatric, cardiopulmonary/cardiovascular, and neurologic. Critical care units such as recovery, emergency, and operating rooms; trauma and burn units; and artificial kidney and coronary care units were not included because of the nature of the work environment and their patient population. Completed questionnaires were returned by 1,238 ICU nurses, a return rate of 60%. Subjects participated on a voluntary basis.

QUESTIONNAIRE

Format

The questionnaire evolved through a series of interviews with ICU nurses and was pilot tested before being administered to the sample. In addition to demographic data, there were free-response and forced-choice questions on the stressors and the satisfiers of ICU nursing. Nurses were asked what initially had attracted them to the unit and why they left, as well as what the sources of greatest satisfaction and greatest stress were for them in the ICU. To corroborate their answers to these questions, nurses were also asked to respond to 43 statements on a Likert-type scale.

The free-response questions relating to why nurses had left their prior critical care unit(s) and the sources of greatest satisfaction and greatest stress were analyzed using category formulation.[14] Responses that were similar were grouped together, although some inferences did have to be made. There was an interrater reliability of 80%.

Results

Demographic data

Over half of the intensive care nurses surveyed were 30 years or younger. The most common age range was 26 to 30; slightly more than 10% were older than 40. Virtually the entire sample were women.

Nearly two thirds of the nurses worked in either an ICU or ICU/CCU, which usually consisted of 7 to 16 beds. Over three fourths of the sample were staff nurses; another 15% identified themselves either as head or charge nurses. Almost 92% of the sample were RNs, nearly two thirds of whom had been nurses for nine years or less.

Seventy percent of the nurses had worked in their present unit for three years or less; half that number had worked there for a year or less. The figures on length of time in the ICU are more dramatic for nurses with prior critical care experience. Nearly 90% of them had three years' experience or less in any one unit; nearly half had a year or less.

Nurses were asked what their basic nursing program had been. Over a third had initially completed an RN diploma program. One fourth held the baccalaureate degree in nursing, and almost that many had the associate degree. The figures for the highest nursing degree presently held were slightly different. More held the baccalaureate degree and associate de-

grees, and fewer retained the diploma. One percent of the sample had received the master's as their highest degree.

Initial attractors to ICU nursing

Nurses ranked the three most important reasons that originally attracted them to ICU nursing as follows: first, opportunities for learning; second, intellectual challenge; and third, proficient use of skills.

Table 1. Sources of greatest satisfaction in the ICU (free responses) $N = 1238$

Category	f	%
I. Patient care	1,563	45.7
Patient improvement, progress, recovery	563	16.5
Close patient contact, patient/nurse ratio	246	7.2
Quality of nursing care	218	6.4
Feeling needed, of having helped	121	3.5
Patient/family contact and support	115	3.4
Emotional/physical support of the patient	112	3.3
Decision-making, autonomy, responsibility	79	2.3
Patient/family thanks	71	2.0
Patient/family teaching	38	1.1
II. Knowledge and skills	1,211	35.5
Opportunities for learning experience	283	8.3
Intellectual challenge, excitement, pace, variety	260	7.6
Use of knowledge and skills	189	5.5
Optimum performance/accomplishment	143	4.2
Learning skills, techniques, theory	125	3.7
Handling emergencies	104	3.1
Satisfactory completion of work	60	1.8
Successfully anticipating situations	32	0.9
Continuing education	15	0.4
III. Interpersonal relationships	616	18.0
Teamwork, working well with others	270	7.8
Recognition, respect	165	4.8
People I work with	138	4.0
Staff development, teaching opportunities	44	1.2
Responsive nursing leadership	9	0.2
IV. Administrative rewards	29	0.8
Pay/benefits	15	0.4
Advancement opportunity	14	0.4
Total Responses	3,419*	100.0

*Each nurse could list as many as three sources of greatest satisfaction in the ICU. Percentages are based on these responses.

312

Reasons for leaving prior critical care units

Nurses were asked about their prior critical care experience and why they had left the unit. Of the 58% who had such experience, over half listed personal reasons for leaving, the most common of which was that the nurse had "moved." Professional reasons made up a third of those cited by the nurses who left. The reason most often given in this category, and second overall, was "desired change, challenge, experience." Few of the responses indicated that the nurse left the unit because of "burnout, stress." The third category of reasons for leaving the unit was administrative, such as no opportunity for "advancement/promotion."

Sources of greatest satisfaction in the ICU

In a free-response question, nurses were asked to list the three sources of greatest satisfaction for them in the ICU, ranking the most satisfying first. (See Table 1.) Almost half of the responses were categorized as patient care. "Patient improvement, progress, recovery" was the single most satisfying aspect of work in the ICU, as indicated by 16.5% of the responses. The opportunities for "close patient contact, patient/nurse ratio" and "quality of nursing care" were also frequently cited. The second greatest source of satisfaction, with over a third of the responses, was knowledge and skills; within that category "opportunities for learning experience" and "intellectual challenge, excitement, pace, variety" were especially rewarding. The third most satisfying aspect of work in the ICU was interpersonal relationships, which

accounted for 18% of the responses. "Teamwork, working well with others" was cited in particular. The least amount of emphasis was placed on administrative rewards, such as pay or opportunities for advancement. Less than 1% of the nurses' responses indicated that these factors provided any satisfaction.

Sources of greatest stress in the ICU

Nurses also were asked to list the three sources of greatest stress for them in the ICU, ranking the most stressful first. (See Table 2.) Management of the unit was the greatest source of stress, with a third of the responses in that category. "Inadequate staffing" was particularly stressful, as was "apathetic, incompetent staff." Almost as stressful as unit management was interpersonal relationships, with one fourth of the responses. "Personality conflicts" with staff, physicians, administrators, residents received a high response rate. "Disagreement with physicians over patient treatment" also was stressful. The third greatest source of stress was patient care, with one fourth of the responses. "Emergencies, arrests" were particular stressors. The remaining categories were much less stressful to nurses.

Forced-choice responses

To further explore the sources of stress and satisfaction for nurses in the ICU, responses were elicited to 43 statements on a four-point Likert-type scale, ranging from "rarely" to "almost always" true. These responses were then grouped into five major categories similar to the ones in

Table 2. Sources of greatest stress in the ICU (free responses) $N = 1238$

Category	f	%
I. Management of the unit	1,175	33.7
Inadequate staffing	440	12.6
Apathetic, incompetent staff	231	6.6
Emergencies, transfers, admissions	169	4.8
Unavailability of physicians	105	3.0
Shifts, scheduling	76	2.2
Interruptions, paperwork	71	2.0
Patients not needing ICU care	35	1.0
Charge position	29	0.8
Floating out of unit	18	0.6
Lack of continuity in patient assignments	1	0.1
II. Interpersonal relationships	936	26.8
Personality conflicts (staff, physicians, administration, residents)	303	8.8
Disagreement with physicians over patient treatment	202	5.8
Unresponsive nursing leadership	143	4.1
Lack of respect from physicians	126	3.6
Lack of teamwork among staff	63	1.8
Communication problems	57	1.6
Lack of teamwork with other departments	37	1.1
III. Patient care	890	25.5
Emergencies, arrests	201	5.8
Unnecessary prolongation of life	169	4.8
Critical, unstable patients	159	4.6
Death of "special" patients	134	3.8
Inability to meet patient needs	96	2.8
Responsibility, decision making	61	1.7
Chronic patients	34	0.9
Uncooperative patients	30	0.9
Routine procedures	6	0.2
IV. Knowledge and skills	236	6.8
Inadequate knowledge	70	2.0
Unfamiliar equipment	50	1.4
Lack of experience and skill	45	1.3
Unfamiliar situations	39	1.1
Inadequate continuing education	30	0.9
Lack of orientation	2	0.1
V. Work environment	222	6.4
Insufficient/malfunctioning equipment	85	2.4
Work space	56	1.6
Noise	32	0.9
General work environment	23	0.6
Lack of supplies	16	0.5
Too many people	9	0.3
Lighting	5	0.1
VI. Life events	17	0.5
Personal	12	0.3
Stamina	4	0.1
Family	1	0.1
VII. Administrative rewards	13	0.3
No opportunity for advancement	7	0.2
Poor pay/benefits	6	0.1
Total responses	3,489*	100.0

*Each nurse could list as many as three sources of greatest satisfaction in the ICU. Percentages are based on these responses.

314

the free-response questions. Briefly, the data can be summarized as follows:

Patient Care

Respondents felt that they could provide quality patient care under pressure, were confident in their ability to meet the patients' physical and emotional needs, and felt comfortable in making patient care decisions. Although nurses rarely were distressed by a fluctuating work pace, work in the ICU was stressful at times. Nurses were upset by the death of patients or major setbacks in patient progress, and by what they perceived as the unnecessary prolongation of patient life.

Interpersonal Relationships

Nurses, however, rarely considered leaving the ICU because of stress and felt quite capable of coping with it. The respondents felt that their expertise was respected by patients; and that their nursing knowledge and judgment were respected by co-workers, the immediate supervisor, and physicians, especially during emergencies. There was a feeling of team spirit on the shift and, to a somewhat lesser degree, between shifts. Time was available to provide emotional support to peers and was provided as well by the families of nurses.

Knowledge and Skills

Nurses felt confident in their abilities and that their knowledge was current. They had sufficient preparation to operate specialized equipment, were not distressed by working with it, and were able to keep up with advances in medical technology.

Management of the Unit

The nurses felt that physicians were available and that there was adequate staff-ing in the unit, which allowed time to give quality patient care, although occasionally the pace in that unit was too rapid. Staffing permitted a satisfying work schedule and relief for lunch and coffee breaks, although not always for attending continuing education events. Opportunities for job advancement were not regarded as being readily available, and group or individual counseling was rarely provided and even less often used. Patients occasionally were on the unit who did not require intensive care and occasionally, too, time prevented nurses from giving emotional support to patients or their families.

Physical Work Environment

Though a lack of work space in the unit was rarely distressing, high noise levels occasionally were. These potential stressors and satisfiers are listed in Table 3.

Discussion

If, as Lazarus and his colleagues[15,16] contend, psychological stress resides neither in the environment nor in the person alone, but depends on the transaction between them, then how a situation is appraised by the individual can be as important as the agent or event itself. Whether the individual will be stressed by interaction with the environment depends on the intensity of its demands, as well as the person's adaptive resources. If environmental demands exceed the ability of the person to cope with them, there will be a stress response. The nature of that response, however, and whether it is perceived as one of harm, threat, or challenge, depends on the cognitive appraisal of the individual. This appraisal can deter-

Table 3. Potential stressors and satisfiers in the ICU (forced choice responses) $N = 1238$

	Response							
	Rarely		Occa-sionally		Fre-quently		Almost always	
Question	f	%	f	%	f	%	f	%
I. Patient care								
I feel confident in meeting patients' physical needs.	5	0.4	29	2.3	394	31.8	788	63.7
I feel comfortable making patient care decisions.	7	0.6	69	5.6	464	37.5	673	54.3
I feel I can provide quality nursing care under pressure.	13	1.1	92	7.4	493	39.8	614	49.6
The unnecessary prolongation of life distresses me.	46	3.7	297	24.0	330	26.7	536	43.3
I am comfortable in my ability to meet patients' emotional needs.	33	2.7	215	17.3	572	46.2	401	32.4
My job is stressful.	95	7.7	462	37.3	466	37.6	184	14.9
I am distressed when patients have major setbacks or die.	89	7.2	591	47.7	385	31.1	154	12.4
Caring for dying patients is extremely upsetting for me.	453	36.6	610	49.3	111	9.0	45	3.6
I am distressed by a fluctuating work pace.	536	43.3	498	40.2	137	11.1	41	3.3
II. Interpersonal relationships								
A feeling of team spirit exists on my shift.	32	2.6	126	10.2	394	31.8	671	54.2
The immediate supervisor respects my judgments.	21	1.7	118	9.5	455	36.8	607	49.0
My expertise is respected by patients.	7	0.6	75	6.1	533	43.1	566	45.7
My knowledge is respected by my immediate supervisor.	20	1.6	140	11.3	485	39.2	558	45.1
I am able to cope with job stress.	18	1.5	115	9.3	558	45.1	528	42.6
My clinical knowledge is respected by co-workers.	6	0.5	133	10.8	603	48.7	466	37.6
My judgments are respected by physicians.	25	2.0	230	18.6	553	44.7	388	31.3
My family provides emotional support for me in my job.	286	23.1	241	19.5	271	21.9	387	31.2
Physicians respect my knowledge.	35	2.8	244	19.7	570	46.1	348	28.1
A feeling of team spirit exists between shifts.	161	13.0	384	31.0	455	36.7	218	17.6
Physicians consider my judgment during emergencies.	82	6.6	371	30.0	527	42.6	210	16.9
I have time to give emotional support to peers.	113	9.1	442	35.7	456	36.8	195	15.8
I consider leaving ICU nursing because of stress.	725	58.6	318	25.7	104	8.4	50	4.0
My clinical judgments are questioned by co-workers.	803	64.9	368	29.7	36	2.9	7	0.6
III. Knowledge and skill								
I feel confident in my abilities.	7	0.6	62	5.0	467	37.7	673	54.4
I have sufficient preparation to operate specialized equipment.	25	2.0	174	14.1	522	42.1	492	39.8
I am able to keep up with technological advances in the ICU.	31	2.5	201	16.2	564	45.6	421	34.0
I feel that my knowledge is current.	11	0.9	142	11.5	686	55.4	381	30.8
Working with specialized equipment distresses me.	840	67.9	321	25.9	55	4.4	8	0.6
IV. Management of the unit								
Physicians are available when I need them.	29	2.3	143	11.5	515	41.6	533	43.1
I have time to give quality patient care.	23	1.9	170	13.7	651	52.6	357	28.8
Staffing permits me to work a satisfying schedule.	141	11.4	306	24.7	415	33.5	342	27.6
Adequate relief is regularly provided for lunch, coffee breaks.	294	23.8	259	20.9	317	25.6	330	26.7
There is adequate staffing in the unit.	156	12.6	322	26.0	473	38.2	260	21.0

Table 3. (Continued)

	Response							
	Rarely		Occa-sionally		Fre-quently		Almost always	
Question	f	%	f	%	f	%	f	%
Staffing allows me to attend continuing education events.	262	21.2	490	39.6	283	22.8	173	14.0
Group or individual counseling is available to me at work.	794	64.1	155	12.5	79	6.4	97	7.8
Time prevents me from giving emotional support to the families of patients.	270	21.8	537	43.4	331	26.7	77	6.2
Patients are in the unit who do not need ICU care.	177	14.3	573	46.3	412	33.3	60	4.8
Opportunities for job advancement are available to me.	558	45.1	452	36.5	116	9.4	55	4.4
Time prevents me from giving emotional support to patients.	304	24.6	582	47.0	303	24.5	29	2.3
The pace in the unit is too rapid.	351	28.4	630	50.9	208	16.8	29	2.3
I participate in group or individual counseling at work.	967	78.1	92	7.4	25	2.0	16	1.3
V. Work environment								
A lack of work space distresses me.	417	33.7	355	28.7	234	18.9	213	17.2
High noise levels distress me.	373	30.1	478	38.6	232	18.7	127	10.3

*Only single-category responses are considered. As a result, responses may total less than 100%.

mine not only the quality and the intensity of the emotional response, but also the coping behaviors that continue to affect it.

This perception may have consequences for mental and physical health. Nurses, for instance, who perceive a situation as difficult, yet manageable, are more likely to be challenged by it than if they were to appraise it as threatening. This was the case, for instance, among the nurses in the present study, who appraised their work in the ICU as challenging. Nearly half of the responses indicated "opportunities for learning" and "intellectual challenge" as reasons that initially attracted nurses to the ICU. The lack of such attractors also was cited as a major reason for leaving the unit.

This sense of being challenged was demonstrated as well by responses about the stressors and the satisfiers in the ICU. Over 90% of the responses indicated that nurses frequently or almost always felt confident in their abilities; almost as many provided quality nursing care under pressure. Nurses were able to cope with job stress and only rarely or occasionally considered leaving the unit because of it. Among the reasons for leaving, only 1.6% of the responses indicated that nurses had left the ICU because of "burnout, stress."

At times, the nurses in the ICU were stressed and unable to adapt to its demands. Since "patient improvement, progress, recovery" was the single most satisfying aspect of working in the ICU, it is not surprising that whatever might thwart that source of satisfaction was a source of stress. "Inadequate staffing" was the single most stressful aspect of the ICU, and "apathetic, incompetent" staffing was the third greatest source of stress.

When asked, however, whether there was adequate staffing, nearly 60% of the nurses responded that, frequently or almost always, there was. For approximately 39%, staffing was only occasionally adequate. This apparent discrepancy can be explained by the fact that situational demands in the ICU frequently are *potential* stressors, which become so only when they exceed the ability of the nurse to cope with them. For most ICU nurses, staffing is adequate; when it is not, there can be considerable stress.

Implications

One of the most important implications in the mediation of stress by cognitive appraisal is whether the consequences of perceiving a situational stressor as challenging or threatening can have different adaptational outcomes in terms of health and illness. Selye has argued that there is no difference in response. Stress is "the nonspecific response of the body to any demand."[17] Every demand made on the body, however specific (eg, fasting, exercise, emotional arousal), elicits a single stereotypic response, which he termed the general adaptation syndrome. Although Selye does distinguish between "good" and "bad" stress effects, the biologic stress response, itself, is nonspecific and a common reaction to all agents that evoke it.

Lazarus and his colleagues disagree with Selye's characterization and emphasize,

instead, that stressors are reactions determined by one's appraisal of the transaction between person and environment. It is not even certain whether there is an absolutely nonspecific stress response. Mason,[18,19] for instance, has found that the body's response to certain types of stressors is stimulus specific and varies from one physical stressor to another, as well as between physiologic and psychological stressors.

If Selye is correct and there is the same somatic response to challenge and threat, nurses in intensive care may be at risk, even though, psychologically, nurses who are challenged by their work should have better morale and be more satisfied. Work satisfaction often requires such a sense of challenge and accomplishment. This has been demonstrated in air traffic control, which, because of the demanding highly complex, often critical nature of the work, is quite similar to intensive care nursing.[20] A major appeal of air traffic control was found to be the challenging, constantly changing work environment; job challenge, in fact, was rated more highly overall than any other factor about work.[21,22] Yet there were physiologic responses elicited by air traffic control that had immediate, as well as long-term, health risks. In that profession, at least, the challenge elicited by air traffic control did not diminish its physiologic consequences.

So great was the discrepancy between the sense of job satisfaction felt by air traffic controllers and the biologic stress responses to their work that one must ask whether differences in appraisal of the same potentially threatening or challenging event may not be a defensive coping process such as denial.

The same question can be asked of ICU

318 nurses. The morale of the nurses in this survey is indicated by their responses. There is a sense that they are confident in their abilities and are challenged to demonstrate them. This is in contrast to studies of ICU nurses often presented in the literature. But if the nurses' ability to cope with the stressors of the ICU seems stronger in this survey, their physiologic vulnerability may be much greater than presently indicated and also should receive attention in the literature.

That consideration will be difficult because of another important implication for the study of nursing stress. In the transaction between person and environment, situational demands have been emphasized. Indeed, that is a necessary first step in determining what exactly does stress the nurse. Such an approach, however, considers only one part of this transaction. The adaptive responses of nurses, themselves, to the potential stressors of the ICU should also be given attention, as has been done by Oskins[23] on the coping methods of ICU nurses.

SUMMARY

A questionnaire survey of 1,238 ICU nurses from 74 San Francisco Bay Area hospitals indicated that the initial attractors to intensive care nursing had been opportunities for learning and intellectual challenge, and that the greatest satisfaction

was inpatient care and individual knowledge and skills. The greatest sources of stress were the management of the unit and interpersonal relationships. Nurses rarely considered leaving the ICU because of stress, however. They felt confident in their knowledge and skill in their ability to deliver quality patient care, and in their working relationships with physicians, staff, and patients.

How these nurses perceive their work in the ICU has important implications for critical care nursing. Whether one perceives a situation as threatening or challenging has an obvious effect on adaptive function, morale, and even health. Yet, in the ICU there may be situational demands so extreme that they exceed the nurses' ability to cope with them, and appraisal of an event may not be able to ameliorate the stress response that it evokes. Although it is still uncertain what the moderating effects of cognitive appraisal are in the adaptive transaction between person and environment, the perception of a situation as challenging, rather than threatening, can have psychological and social benefits. Because of greater confidence, there should be higher morale, increased motivation, and better ability to work under pressure. Whether these benefits, however, outweigh the possible noxious physiologic consequences that Selye has contended are the result of stress is another question, and one that the nursing literature should attempt to answer.

REFERENCES

1. Bilodeau CB: The nurse and her reactions to critical-care nursing. *Heart Lung* 2:358-363, 1973.
2. Cassem NH, Hackett TP: Stress on the nurse and therapist in the intensive-care unit and the coronary-care unit. *Heart Lung* 4:252-259, 1975.
3. Eisendrath SJ, Dunkel J: Psychological issues in intensive care unit staff. *Heart Lung* 8:751-758, 1979.
4. Gentry WD, Foster SB, Froehling S: Psychologic

response to situational stress in intensive and nonintensive nursing. *Heart Lung* 1:793-796, 1972.

5. Hay D, Oken D: The psychological stresses of intensive care nursing. *Psychosom Med* 34:109-118, 1972.

6. Huckabay LMD, Jagla B: Nurses' stress factors in the intensive care unit. *J Nurs Adm* 9(2):21-26, 1979.

7. Jacobson SP: Stressful situations for neonatal intensive care nurses. *MCN* 3:144-150, 1978.

8. Koumans AJR: Psychiatric consultation in an intensive care unit. *JAMA* 194:163-167, 1965.

9. Michaels DR: Too much in need of support to give any? *Am J Nurs* 71:1932-1935, 1971.

10. Simon NM, Whitely S: Psychiatric consultation with MICU nurses: The consultation conference as a working group. *Heart Lung* 6:497-504, 1977.

11. Strauss A: The intensive care unit: Its characteristics and social relationships. *Nurs Clin North Am* 3:7-15, 1968.

12. Vreeland R, Ellis GL: Stresses on the nurse in an intensive-care unit. *JAMA* 208:332-334, 1969.

13. Steffen S, Bailey J: Sources of stress and satisfaction in ICU nursing. *Focus* 6(6):26-32, 1979.

14. Bailey JT: The critical incident technique in identifying behavioral criteria of professional nursing effectiveness. *Nurs Res* 5:52-64, 1956.

15. Lazarus RS, Launier R: Stress-related transactions between person and environment. In Pervin LA, Lewis M (eds): *Perspectives in Interactional Psychology.* New York, Plenum Publishing Corp, 1978, pp 287-327.

16. Lazarus RS, Cohen JB, Folkman S, et al: Psychological stress and adaptation: Some unresolved issues. In Selye H (ed): *Selye's Guide to Stress Research.* New York, Van Nostrand Reinhold Co, 1980, vol 1, pp 90-117.

17. Selye H: *Stress in Health and Disease.* Boston, Butterworths Publishers Inc, 1976, p 15.

18. Mason JW: A re-evaluation of the concept of "nonspecificity" in stress theory. *J Psychiatr Res* 8:323-333, 1971.

19. Mason JW: Specificity in the organization of neuroendocrine response profiles. In Seeman P, Brown GM (eds): *Frontiers in Neurology and Neuroscience Research.* Toronto, University of Toronto Press, 1974, pp 68-80.

20. Grout JW: Occupational stress of intensive care nurses & air traffic controllers: Review of related studies. *JNE* 19(6):8-14, 1980.

21. Smith RC: Comparison of the job attitudes of personnel in three air traffic control specialties. *Aerospace Med* 44:918-927, 1973.

22. Smith RC, Cobb BB, Collins WE: Attitudes and motivations of air traffic controllers in terminal areas. *Aerospace Med* 43:1-5, 1972.

23. Oskins SL: Identification of situational stressors and coping methods by intensive care nurses. *Heart Lung* 8:953-960, 1979.

Selected Bibliography on Stress

Ageulera, D. and Messick, J. *Crisis Intervention* (St. Louis: C.V. Mosby Co., 1978, 3rd ed).

Anderson, R. *Stress Power: How to Turn Tension into Energy* (New York: Human Science Press, 1978).

Antonovsky, A. *Health, Stress and Coping: New Perspectives on Mental and Physical Well-Being* (San Francisco, Jossey-Bass Publishers, 1979).

Benson, H. *The Relaxation Response* (New York: William Morrow & Co., 1977).

Benson, H. *The Mind/Body Effect* (New York: Simon & Schuster, 1979).

Bernstein, D. and Borkovec, T. *Progressive Relaxation Training: A Manual for the Helping Professions* (with record) (Chicago: Research Press, 1973).

Brown, B. *New Mind, New Body* (New York: Harper & Row, 1975).

Brown, B. *Stress and the Art of Biofeedback* (New York: Harper & Row, 1977).

Carrington, P. *Freedom in Meditation* (New York: Anchor Press/Doubleday, 1977).

Chan, P. *Finger Acupressure* (New York: Ballantine Books, 1974).

Cooper, K. *Aerobics* (New York: Bantam Books, 1972).

Cooper, K. *New Aerobics* (New York: Bantam Books, 1970).

Cooper, M. and Cooper, K. *Aerobics for Women* (New York, Bantam Books, 1974).

Deutsch, M. *The Resolution of Conflict* (New Haven, Conn.: Yale Univ. Press, 1973).

DeVries, H. *Vigor Regained* (Englewood Cliffs, N.J.: Prentice-Hall, 1974).

Ellis, A. and Harper, R.A. *A New Guide to Rational Living* (Englewood Cliffs, N.J.: Prentice-Hall, 1975).

Emmons, M.L. "Assertion Training within an Holistic-Eclectic Framework" in *Assertiveness: Innovations, Applications, Issues* by Robert E. Alberti (ed) (San Luis Obispo, Calif.: Impact Publishers Inc., 1977).

Ferguson, T. (ed). *Medical Self-Care: Access to Medical Tools* (New York: Summit Books, 1980).

Flynn, P. *Holistic Health: The Art and Science of Care* (Bowie, Md.: Robert J. Brady Co., 1980).

Friedman, M. *Type A Behavior and Your Heart* (New York: A. Knopf, 1974).

Garfield, C. *Stress and Survival: The Emotional Realities of Life Threatening Illness* (St. Louis: C.V. Mosby Co., 1979).

Gemderson, E. and Rake, R.H. (eds). *Life Stress and Illness* (Springfield, Ill.: Charles C Thomas, 1974).

Girdano, D. and Everly, G. *Controlling Stress and Tension: A Holistic Approach* (Englewood Cliffs, N.J.: Prentice-Hall, 1979).

Green, E. and Green, A. *Beyond Biofeedback* (New York: Dell Publishing Co., 1977).

Gunderson, E.K. and Rahe, R.H. (eds). *Life and Stress Illness* (Springfield, Ill.: Charles C Thomas, 1974).

Hettleman, R. *Yoga* (New York: Bantam Books, 1969).

Jacobson, E. *You Must Relax: Practical Methods for Reducing the Tensions of Modern Living* (New York: McGraw-Hill Paperbacks, 5th ed., 1978).

Karlins, M. and Andres, L. *Biofeedback: Turning on the Powers of Your Mind* (New York: Warner Books, 1974).

Kreiger, D. *The Therapeutic Touch: How to Use Your Hands to Help or Heal* (Englewood Cliffs, N.J.: Prentice-Hall, 1979).

Kurland, H. *Quick Headache Relief: Without Drugs* (New York: Ballantine Books, 1977).

Kutash, I., Schlesinger, L.D., et al. *Handbook on Stress and Anxiety: Contemporary Knowledge, Theory and*

322

Treatment (San Francisco: Jossey-Bass Publishers, 1981).

Lakein, A. *How To Get Control of Your Time and Your Life* (New York: Peter H. Wyden, 1973).

Lamott, K. *Escape from Stress* (New York: J.P. Putnam, 1975).

Lande, N. *Mindstyles, Lifestyles* (Los Angeles: Price/Stern/Sloan Publishers, 1976).

Lappe, F. *Diet for a Small Planet* (New York: Ballantine Books, 1971).

Lecker, S. *The Natural Way to Stress Control* (New York: Grusset, Dunlap, 1978).

LeShan, L. *You Can Fight for Your Life: Emotional Factors in the Causation of Cancer* (New York: M. Evans, 1980).

Lindemann, H. *Relieve Tension the Autogenic Way* (New York: Peter H. Wyden, Inc., 1973).

Luthe, W. (ed). *Autogenic Therapy* (New York: Grune & Stratton, 1969).

Mann, F. *Acupuncture of Many Diseases* (New York: Tao of Books, 1972).

Mayer, J. *A Diet for Living* (New York: Pocket Books, 1977).

McQuadi, W. and Aikman, H. *Stress* (New York: Bantam Books, 1974).

Miller, N.E. et al. (eds). *Biofeedback and Self-Control* (Chicago: Aldine-Atherton Publishers, 1973).

Mitchell, C. *The Perfect Exercise. The Hop, Skip and Jump Way to Health* (New York: Simon & Schuster, 1976).

Moyer, K. *The Physiology of Hostility* (Chicago: Markham Publishing, 1971).

National Association for Human Development, *"Basic Exercises," "Moderate Exercises," "Advanced Exercises"* (Washington, D.C.)

Nursing Skillbook Series. *Using Crisis Intervention Wisely* (Horsham, Pa.: InterMed Communications, Inc., 1979).

Pelletier, K. *Mind as Healer, Mind as Slayer: A Holistic Approach to Preventing Stress Disorders* (New York: Delacorte, 1977).

Pelletier, K. *Holistic Medicine* (New York: Dell Publishing Co., 1980).

Rosa, K. *You and AT: Autogenic Training* (New York: Saturday Review Press, 1973).

Samuels, M. and Bennett, H. *The Well Body Book* (New York: Random House, 1973).

Shapiro, D. et al. (eds). *Biofeedback and Self-Control* (Chicago: Aldine-Atherton Publishers, 1972).

Shealy, C.N. *Ninety Days to Self-Health* (Millbrae, Calif.: Celestial Arts, 1976).

Selye, H. *Stress without Distress* (Philadelphia: J.B. Lippincott/Signet, 1975).

Selye, H. *The Stress of Life* (New York: McGraw-Hill, 2nd ed., 1978).

Simonton, C. and Matthews-Simonton, S. and Creighton. *Getting Well Again: A Step by Step, Self-Help Guide to Overcoming Cancer for Patients and Their Families* (Los Angeles: J.P. Tarcher, Inc., 1978).

Stern, F. and Hock, R. *Mind Trips to Help You Lose Weight* (New York: Playboy Press Paperbacks, 1976).

Sutterley, D. and Donnelly, G. *Perspectives in Human Development* (Philadelphia: J.B. Lippincott, 1973).

Tanner, O. (ed). *Stress, Human Behavior Series* (New York: Time-Life Book, 1976).

Toffler, A. *Future Shock* (New York: Random House, 1970).

Travis, J.W. *Wellness Inventory*. Wellness Resource Center—Wellness Workbook (1/2 Miller Avenue, Mill Valley, Calif.).

United States—Congress.—The Senate Select Committee on Nutrition and Human Needs. *Dietary Goals for the United States and Nutrition Research Alternatives* (Washington, D.C.: U.S. Government Printing Office, 1977).

Warren, F.Z. *Freedom from Pain through Acupressure* (New York: Frederick Fell Publisher, 1976).

Watson, W. *Stress and Old Age* (Brunswick, N.J.: Transaction Books, 1980).

White, J. and Fadiman, J. (eds). *How You Can Feel Better, Reduce Stress and Overcome Tension* (New York: Dell Books, 1976).

Woolfolk, R.L. and Richardson, F.C. *Stress, Sanity and Survival* (New York: Monarch Press, 1978).

Index

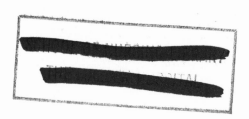